American Medical Association
Physicians dedicated to the health of America

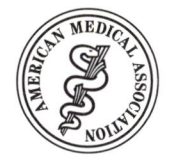

Reader's Guide to

Alternative Health Methods

An analysis of more than 1,000 reports on unproven, disproven, controversial, fraudulent, quack, and /or otherwise questionable approaches to solving health problems.

John F. Zwicky, PhD
Arthur W. Hafner, PhD
Stephen Barrett, MD
William T. Jarvis, PhD

615.5 R286z

Reader's guide to
alternative health methods

This book was designed by Arthur W. Hafner and Stephen Barrett and typeset on a Macintosh computer using Pagemaker 4.2. The typefaces are Helvetica Black for headings and Garamond Book Condensed for the text.

ISBN 0-89970-525-1
AMA order number OP 313792

Copyright ©1993 American Medical Association. All rights reserved.

Arthur W. Hafner, Ph.D., is the editor-in-chief for this book.

Additional copies may be ordered from:
Book and Fulfillment OP 313792
American Medical Association
P.O. Box 2964
Milwaukee, WI 53201-2964

Or call 800 621-8335

No part of this publication may be stored in a retrieval system, transmitted, or reproduced in any way, including but not limited to photocopy, photograph, magnetic or other record, without the prior agreement and written permission of the publisher.

Printed in the United States of America.

Library of Congress Cataloging-in-Publication Data

Reader's guide to alternative health methods / Arthur W. Hafner,
 editor ... [et al.].
  p. cm.
 "An analysis of more than 1000 reports on unproven, disproven, controversial, fraudulent, quack, and/or otherwise questionable approaches to solving health problems."
 Includes bibliographical references.
 ISBN 0-88970-525-1
 1. Alternative medicine—evaluation. 2. Alternative medicine—Bibliography.˙ I. Hafner, Arthur Wayne, 1943- . II American Medical Association. III Title: Alternative health methods.
R733.R4 1992
615.5—dc20   92-31144
                                                            CIP

Contents

About the Authors ix

Acknowledgments x

Part I: Overview
A Scientific Perspective 3
   How medical truths are determined, 3
   Definitions related to unscientific methods, 4
   Misconceptions about quackery, 7
   The lure of "alternative" methods, 9
   Examples of dubious products, 10
   History of the AMA's concern with health fraud, 11
Health fraud and quackery 13
   History of quackery, 13
   How quackery sells, 15
   General literature, 16
   Dubious dentistry, 27
   Mail fraud, 29
   Government regulation, 30
   Organizations promoting "alternative methods," 32
   Antiquackery activities, 33

Part II: "Alternative" Healing Systems
Acupuncture 39
Ayurvedic medicine 45
Chiropractic 47
Christian Science 58
Faith healing 63
Folk (traditional) medicine 69
Herbs 74
"Holistic medicine" 81
Homeopathy 85
Iridology 94
Natural Hygiene 97
Naturopathy 100
"New Age" and occult practices 104

Part III: Major Diseases

Questionable cancer treatment 113
  General information about cancer, 113
  Characteristics of questionable methods, 114
  Diet and cancer prevention, 124
  Antineoplastons, 126
  Gerson cancer therapy, 127
  Greek cancer cure, 128
  Hoxsey cancer treatment, 130
  Immunoaugmentative therapy (IAT), 131
  Laetrile, 135
  Livingston-Wheeler therapy, 139
  Metabolic cancer therapy, 140
  "Psychic surgery," 142
  Unproven psychological approaches, 142
  Revici method, 144
  High-dosage vitamin C, 145
  Miscellaneous methods, 146
  Proponent organizations, 147
  Proponent literature, 148
Unproven AIDS remedies 150
Chelation therapy 157
Unproven approaches to arthritis 163

Part IV: Diet and Nutrition

Vitamins and "health" foods 173
  General information, 173
  Food faddism, 175
  "Nutrition insurance," 176
  "Organic foods," 178
  "Orthomolecular medicine," 180
  Health food stores, 184
  Dubious nutrition consultants 187
  Life-extension claims, 190
  Gerovital, 191
  Raw (unpasteurized) milk, 193
  "Ergogenic aids," 194
  Miscellaneous products, 195
  Adverse case reports, 199
  Criticism of individual proponents, 202
  Health food industry organizations and activities, 205
  Proponent literature, 206

Dubious diagnostic tests 208
   Applied kinesiology, 208
   Commercial hair analysis, 209
   Electroacupuncture, 215
   Herbal crystallization analysis, 216
   Lingual vitamin C test, 216
   Live-cell analysis, 217
Fad diagnoses 218
   "Environmental illness," 218
   "Candidiasis hypersensitivity," 225
   Chronic fatigue syndrome, 228
   "Hypoglycemia," 229
   "Mercury-amalgam toxicity," 230
   Proponent literature, 232
Dubious allergy concepts and practices 234
   General discussions, 234
   Cytotoxic testing, 236
   Misdiagnosis of food allergies, 237
   Carotid body resection, 238
Diet and behavior 240
   General literature 240
   Feingold diet 242,
   Diet and criminal behavior, 244
   Sugar and hyperactivity, 245
Macrobiotic diet 247
Multilevel marketing 253
Vegetarianism 258
Questionable approaches to weight control 264

Part V: Other "Alternative" Approaches
Aromatherapy 279
Baldness remedies 282
Biofeedback 285
Cellular therapy 290
Colonic irrigation 293
Dimethyl sulfoxide (DMSO) 296
Questionable approaches to mental and emotional help 300
   General literature, 300
   Astrologic counseling, 301
   Firewalking, 301
   Meditation, 302
   Neural organizational technique, 303

Questionable approaches to mental and emotional help (cont'd.)
   Past-life therapy, 303
   Reichian therapy (orgone therapy), 304
   Self-help books, 304
   Subliminal tapes, 305
Therapeutic touch 306

Part VI: Appendices
1. Organizations skeptical of "alternative" methods 311
2. Publications skeptical of "alternative" methods 316
3. Organizations that promote "alternative" methods 319
4. Publications that promote "alternative" methods 321
5. Glossary of "alternative" methods and terms 325

Index 339

Notice

The information in this book reflects the opinions of its authors and the sources they cite and does not represent the official policy of the American Medical Association unless this is clearly specified.

About the Authors

• John F. Zwicky, PhD, is a technical librarian in the AMA Division of Library and Information Management. Prior to his employment with the Association, he worked for the Social Security Administration for twelve years. He then returned to graduate school to complete his PhD in history from Loyola University (Chicago). Dr. Zwicky has taught courses in American history and Western civilization at Loyola University and DePaul University.

• Arthur W. Hafner, PhD, is Director of the AMA Division of Library and Information Management. He is a distinguished member of the Academy of Health Information Professionals and holds the certified association executive (CAE) designation awarded by the American Society of Association Executives. He received his PhD and MA degrees in library sciences and his MS degree in mathematics from the University of Minnesota. He writes and lectures on a broad range of information issues including the American public library and freedom-of-expression issues, medical information and professional liability, and evaluation of library outcomes and staff performance. He is a consultant to libraries and publishers and teaches many seminars and workshops in descriptive statistics for library managers. He is adjunct professor of library science at Rosary College, River Forest, Illinois and clinical associate professor at the University of Minnesota School of Medicine Duluth campus. Before coming to the American Medical Association he was Director of Library Services and Associate Professor of Library Science for the Chicago College of Osteopathic Medicine.

• Stephen Barrett, MD, who practices psychiatry in Allentown, Pennsylvania, is a nationally renowned author, editor, and consumer advocate. He edits and publishes *Nutrition Forum Newsletter* and is medical editor of Prometheus Books. He is a board member of the National Council Against Health Fraud and chairs its Task Force on Victim Redress. He is a scientific and editorial advisor to the American Council on Science and Health and a Fellow of the Committee for the Scientific Investigation of Claims of the Paranormal (CSICOP). His thirty-two books include *Health Schemes, Scams, and Frauds*; *Vitamins and "Health" Foods: The Great American Hustle*; and four editions of the college textbook *Consumer Health: A Guide to Intelligent Decisions*. In 1984 he won the FDA Commissioner's Special Citation Award for Public Service in fighting nutrition quackery. In 1986 he was awarded honorary membership in the American Dietetic Association. In 1987 he began teaching health education at The Pennsylvania State University.

- William T. Jarvis, PhD, is an expert on the psychology and epidemiology of quackery. He is Professor of Health Promotion and Education at Loma Linda University, where he teaches courses dealing with controversial health practices. He founded and is president of the National Council Against Health Fraud. He is a scientific advisor to the American Council on Science and Health, an associate editor of *Nutrition Forum,* and co-chairman (with Dr. Barrett) of the paranormal health claims subcommittee of the Committee for the Scientific Investigation of Claims of the Paranormal. He is a member of the American Cancer Society's committee on questionable methods and wrote the society's booklets, "Questionable Methods of Cancer Management" and "Helping Your Patients Deal with Questionable Cancer Treatments." He has been a featured speaker at national health-fraud conferences and testifies in court and at government hearings on controversial health matters.

Acknowledgments

The authors express their appreciation to M. Roy Schwarz, MD, American Medical Association, Senior Vice President, Medical Education and Science, for his support and encouragement for this project and for the editors to engage in research. Thanks is expressed to B.J. Anderson, JD, American Medical Association, Office of the General Counsel, for her help, technical advice, and willingness to provide direction.

Thanks are also due to Association personnel: Julie W. Breo, Director of Marketing Management and Development, Rhonda Taira, Director of the Department of Marketing Services, and Herbert L. Hinkelman, Department of Marketing Services, all of whom were instrumental in seeing the manuscript through its production and printing.

Special thanks is due to several Library and Information Management staff members: Cheryl M. Steffen for her many contributions in proofreading the manuscript and to Valerie M. Camarigg and Sandra R. Schefris for their review of written materials.

We thank Senior Research Associate Anne White-Michalski and Research Associate Lorri A. Zipperer for performing a variety of literature searches to identify potential articles for inclusion in this book. We thank the division's Technical Service Assistants Maurice Bell, Richard W. Padbury, Jr., and Mary Sugrue, who retrieved articles from journals, magazines, newsletters, and newspapers, and Yolanda Davis who obtained many articles for the editors via interlibrary loan document delivery.

We thank Saul Green, PhD, a scientific consultant in New York City, for his help with the chapter on chelation therapy and Bruce J. Masek, PhD, Assistant Professor of Psychology in Psychiatry, Harvard Medical School and Director, Pediatric Behavioral Medicine, Children's Hospital and Massachusetts General Hospital, for his review of the chapter on biofeedback training.

We thank Stuart B. Schapiro for his assistance in solving technical and computer-related problems. And finally, we express our appreciation to C. Diane Holtz, Rye Free Reading Room, Rye, New York, for her many helpful comments in completing this project.

Part I: Overview

A Scientific Perspective

The purpose of this book is to provide information with which to evaluate health-care approaches that are not based on established scientific knowledge. These approaches are commonly referred to as "alternatives" by their promoters and "quackery" or "health frauds" by their critics. The first edition of this book, published in 1988 as *Alternative Therapies, Unproven Methods & Health Fraud*, covered eighteen topics in its forty-seven pages. This edition contains more than eight times as much information.

The book's objective continues to be to identify and shed light on "alternative" therapies and their promoters. Most topics selected for inclusion are those about which the American Medical Association's Division of Library and Information Management receives the most inquiries. The sources include clinical and nonclinical articles from medical and scientific journals, consumer magazines, newsletters, newspapers, medical and other professional association statements, and books.

Our handling of information contrasts starkly with that of the general media. During the past few years, many articles and broadcasts addressed to the public have given what we believe is a very distorted view of "alternative" health-care methods. Most of these reports are marked by a complete absence of critical thinking and merely echo the views of proponents and their satisfied clients.

In selecting material for this book, we have tried to identify key articles that can help readers make educated decisions. Each section begins with an overview that reflects our beliefs and is followed by citations to literature that we consider reliable. For some methods, we also identify literature containing proponents' viewpoints "in the raw."

Since number of critical articles greatly exceeds the number of proponent articles, the advocates of "alternative" methods may complain that this book is one-sided and biased against "competing methods of health care." The facts are otherwise, however. The only commitment we have is to scientific truth.

How Medical Truths are Determined

How is it possible to determine whether a method works? For more than a century, scientists throughout the world have been applying agreed-upon rules to answer this question. These rules, known collectively as the "scientific" or "experimental" method, are embraced by all fields of science, not just those related to health care.

The scientific method provides a way to test hypotheses by carefully collecting data and interpreting them with appropriate statistical analysis. If observations or experimental results appear significant, they are normally submitted to peer-reviewed scientific journals for publication. Well-written reports contain enough detail that other scientists can judge for themselves whether the experiments were properly designed and whether the conclusions are supported by the data.

Astronomer Carl Sagan has said that "science is a way of thinking much more than it is a body of knowledge." Scientific medicine determines safety and effectiveness from peer-reviewed clinical research, epidemiological studies, consensus conferences, and by adhering to standards prescribed by the U.S. Food and Drug Administration. The "gold-standard" of medical research is the double-blind controlled clinical trial in which people receiving treatment are compared with similar subjects getting no treatment or a placebo. In such a study, neither the experimenters nor the people being tested know who is getting which. Enough data must be gathered to make it unlikely that the outcome occurs merely by chance. Blinding is necessary to ensure that neither patients nor experimenters allow any biases to interfere with accurate observation. To gain acceptance by the scientific community, experiments must be repeatable by other researchers.

Instead of testing their methods to determine whether they work, "alternative" practitioners rely mainly on personal observation and testimonials. Unfortunately, the fact that an individual recovers after doing something is rarely sufficient to demonstrate that the recovery was caused by the action taken and is not simply coincidental. Moreover, reports of personal experiences can be biased, inaccurate, or even fraudulent. Well-designed experiments involving many people are needed to establish that a treatment method is effective.

Definitions Related to Unscientific Methods

Methods that are not based on established scientific knowledge have been called many things. Their critics most often choose among unproven, unconventional, unorthodox, unscientific, nonscientific, questionable, dubious, cult, faddism, fraudulent, quack, and quackery. Their proponents prefer the terms nontraditional, complementary, holistic, and alternative. Although these terms are often used interchangeably, they have significant differences.

- *Quack* originated during the Renaissance when quicksilver or mercury was a popular remedy for syphilis. Wandering peddlers known as "quacksalvers" sold mercury ointment. They would claim that their agents would cure all diseases. The term was later shortened to "quacks," who became a symbol of evil medical practice. Dictionaries generally define "quack" as a pretender to special health-related skills. This definition implies an intent to deceive, which would not fit promoters of unproven methods who believe in what they are doing. In 1984 the late Congressman Claude Pepper and his staff defined a "quack" as "anyone who promotes medical schemes or remedies known to be false, or which are unproven, for a profit." This definition eliminates the question of intent.

- *Quackery* is the promotion of an unproven product or service. The operant word is promotion rather than intent. (Quacks quack!)

- *Fraud* is defined in dictionaries as an intentional perversion of truth for gain. The FDA has defined health fraud as promotion of an unproven remedy for profit. Although the FDA definition eliminates the question of intent, some people object to its use because ordinary use of the term fraud implies an intent to deceive.

- *Unscientific* means contrary to scientific evidence.

- *Nonscientific* means not based on a scientific approach.

- *Unconventional* and *unorthodox* are used to avoid denunciation of the method under consideration. Both of these words may falsely imply that medical science is wed to established doctrine and is too rigid.

- *Cult* is a health system based on dogma set forth by its promoter.

- *Faddism* is a generic term used to describe nutrition nonsense. Food faddists are characterized by exaggerated beliefs in the role of diet and nutrition in health and disease.

- *Unproven* has fewer negative connotations than most of the other terms. It correctly implies that, under the rules of science, proponents have the burden of proving that their methods work. Unproven methods that appear logical and consistent with established knowledge carry no connotation of quackery. However, methods that appear illogical and in conflict with established knowledge deserve to be looked at with great suspicion.

- *Questionable* and *dubious* generally mean unproven but inconsistent with established facts. The American Cancer Society, which for years maintained a list of "unproven methods of cancer management," recently switched to the word "questionable," which it defines as an unproven method promoted for general use (rather than experimental use). The word "dubious" is used by critics who wish to make it clear that they have a low opinion of the method under consideration.

- *Nontraditional* incorrectly suggests that an unscientific method is innovative, while falsely suggesting that the scientific community is traditional (meaning staid, rigid and close-minded). Actually, science is an antagonist of traditional medicine as it destroys old myths and establishes new approaches to healing. "Traditional" is correctly used in reference to folk medicine. Folk healers, not scientific healers, are the traditional ones. A considerable amount of quackery stems from the commercialization of traditional folk medicine and ancient dogma.

- *Complementary* is claimed to be a synthesis of orthodox and alternative methods put together to integrate the best of both. However, no published data indicate the extent to which "complementary" practitioners actually use proven methods or the extent to which they burden patients with useless methods. Typically these practitioners employ a "heads-I-win, tails-you-lose" strategy in which they claim credit for any improvement experienced by the patient and blame standard treatments for any negative effects. The result may be to undermine the patient's confidence in standard care, reducing compliance or having the patient wish to abandon it altogether.

- *Holistic* implies that an approach is special and more complete because it treats the "whole patient" and not just the disease. However, good physicians have always paid attention to patients' social and emotional concerns as well as their physical problems.

- *Alternative* has two possible meanings. Correctly employed, it refers to methods that have equal value for a particular purpose. (An example would be two antibiotics capable of killing a particular organism.) When applied to unproven methods, however, the term can be misleading because methods that are unsafe or ineffective are not reasonable alternatives to proven treatment. To emphasize this fact, we place the word "alternative" in quotation marks throughout this book whenever it is applied to methods that are not based on established scientific knowledge.

The British Medical Association's Board of Science and Education, which carried out an extensive study published in 1986, has proposed an important distinction between "alternative medicine" and "alternative therapy":

"Some of the procedures . . . for example, chiropractic and acupuncture, stem from particular beliefs about the nature and causation of disease. Their proponents reject the views of orthodox medicine, and may be said to offer alternative medical systems. These systems are incompatible with the corpus of scientific knowledge, and must be rejected by anyone who accepts the validity of the latter.

"What constitutes an alternative therapy is not so clear. Some procedures, such as manipulation, are already part of the orthodox repertoire, and are only regarded as 'alternative' when claims for their value are greatly extended. Others are not at present used by registered practitioners, but there would be no bar to their adoption should good evidence of their efficacy be forthcoming."

Most nonscientific health care is rooted in *vitalism,* the concept that the functions of an organism are due to a vital principle or "life force" distinct from the physical forces explainable by the laws of physics and chemistry. Nonscientific health systems based on this philosophy maintain that diseases should be treated by "stimulating the body's ability to heal itself" rather than by "treating symptoms." Homeopaths, for example, claim that illness is due to a disturbance of the body's "vital force," which they can correct with special remedies, while acupuncturists claim that disease is due to imbalance in the flow of "life energy" (Chi or Qi), which they can balance by twirling needles in the skin. Chiropractors claim to assist the body's "Innate Intelligence" by adjusting the patient's spine. Naturopaths speak of "Vis Medicatrix Naturae." Followers of Wilhelm Reich refer to "orgone energy." Hindus refer to "prana." And so on.

Although vitalists often attempt to gain status by making a pretense of being scientific, deep down they reject the scientific method with its basic assumptions of material reality, mechanisms of cause and effect, and provability. Vitalistic healing philosophies transcend mere physical realities and allow for magic and the supernatural. To proponents of vitalism, personal experience, subjective judgment and emotional satisfaction are preferable to objectivity and hard evidence.

Cooperation with "alternative" practitioners poses both legal and ethical dilemmas for responsible health-care providers. Methods that have not been proven safe or effective cannot be employed without risk of physical or psychological harm.

Misconceptions about Quackery

Although many Americans are harmed to some extent by quackery, few seem to perceive it as a serious problem in our society and even fewer seem interested in trying to do anything about it. The following misconceptions contribute to this apathy:

• *Quackery is easy to spot.* Quackery is far more difficult to spot than most people realize. Modern promoters use scientific jargon that can fool people not familiar with the concepts being discussed. Even health professionals can have difficulty in separating fact from fiction in fields unrelated to their expertise. Many victims of quackery never realize they have been duped.

• *Personal experience is the best way to tell whether something works.* When someone feels better after having used a product or procedure, it is natural to credit whatever was done. This can be misleading, however, because most ailments resolve themselves and those that persist can have variable symptoms. Even serious conditions can have sufficient day-to-day variation to enable quack methods to gain large followings. In addition, taking action often produces temporary relief of symptoms (a placebo effect). People who are not aware of these facts tend to give undeserved credit to "alternative" methods.

• *Most victims of quackery are easy to fool.* The majority of quackery's victims are merely unsuspecting. People tend to believe things they hear repeatedly, and quack ideas—particularly regarding nutrition—are everywhere. Many other victims have serious or chronic diseases that make them feel desperate enough to try anything that offers hope. Alienated people—many of whom are paranoid—form another victim group. These people tend to believe that our food supply is unsafe, that drugs do more harm than good, and that doctors, drug companies, large food companies and government agencies are not interested in protecting the public. Such beliefs make them vulnerable to those who offer foods and healing approaches alleged to be "natural."

• *All quacks are frauds and crooks.* This is untrue. Many promoters of quackery are true believers, zealots and devotees whose problem is failure to apply skepticism to the favored therapy, very much like a religious fanatic who blindly accepts "the faith." Their apparent sincerity and self-confidence help persuade people to try their methods and discourage those who become disillusioned from trying to seek justice.

• *"Minor" forms of quackery are harmless.* Quackery involving small sums of money and no physical harm is often viewed as harmless. Examples are "nutrition insurance" with vitamin pills and wearing a copper bracelet for arthritis. But their use indicates confusion on the part of the user and vulnerability to more serious forms of quackery. There is also harm to society. Money wasted on quackery would be better spent for research, but much of it goes into the pockets of people (such as vitamin pushers) who are spreading misinformation and trying to weaken consumer protection laws.

• *Government protects us.* Although many government agencies are involved in fighting quackery, most do not give it sufficient priority to be effective. Moreover, these agencies lack a coordinated plan to maximize their effectiveness.

• *Quackery's success represents medicine's failure.* It is often suggested that people seek "alternatives" because doctors are brusque, and that if doctors were more attentive, their patients would not turn to quacks. Doctors sometimes pay insufficient attention to the emotional needs of their patients. But blaming the medical profession for quackery's success would be like blaming astronomers for the popularity of astrology. Some people's needs exceed what ethical, scientific health care can provide. And many types of quackery have nothing to do with doctor-patient relationships. The main reason for quackery's success is its ability to seduce people who are unsuspecting or desperate.

The Lure of "Alternative" Methods

The reasons why people choose "alternative" methods instead of, or in addition to, conventional methods include the following:

• Proponents promote their methods vigorously, through the media as well as person-to-person. Many have developed effective sales pitches that promise relief and exploit fears.

• Patients who fear that conventional treatment has unpleasant side effects are attracted by promises that "alternative" treatment is painless and nontoxic.

• People with chronic, painful, disabling, or life-threatening illnesses may become desperate enough to try anything said to offer hope.

• Sincerity, sympathy, and self-confidence exhibited by proponents can inspire confidence in prospective clients.

• Many "alternative" approaches are appealing because they seem simple and use everyday terms. For example, proponents may attribute an illness to "buildup of toxins," and describe their treatment as "detoxification."

• "Alternative" approaches that involve active participation by the patient (such as preparation of special foods) can make people feel more in control of their life.

- Many people learn about an unproven method from a trusted friend who believes in the method.

- Some people feel alienated toward the medical profession as a result of bad experiences they or people close to them have had as patients.

- Some people follow a "miss-no-bets" strategy in which they use both proven and unproven methods.

- Some immigrants and culturally isolated groups continue to use traditional practices of folk medicine.

Examples of Dubious Products

In 1984, the House Subcommittee on Health and Long-Term Care (chaired by Representative Claude Pepper) reported that almost every substance imaginable has been touted as a cure and sold to the desperate and unwary. The subcommittee identified quacks who advertised cures composed of distilled water, seaweed extracts, ground-up diamonds, mistletoe extracts, ground warts from horses, vegetable oil, serums from urine and fecal matter, grape diets, clam extracts, and others. Arthritis cures ranged from the venoms of snakes and ants to diets involving honey, liver, and herbs. Extracts of other plants, like alfalfa, basil, caraway seeds, cayenne pepper, and parsley were also sold as cures.

People with arthritis have been advised to bury themselves in uranium-bearing soil, to sit in an abandoned mine shaft, or to stand naked under a 1000-watt light bulb during the full moon. They have been wrapped in manure, soaked in mud, and bathed in cod liver oil, kerosene, and peppermint oil. Sufferers of cancer and other diseases have been subjected to colonic irrigations. These are enemas performed by inserting a rubber tube into the rectum and then pumping as much as twenty gallons of water into the intestines. Some healers subject their patients to multiple coffee enemas daily as part of their treatment to "cleanse the body of environmental pollutants." Other patients receive kelp and seaweed injections to fight cancer. To allegedly remove deposits from clogged arteries, some people undergo chelation therapy, which involves intravenous administration of a synthetic amino acid. Some products the subcommittee reviewed were narcotics and caused addiction. Others could cause nervous conditions, cirrhosis of the liver, cancer, convulsions, cataracts, hemorrhaging, heart palpitations, and insulin shock in diabetics. By comparison, vitamin and mineral supplements and pills, powders, and herbal teas claimed to cause weight loss without dieting or exercising may seem harmless. But these products cause their share of injuries and bring billions of dollars a year to the coffers of "alternative" promoters.

History of the AMA's Concern with Health Fraud

The American Medical Association was founded in 1847, in part "for enlightening and directing public opinion in regard to the duties, responsibilities, and requirements of medical men." The Proceedings of the 1846 and 1847 National Medical Conventions, during which the Medical Code of Ethics was established, offer a glimpse of the Association's first statements regarding medical practices. For one thing, holding pharmaceutical patents was deemed unethical because "if such nostrum be of real efficacy, any concealment regarding it is inconsistent with beneficence and professional liberality; and, if mystery alone give it value and importance, such craft implies either disgraceful ignorance, or fraudulent avarice." Physicians, consequently, were advised "to discourage druggists and apothecaries from vending quack or secret medicines, or from being in any way engaged in their manufacture and sale."

Similarly, the AMA's new code called upon physicians to expose frauds and empirics to the public because victims and lay medics could not be expected to have knowledge of potential hazards: "It is the duty of physicians, who are frequent witnesses of the enormities committed by quackery, and the injury to health and even destruction of life caused by the use of quack medicines, to enlighten the public on these subjects, to expose the injuries sustained by the unwary from the devices and pretensions of artful empirics and impostors." Thus, since its establishment, the American Medical Association has expressed a concern for exposing and publicizing fraudulent medical practices. Today's AMA continues to set ethical standards to help physicians provide appropriate, compassionate patient care, and to help all Americans lead a healthier and more productive life.

In 1906, the Association's documentation of fraudulent medical practices in the United States began in earnest when Arthur J. Cramp, MD, joined the editorial staff of the *Journal of the American Medical Association* and regularly published items concerning health fraud and quackery. In 1913, the Association formally established a separate "Propaganda Department" to gather and disseminate information concerning health fraud and quackery. This department grew and became the Bureau of Investigation (1925) and later the Department of Investigation (1958). For many years, the Department of Investigation answered inquiries from physicians, local Better Business Bureau offices across the United States, the news media, and members of the public. While preparing answers to these inquiries, the Department also corresponded with federal and state regulatory agencies, state and county medical societies, and experts in the field, to evaluate the legitimacy of promoters' claims.

In 1975, the Association closed the Department of Investigation. The correspondence, investigative statements, advertisements, books, newspapers, clippings, promotional literature, court testimonies, journals, photographs, and patent descriptions that had amassed were transferred to the Association's Department of Archives, History, and Policy Information, an organizational unit of the Division of Library and Information Management. These materials, now called the Historical Health Fraud and Alternative Medicine Collection, include information on more than 3,500 fraudulent or alternative health practitioners, products, and practices that were the subjects of inquiries to and/or investigations by the American Medical Association.

In 1988, a two-year Project Grant from the National Library of Medicine helped to support an effort to organize and catalog this collection. This project was completed in mid-1991 and published in early 1992 as the *Guide to the American Medical Association Historical Health Fraud and Alternative Medicine Collection.*

Although the AMA no longer has a special department to combat quackery, other arms of the organization continue to play an important role in evaluating and opposing questionable health matters. The AMA Council on Scientific Affairs drafts position papers, which, when accepted by the House of Delegates, shape AMA policy toward the issues involved. The AMA Diagnostic and Therapeutic Technology Assessment (DATTA) project polls experts on the safety and effectiveness of major technologies and publishes its results. *JAMA; Journal of the American Medical Association*, other AMA journals, and *American Medical News* keep the medical community and news media informed of scientific findings when "alternative" methods are tested.

Health Fraud and Quackery

Fraudulent and quack methods can be divided into three categories according to the degree of danger they pose. The first category is for methods that cause direct harm. The second category contains methods that cause indirect harm by diverting people away from effective care. The third category is "economic frauds," which can cause no physical harm but rob people of money. The dollar cost of quackery is unknown, but it is at least $10 billion a year, with at least $3 billion wasted on unnecessary or inappropriate vitamin supplements. The costs in terms of death, discomfort, and disability are also unknown and are even more difficult to tabulate.

The publications listed below identify many types of health fraud and quackery, list ways to distinguish between bogus and scientific claims, and discuss ways that physicians can help patients to avoid being "quacked."

History of Quackery

American Medical Association: Nostrums and quackery
Chicago, American Medical Association Press, 1911, 1921, 1936.
A three-volume set describing hundreds of fraudulent products and promotions. Contains reproductions of many ads and product labels.

Young JH: The toadstool millionaires.
Princeton, Princeton University Press, 1961.
Traces the history of patent medicines in America from colonial times through passage of the Pure Food and Drugs Act of 1906. Notes, however, that quackery was still thriving half a century later.

Ellerbroek WC: The unicorn: A paradigm of human thought.
JAMA 204:131–134, April 1, 1968.
Traces the origin of myths about the unicorn, noting that a market for its horn existed for several hundred years. States that during the sixteenth century the horn was advised for epilepsy, barrenness, worms and the plague, as well as for smallpox and other assorted ills. Since pieces of "genuine" horn brought up to ten times their weight in gold, counterfeit horn was common and water in which a horn was placed (thereupon transferring its power) was available to the poor. Concludes that "unicorn horn" worked its wonders through what we now recognize as the placebo effect.

McNamara B: Step right up.
Garden City, NY, Doubleday & Co., 1975.
An illustrated history of the American medicine show, which combined flamboyant entertainment with pitches for cure-alls and other snake oils.

Deutsch R: The new nuts among the berries: How nutrition nonsense captured America.
Palo Alto, Bull Publishing Co., 1977.
Describes the history of food faddism in America as promoted by the Kellogg brothers, Adelle Davis, Carlton Fredericks, Gayelord Hauser, Horace Fletcher, Bernarr Macfadden, and many others.

Roth J: Health purifiers and their enemies.
New York, Prodist, 1977.
An overview of the "natural health" movement and its critics. Notes interesting parallels in the ways that scientific practitioners and "natural healthers" are organized.

Wharton J: Crusaders for Fitness: A History of American health reformers.
Princeton, Princeton University Press, 1982.
Describes the life and times of William Alcott, Jennie Chandler, Horace Fletcher, Sylvester Graham, Luther Gulick, Alexander Haig, G. Stanley Hall, Martin L. Holbrook, Woods Hutchinson, John Harvey Kellogg, Bernarr Macfadden, and Mary Gove Nichols. Suggests that it is better to describe the devotion and zeal of such people as "hygienic religion" rather than "faddism," because "faddism" implies that their activity is little more than short-lived foolishness.

Baeke JL, Payer L: "The apotheosis of quackery."
MD 29:89–91, 107, 109, August 1985.
Describes the life and work of John R. Brinkley, who, during the 1920s and early 1930s, made millions of dollars by surgically implanting tissue from the testicles of goats in thousands of people for such problems as varicose veins, hemorrhoids, premature ejaculation, poor vision, acne, dizzy spells, and melancholia. He made additional millions by selling "tonics" through a network of drugstores, which he advertised on his own radio stations.

Burnham JC: How superstition won and science lost.
New Brunswick, NJ, Rutgers University Press, 1987.
Describes how the mass media and advertising have promoted and perpetuated misinformation related to health, nutrition, and psychology. States that scientists became less willing to speak out against magical ideas and superstitions.

Ver Berkmoes R: Don't touch that dial!
American Medical News 33:9–11, September 21, 1990.
Describes many items on exhibit at the Museum of Questionable Medical Devices, maintained in Minneapolis by Bob McCoy.

Young JH: The medical messiahs.
Princeton, NJ, Princeton University Press, 1992.
Traces the history of the government struggle against quackery during the twentieth century. Describes the development of federal regulation by the FDA, the FTC, and the U.S. Postal Service. Details the activities of Ruth Drown, Harry Hoxsey, Adolphus Hohensee, and many other leading entrepreneurs.

Young JH: American health quackery.
Princeton, NJ, Princeton University Press, 1992.
Presents a compendium of essays by James Harvey Young, foremost expert on the history of health fraud and quackery. Covers a broad range of bogus remedies and their promoters, noting that quackery in the 1990s seems even more extensive than it was in earlier and allegedly more naive eras.

Hafner AW, Carson JG, Zwicky JF: Guide to the American Medical Association historical health fraud and alternative medicine collection.
Chicago, American Medical Association, 1992.
Describes the AMA's files of archival material on more than 3,500 fraudulent or alternative health practitioners, products, and practices that were the subjects of inquiries and/or investigations by the AMA.

How Quackery Sells

Freireich EJ: Unproven remedies: lessons for
improving techniques of evaluating therapeutic efficacy.
In Cancer chemotherapy – fundamental concepts and recent advances.
Chicago, Year Book Medical Publishers, 1975.
Contains a tongue-in-cheek description of the "Freireich Experimental Plan," which assures that when proper research methods are not used, any remedy with no obviously harmful side effects can be "proven" effective for virtually all patients with serious disease. The essential elements are: (1) pick a disease that has natural variability, (2) apply the "treatment" when the patient's disease is getting progressively worse; (3) if the patient's condition improves or stabilizes, take credit, then stop the treatment or decrease the dosage; (4) if the patient's condition worsens, say that the dosage must be increased or that the treatment was stopped too soon; and (5) if the patient dies, say that the treatment was applied too late.

Barrett S: The health quack: supersalesman of the seventies.
Archives of Internal Medicine 138:1065–1066, 1978.
Describes the modern health quack as a supersalesman with an endless list of products. Describes how quacks reach people emotionally by playing on fears, catering to hopes, appealing to vanity, and attacking the medical profession, the food and drug industries, and consumer protection agencies.

Miller RW: Voice of the quack.
FDA Consumer 14:24–25, October 1980.
Identifies dozens of adjectives and phrases used in sales pitches that should tip people off that a health product will not live up to its advertising claims.

Quacks sell hope, not health care.
Wisconsin Medical Journal 87:25–26, November 1988.
Examines the appeal of quackery. Describes methods used by quacks to sell worthless products. Notes that a few physicians turn to quackery and lists reasons why. Lists methods used by quacks to promote themselves and enhance their appeal. Mentions examples of unproven methods promoted by "alternative practitioners." Urges physicians to fight quackery by communicating more with their patients.

Barrett S, Jarvis WT: How quackery sells.
Nutrition Forum 8:9–13, March/April 1991.
Describes a wide variety of emotional appeals and propaganda tricks used to promote unnecessary or unproven products and services. Included are appeals to vanity, testimonials, scare tactics, seductive tactics, and ploys used to undermine confidence in scientific medical care. States that self-confidence is probably the most important characteristic to which the success of quacks can be attributed. Also discusses how quacks use the concept of "health freedom" to divert attention away from their improprieties and to arouse their followers to oppose government regulation.

General Literature

FDA: A study of health practices and opinions (Publication 210978).
Springfield, VA, National Technical Information Service,
U.S. Dept. of Commerce, 1972.
Classic study of 2,839 adults who were interviewed with an extensive questionnaire about their use of dietary supplements, "health foods," weight-reduction practices, laxatives, quit-smoking aids, and various other products. They were also asked about their choice of health practitioners and their tendencies toward self-diagnosis and self-treatment.

Young JH: The persistence of medical quackery in America.
American Scientist 60:318–326, 1973.
Notes that many people have predicted that quackery would vanish when the public acquires more education, when stronger laws are enacted, and when science expands its horizons. Discusses various characteristics of patients, orthodox practitioners, and quacks that contribute to quackery's persistence. Notes that quacks have a competitive advantage because they lack ethical restraints against false promises. Expresses concern that many young people have turned against science and are flirting with occult practices.

Health frauds and quackery.
FDA Consumer 11:12–17, November 1977.
Interviews Stephen Barrett, MD, who discusses various problems with laetrile, acupuncture, chiropractic, fad diagnoses, and excessive use of placebos (by medical doctors). Also covers how publicity promotes quackery, how promoters of quackery are attempting to curb FDA enforcement powers, and where reliable health information can be obtained.

Barrett S (ed.): The health robbers: how to protect your money and your life.
Philadelphia, George F. Stickley Co., 1980.
Comprehensive exposé of health frauds and quackery. Covers mistreatment of arthritis, acupuncture, chiropractic, ineffective nonprescription drugs, faith healing, medical impostors, nutrition quackery, "hypoglycemia," the campaign against fluoridation, diet fads and facts, nutrition for athletes, why quackery persists, government regulatory actions, cigarette company deception, where to get accurate information, and how to communicate effectively with one's doctors.

Health quackery: Consumers Union's report on false health claims, worthless remedies, and unproven therapies.
Mt. Vernon, NY, Consumers Union, 1980.
Updated compendium of articles previously published in *Consumer Reports* magazine. Covers arthritis quackery, laetrile, antifluoridation propaganda, "organic" and "health" foods, chiropractic, vitamin E, mail-order frauds, and government regulatory action.

Jarvis WT: Quackery and you.
Washington DC, Review and Herald Publishing Company, 1983.
Identifies promotional methods, signs, and dangers of quackery. Describes "fountain-of-youth" products, food myths, weight-reduction quackery, mail frauds, diploma mills, cosmetic quackery, person-to-person sales methods, mental health quackery.

Doyle RP: The medical wars.
New York, William Morrow and Company, 1983.
Provides a lucid analysis of the scientific method and its application to such controversial topics as diet and hyperactivity, laetrile, orthomolecular medicine, water fluoridation, and the alleged dangers of sugar.

Pepper C et al.: Quackery, A $10 billion scandal.
Washington, D.C., U.S. Government Printing Office, May 31, 1984.
Reports on a four-year investigation by the staff of the Subcommittee on Health and Long-Term Care of the House of Representatives Select Committee on Aging. States that quackery costs consumers at least $10 billion a year. Comments on a large number of bogus arthritis and cancer cures, quack devices, diploma mills, and many other problems. Analyzes the resources and enforcement efforts of the FDA, FTC and U.S. Postal Service. Concludes that: (1) the FDA has the broadest authority to control quackery but has given it little priority, (2) the FTC's impact on quackery is "imperceptible," and (3) the Postal service had targeted resources and been continuously involved in attacking mail frauds.

Hearing before the Subcommittee on Health and Long-Term Care of the Select Committee on Aging, House of Representatives, May 31, 1984.
Washington, DC, U.S. Government Printing Office, 1984.
Contains testimony and exhibits submitted by victims of quackery (or their survivors), government regulators, antiquackery activists, a former mail-fraud operator who was imprisoned, and the lobbyist for the National Health Federation, a group espousing minimum regulation of the health marketplace.

Miller RW: Critiquing quack ads.
FDA Consumer 19:10–13, March 1985.
Reports that during a one-month period, the FDA collected 435 questionable ads from newspapers and magazines. Notes that the most common items were weight-loss products (249 ads, 218 of which were for pills) and hair restorers (42 products and 47 clinics). Mentions FDA actions against firms marketing body-wrap products and grapefruit pills.

Donnelly WJ, Spykerboer, Thong YH: Are patients who use alternative medicine dissatisfied with orthodox medicine?
Medical Journal of Australia 142:539–541, 1985.
Reports on the results of a survey of families with a child who had been admitted to a hospital with either asthma (128 families) or a minor surgical complaint (110 families). Notes that slightly fewer than half of each group had consulted an

"alternative" practitioner at some time and that only 7 percent of these families had been dissatisfied with their conventional care.

Santich K: Nevada's medical dilemma.
Reno Gazette Journal, January 19–25, 1986.
A 7-part series which states that "with lax licensing standards and little policing, unorthodox medicine in Nevada has attracted both people truly dedicated to holistic medicine as well as get-rich-quick hucksters." Notes that in 1973 Nevada became the first state to legalize the practice of acupuncture by laypersons, and that it subsequently legalized laetrile and Gerovital and set up licensing boards for naturopaths [later repealed] and homeopaths. Describes allegations of bribery surrounding passage of the bill to legalize Gerovital. Describes the criminal prosecutions of a naturopath (for murdering a patient) and the operator of a clinic that administered intravenous DMSO (for insurance fraud).

Payne JP et al: Alternative therapy.
London, British Medical Association, 1986.
Detailed report on "alternative" therapies and how they can be scientifically evaluated. Includes summary of a 1981 report by a Dutch commission on alternative medical systems.

Herbert V, Barrett S: Twenty-one ways to spot a quack.
Nutrition Forum 3:65–68, September 1986.
Identifies the sales pitches and antimedical propaganda typical of promoters of quackery, including scare tactics, false promises of cure, and opposition to public health measures.

Fuerst ML: The growth of health fraud and unproven therapies.
Generics 7:31-37, Fall 1986.
Notes the increasingly high cost of health fraud. Examines reasons for the increasing popularity of unproven therapies and the decline in government action against them. Reviews governmental and private efforts to combat health fraud. Discusses a cancer clinic which dispenses dimethyl sulfoxide (DMSO), Dr. Burzynski's cancer clinic, and the Livingston-Wheeler cancer therapy. Describes the harmful results suffered by some patients who resort to alternative therapies. Suggests ways of combating health fraud, mainly through patient education.

Budiansky S: New snake oil, old pitch.
U.S. News & World Report 101:68–70, December 8, 1986.
Notes the heavy volume of unproven remedies being peddled and the difficulty that

government agencies have in fighting them. Discusses nutrition fads and the promotion of unnecessary and often worthless vitamins and food supplements. Mentions immunoaugmentive therapy (IAT), dimethyl sulfoxide (DMSO), vitamin supplements, "candidiasis hypersensitivity," chelation therapy, and unwarranted replacement of mercury-amalgam filings.

Iowa Department of Public Health: Iowa: The victim state.
Iowa Medicine 77:37–40, January 1987.
Notes that Iowans have been a good market for questionable products. Suggests ways in which physicians can monitor their patients' use of potentially harmful alternative remedies. Describes the marketing of various fraudulent products.

Fuerst, ML: The promotion has gone high-tech; the results haven't.
Medical World News 28:34-36, 39-42, 48, 50, 53, May 11, 1987.
Explores the world of health fraud, noting the emphasis on pseudoscientific information to sell fraudulent products and services. Discusses live-cell therapy, cytotoxic testing, hair analysis, electrodiagnosis by homeopaths, chelation therapy, clinical ecology, candidiasis hypersensitivity, and immunoaugmentive therapy (IAT), pointing out flaws of these practices. Reviews antifraud activities by government agencies and the National Council Against Health Fraud. Notes popular attitudes that contribute to the spread of quackery. Mentions costs of health fraud.

Barrett S: Common misconceptions about quackery.
Nutrition Forum 4:41–44, June 1987.
Defines quackery as "anything with false claims in the field of health." Discusses seventeen misconceptions about health fraud and quackery. Focuses on mistaken ideas about victims of quackery, promotion and advertising of quackery, and the harmlessness of quackery. Discusses the role of government, the media, and medical doctors in fighting quackery and mentions the risks involved in fighting quackery.

Lowell JA: Health hoaxes and hazards.
Tucson, Nutrition Information Center, 1987.
A referenced anthology covering questionable weight-reduction products, vitamin and mineral supplements, questionable cancer regimens, miscellaneous irrational remedies, nutrition misinformation, clues to quackery, questionable nutrition assessments, diet and behavior, quackery and the elderly, dangerous products, and colonic enemas.

Health survey: the results
New Age Journal 3:57–59, September/October 1987.
Reports that almost 100 percent of readers who responded to a questionnaire had

used "alternative" health methods and that 97 percent would be willing to choose such methods for treatment of a potentially life-threatening illness. The respondents reported using the following methods with mostly satisfactory results: acupuncture (used by 33 percent), acupressure (42 percent), chiropractic (56 percent), crystal healing (25 percent), colonics (21 percent), energy therapy (25 percent), Feldenkrais bodywork (13 percent), aromatherapy (26 percent), herbal medicines (47 percent), homeopathy (47 percent), mental imagery (70 percent), iridology (19 percent), macrobiotic diet (26 percent), meditation (85 percent), polarity therapy (24 percent), reflexology (38 percent) rolfing (19 percent), and yoga (53 percent). Despite the popularity of these methods, 73 percent of the respondents said that an "alternative" practice had been harmful and 57 percent felt that closer regulation was needed—preferably by "experts in various holistic therapies." The methods most often judged harmful were chiropractic, acupuncture, colonics, fasting, and various "natural" diets. Almost all of the respondents felt that "maintaining an emotional, physical, and spiritual balance" and "maintaining a positive attitude" were vital to good health, but only 57 percent thought it was important to have regular checkups by a medical doctor.

Quackery targets teens.
FDA Consumer 22:24-27, February 1988.
Discusses breast developers, weight loss pills and devices, steroids, and growth hormones, tanning and tanning pills, body hair removal, and hair-growth products. Notes the dangers of so-called "look-alike" drugs, which look like illegal drugs, but are actually dangerous and illogical combinations of decongestants and stimulants. Lists ways to recognize quackery.

Nelson MV: Health professionals and unproven medical alternatives.
Journal of Pharmacy Technology, pp. 60–69, March/April 1988.
Summarizes problems with acupuncture, auriculotherapy, inappropriately administered biofeedback, cellular therapy, chelation therapy, chiropractic, colonic irrigation, faith healing, hair analysis, herbal medicine, holistic medicine, homeopathy, iridology, naturopathy, unproven nutrition practices, orthomolecular psychiatry, unproven cancer remedies, and several other unproven practices. Urges pharmacists to prepare themselves to answer questions about these subjects.

Quackery: It's alive and well, but threatening your health and your pocketbook.
Mayo Clinic Health Letter, Medical Essay, June 1988.
Compares and discusses scientific medicine, unproven treatments, and quackery. Lists ways to spot quackery. Discusses problems caused by quackery. Examines the popularity of fraudulent methods, noting ways in which quacks take advantage of

strains in the doctor-patient relationship. Mentions some examples of quackery, pointing out how they can be harmful. Reviews sources of information on quackery and ways of fighting quacks.

Skrabanek P: Paranormal health claims.
Experimentia 44:303–309, 1988.
States that in medical quackery, inventiveness seems to be limitless. Provides insights into the nature and development of faith healing, Christian Science, psychic surgery, radionics, homeopathy, Bach flower remedies, chiropractic, and acupuncture.

Grigg W: Quackery: It costs more than money.
FDA Consumer 22:30–32, July/August 1988.
Mentions varying estimates about the cost of health fraud. Notes social costs in lives lost or injured by fraudulent cures. Discusses how many unproven remedies, such as immunoaugmentive therapy (IAT), are extended to new diseases such as AIDS. Urges consumers to seek medical advice before trying an unproven method.

Michelmore P: Beware the health hucksters.
Reader's Digest 122:114–118, January, 1989.
Describes the death of three victims of quackery and the disfigurement of a fourth. Criticizes chelation therapy, cytotoxic testing, iridology, and two types of cancer quackery. Provides several tips on how to spot a quack.

Johnson GC, Gottesman RA: The health fraud battle.
Postgraduate Medicine 85:289-293, June 1989.
Focuses on fraudulent devices, some of which are merely economic hazards, others of which are harmful. Notes that purveyors of fraudulent products often market their products without prior FDA approval. Offers tips on how to recognize health fraud. Advises what physicians can do if they suspect that a patient is using a fraudulent product.

Barrett S: Truth or trash? Health-related information in the tabloids.
Priorities, pp., 27–30, Summer 1989.
Describes the author's analysis of 323 articles about health, nutrition, or psychology published during 1987 in the *National Enquirer, Globe, National Examiner, Sun,* and *Weekly World News*. Concludes that fewer than half of the articles on these topics were reliable, with nutrition-related articles scoring especially poorly. Also notes that 239 out of 247 articles involving occult or supernatural beliefs presented occult events as factual, and that all of the tabloids carried ads for dubious mail-order health products.

The Editors of Consumer Reports Books: The new medicine show.
Mount Vernon, NY, Consumer Reports Books, 1989.
Separates fact from hype about nonprescription products marketed for the treatment of common ailments. Covers pain relievers, cough and cold products, allergy treatment, antacids, laxatives, antidiarrheals, sleep aids, vitamins, acne remedies, baldness remedies, and a variety of other topics.

Top 10 health frauds.
FDA Consumer 23:29–31, October 1989.
Briefly discusses fraudulent remedies for arthritis, AIDS, quack baldness remedies and other appearance modifiers, questionable cancer clinics, weight-loss schemes, fraudulent sexual aids, false nutritional schemes, chelation therapy, unproven use of muscle stimulators, and treatments for "candidiasis hypersensitivity." Offers additional tips on how to spot a quack and obtain redress for injury.

Skelly FJ: Beyond conventional medicine.
American Medical News, Vol. 32, November 3, 10, 17, 1989.
Three-part series deals with why unproven therapies appeal to patients and how physicians can counsel patients who want to try them.

Davant C III: No medical degree, no license? Come practice here.
Medical Economics 66:70-71, 74, 77, 81, 85, December 18, 1989.
Relates the story of a naturopath who claimed to be a medical doctor and practiced in a small community in North Carolina. Describes the efforts of local physicians to persuade reluctant licensing boards to investigate the naturopath and force him to cease practicing medicine. Discusses some licensing requirements. Notes questionable practices utilized by the naturopath. Warns that while the naturopath was finally forced to leave his practice, he could relocate to another state and set up practice.

Lowell J: Quackery and the elderly.
New York, American Council on Science and Health, 1990
Contains general information on health frauds, with emphasis on antiaging products and dubious remedies for cancer, heart disease, and arthritis.

Nishiwaki R, Morton A, Bouchard C, et al: Perceived health quackery use among patients.
Western Journal of Medicine 152:87–89, 1990.
Reports on responses by 417 physicians to a mail survey. Indicates that 51 percent thought that quackery was a major problem, and 10 percent had taken a course

about quackery. Seventy percent had encountered a patient using some form of quackery, but only 7 percent of them had reported the problem to an appropriate agency. The reasons given for not reporting were uncertainty about where to make the report, lack of faith in government effectiveness, concern about possible litigation, and insufficient time to report. The most common problems for which quack treatments were involved were cancer (200 listed by physicians), arthritis (106), obesity (91), and heart disease (63). The authors urge physicians to become more knowledgeable and to report instances of fraud to appropriate agencies.

Fairfield PB, Hachadorian C Jr: Medical quackery in Rhode Island: The perspective of state and federal drug control agencies. Rhode Island Medical Journal 73:145–147, 1990.
Discusses efforts by federal and state agencies to curtail health fraud and quackery in Rhode Island. Lists priorities in determining targets of investigation and possible enforcement actions. Explains the function of specific agencies in attacking health fraud. Describes various products being sold in Rhode Island which are considered worthless and fraudulent, and, in some cases, unsafe.

Hollmann PA: Quackery and the elderly. Rhode Island Medical Journal 73:149–51, April 1990.
Examines the problem of health fraud as it affects the elderly. Notes that people are more likely to embrace unproven therapies when their affliction is incurable or life-threatening. Reviews special health problems of the elderly, especially as they relate to susceptibility to questionable therapies. Discusses the role of physicians in dealing with the elderly.

Rubin BK, LeGatt, DF, Audette RJ: The Mexican asthma cure; systemic steroids for gullible gringos. Chest 97:959-961, 1990.
Describes an asthma clinic in Mexico that sells a steroid-containing medication though the Mexican physicians in charge deny that it contains a steroid and tell patients it is "a bronchodilator medication unavailable in the United States." Notes that although systemic steroids can provide dramatic relief of asthma, they can produce hirsutism, weight gain, easy bruising, lowered resistance to infections, and adrenal suppression and failure, which can be fatal if the supply of the steroid runs out.

Renner J: Health smarts HealthFacts Publishing, Inc., Kansas City, MO, 1990.
Identifies and debunks a wide variety of fads, fallacies, and dubious treatments. Provides strategies for getting effective health care and avoiding quackery.

Holt G, Morici J: Hazardous health "cures."
Family Circle 175:27, 29–30, May 15, 1990.
Describes the death of a 23-year-old man who developed anaphylactic shock after taking a useless bodybuilding supplement. Criticizes bogus arthritis aids, phony cancer cures, diet patches, bogus appearance-enhancers, allergy scams, chelation therapy, and "effortless" exercise machines. Advises people who have been "scammed" to complain to their Congressional representatives. Sidebar dissects the claims for a phony "diet pill."

Skrabanek P, McCormick J: Alternative medicine.
In Skrabanek P, McCormick J: Fads & fallacies in medicine, pp. 103–120.
Buffalo, Prometheus Books, 1990.
Describes five groups of "alternative" therapies as mind cures, medication, manipulation, occultism, and quack devices. Notes that many people who do not believe in magic are prepared to accept magic when it is packaged as science. Describes the uncritical acceptance of homeopathy, Bach flower remedies, acupuncture, "electroquackupuncture," chiropractic, faith healing, Christian Science, psychic surgery, and radionics.

Baron-Faust R. Dangerous doctors & phony cures.
Redbook 175:54, 57–59, October 1990.
Describes the case of Ruth Conrad, who had much of her face burned off by a skin cream prescribed by a self-proclaimed naturopath for a blemish he diagnosed as cancer. Debunks the myth of "detoxification," and warns against chelation therapy and allergy scams.

Barrett S and the editors of Consumer Reports:
Health schemes, scams, and frauds.
New York, Consumer Reports Books, 1990.
Covers frauds and quackery related to vitamins, misbranded "food supplements," fad diagnoses, cancer and arthritis quackery, bogus allergies, chiropractic, homeopathy, water purifiers, and weight control. Describes "38 ways to avoid being quacked."

Jarvis WT: What is quackery, and why health professionals become quacks.
Louisville Medicine 10:5, 7–8, February 1991.
Explains why promotionalism is the essence of quackery. Discusses the difference between scientific testing of an unproven method and the quack marketing of an unproven method with false claims and without informed consent. States that boredom, low self-esteem, fear of death, underlying supernatural beliefs, the profit

motive, a desire for adulation, psychopathic personality disorders, and spiritual conversion phenomena are common factors in the making of quacks.

Barrett S: Quack, Quack.
American Health 10:59-63, March 1991.
Lists thirty ways in which consumers can avoid quackery. Identifies various types of dubious practitioners and explains why they should be avoided. Mentions various misconceptions about devices, diets, and nutrition. Cautions against claims made in advertising, testimonials, and several other forms of promotion.

Frazier K (ed.): The hundredth monkey and other paradigms of the paranormal.
Buffalo, Prometheus Books, 1991.
An updated anthology of articles originally published in *Skeptical Inquirer*. Includes discussions of fringe medicine, homeopathy, folk remedies, astrology, chiropractic, firewalking, the Kirlian effect, Qigong, and past-life regression.

Barrett S (ed.) et al: Quackery and fraud in the health-care industry.
Healthline (special issue), October 1991.
Covers nutrition quackery, heart-related quackery, dubious dentistry, evaluation of weight-loss promotions, dubious cancer treatments, and insurance fraud involving chiropractors.

Murray RH, Rubel AJ: Physicians and healers, unwitting partners in health care.
New England Journal of Medicine 326:61-64, 1992.
Notes that there is no recognized system of classification for "alternative medicine." Suggests that most types can be grouped into four categories: (1) spiritual and psychological, (2) nutritional, (3) drug and biologic, and (4) physical forces and devices. States that alternative practices are widespread. Identifies reasons why people choose them and the dangers that may be involved. Suggests that scientific physicians become informed and attempt to have frank discussions with patients using alternative methods. Expresses hope that a panel of representatives of conventional and alternative medicine can be created to negotiate standards for diagnosis, treatment, and controlled clinical trials.

Einterz EM: The poor need no more charlatans.
Lancet 339:795–796, 1992
Gives examples of charlatanism, which the author believes is growing rapidly throughout Africa. Notes that while traditional healers believe they have the power to cure, charlatans rely on trickery. States that even medical professionals are being

lured by profit to prescribe unnecessary injections and other treatments that they know are ineffective, in part because patients request them. Urges greater recognition and more effort to end exploitative practices.

Jarvis WT: Quackery: A national scandal.
Clinical chemistry 38:1574–1586, 1992.
Defines quackery and focuses on our society's failure to control it. Notes inadequacies in consumer protection laws and their enforcement. Notes that the FDA requires over-the-counter medicines to be proven safe and effective in order to remain marketable, but it does not require herbs or homeopathic remedies to meet the same standards. Notes that state legislatures have failed to compel health-care providers to base their practices on science in order to achieve licensure. Notes that the U.S. Office of Education does not require schools that train health-care practitioners to base their teachings on science in order to achieve accreditation. Outlines the origins and current practices of acupuncturists, chiropractors, homeopaths, naturopaths, and ayurvedic physicians. Urges scientists to do more to oppose quackery. Concludes that "only trustworthy people should be granted the privilege of providing health products and services, because like those who are granted the privilege of piloting airliners, they hold the lives of strangers in their hands."

Sibley WA: Therapeutic claims in multiple sclerosis, 3rd edition.
New York, Demos Publications, 1992.
Presents a comprehensive picture of multiple sclerosis (MS) and the past and recent claims made for various treatment approaches. Describes how clinical trials must be designed to avoid being misled by the variable course of MS.

Cornacchia HJ, Barrett S: Consumer health: A guide
to intelligent decisions, 5th edition.
St. Louis, Mosby Year Book, 1993.
College textbook covering all aspects of consumer decisions about health care. Contains extensive discussions of nonscientific practices, quackery, and consumer protection agencies. Provides detailed information on sources of reliable information.

Dubious Dentistry

Fluoridation.
Consumer Reports 43:392–396, 480–482, July, August 1978.
Describes how fluoridation has been attacked with false claims that it causes cancer

and other serious diseases. Notes how the National Health Federation, which coordinated antifluoridation activity, was rooted in quackery. Concludes: "The simple truth is that there's no 'scientific controversy' over the safety of fluoridation. The practice is safe, economical, and beneficial. The survival of this fake controversy represents one of the major triumphs of quackery over science in our generation."

Greene CS: Where does the holistic end and the quackery begin?
Journal of the American Dental Association 102:25–27, 1981.
Discusses "holistic dentistry," noting that it professes to look beyond the local pathology of the moment and consider the overall physical and mental health of each patient. Notes, however, that "it includes an astonishing variety of unconventional treatment methods that are supposed either to prevent disease or cure it"— including acupuncture, oriental medicine, herbology, homeopathy, cranial osteopathy, biomagnetic therapy, electroacupuncture by Voll, balancing body chemistry, and megavitamin therapy. States that the medical profession labels most of these quackery, that it is obvious that most of these treatments do not even have remote dental applications, and that even in nondental situations their use is not based on substantial scientific evidence. Expresses concern that holistic dentistry appears to be more than a passing fad.

Remba Z: Beyond dentistry: how far is too far?
AGD Impact 12:1,6–8, August 1984.
Describes and severely criticizes holistic dentistry. States that the rhetoric of holistic dentistry is difficult to disagree with, but that for some dentists the banner of holism has become a license to use unproven diagnostic and treatment techniques and to sell vitamin supplements, minerals, herbal products, and other trappings of the so-called "wellness" movement. Discusses several questionable practices and practitioners. Presents criticisms, defensive statements by advocates, and the ultimate legal question of how far a dentist can go before exceeding the legal scope of practice.

Dodes JE: The dentist and nutrition quackery.
Nutrition Forum 2:78–80, October 1985.
Describes the activities of several promoters of unscientific nutrition practices used by dentists. Criticizes several theories and practices of dentists who call themselves "holistic." States that dentists should not be doing "nutrition counseling." Concludes that "courses in skeptical thinking are needed at every dental school."

Berry J: Questionable care: What can be done about quackery?
Journal of the American Dental Association 115:679–685, 1987.
States that far too many dentists are involved in nutrition quackery, inappropriate

temporomandibular joint (TMJ) therapy, "mercury-amalgam toxicity," cranial osteopathy, antifluoridation, applied kinesiology, reflexology, acupuncture, and various unscientific approaches that they label "holistic." Notes that several dental schools and dental societies have provided a forum for promoters of quackery. Lists tips on spotting a quack. Quotes dental leaders who believe the American Dental Association should be more aggressive in identifying frauds and that dental schools should make more effort to teach their students how to evaluate health claims.

Wulf C et al: Abuse of the scientific literature in an antifluoridation pamphlet, 2nd edition.
Columbus, Ohio, 1988, American Oral Health Institute.
Analyzes the *Lifesavers Guide to Fluoridation*, a pamphlet written by John Yiamouyiannis, PhD, fluoridation's most active opponent. Although the pamphlet cites 250 references to back its claims, experts from the Ohio Department of Health found that almost half had no relevance to community water fluoridation and that many others actually supported fluoridation but were selectively quoted and misrepresented.

Dodes JE: Dubious dental care.
New York, American Council on Science and Health, 1991.
Criticizes Sargenti root canal therapy, the Keyes technique for gum disease, inappropriate temporomandibular joint (TMJ) therapy, do-it-yourself tooth bleaching, the sale of nutritional supplements by dentists, applied kinesiology, cranial osteopathy, auriculotherapy (acupuncture of the ear), reflexology, and false claims about mercury-amalgam toxicity. States that dental schools and organizations are not doing enough to combat quackery. Describes how the news media sometimes promote quackery by not investigating thoroughly. Concludes that "dubious dentistry poses a substantial risk for the American public." States what consumers, dental educators, state dental boards, legislators, and dental organizations can do about the problem.

Mail Fraud

Delusions of vigor: better health by mail.
Consumer Reports 44:50-54, January 1979.
Notes that a Pennsylvania Medical Society study of 500 nationally circulated magazines had found that about a fourth of them had carried ads for mail-order health products and that every ad was misleading. Reports on various fraudulent ads and products. Notes that some publishers claimed to be concerned about the problem but very few screened out misleading ads. Suggests ways that Postal laws could be strengthened.

Kelley HE: In a plain brown wrapper – Quackery by mail.
ACSH News & Views 3:1, 5, 13–14, November/December 1981.
Describes a large number of bogus mail-order products ordered by the author. States that there appeared to be an inverse relationship between the stature of a publication and the number of ads for fraudulent products, with pulp magazines having the greatest number of such ads.

Shearing the suckers
Consumer Reports 51:87-94, February 1986.
Notes that postal laws had been strengthened since the previous report. Describes "rogues gallery" of several companies engaged in multiple swindles. Provides several tips to avoid mail-order victimization.

Folkenberg J, Modeland V, Segal M: Australian Convicted In 'Cho Low' Fraud.
FDA Consumer 23:35, December 1989/January 1990.
Describes the activities of Peter Foster, an Australian who ran many newspaper ads claiming that "Cho Low Tea" was "as effective as medically prescribed drugs in lowering cholesterol" and "has kept Chinese families slim and healthy for centuries." Reports that Foster was arrested and sentenced to 120 days in prison and that law enforcement authorities were able to return the checks sent in response to the ads. Indicates that a search of Foster's house found ordinary Chinese black tea, but no "Cho Low Tea." States that Foster was involved in other schemes in Australia and England.

Barrett S: Quackery by mail.
New York, 1991, American Council on Health.
Comprehensive report of the mail-order health marketplace. Includes the author's survey of 463 magazines obtained during the spring and summer of 1990. Of these, 79 (18 percent) carried ads for health-related mail-order products, only one of which (a device used to reduce sweating) could live up to its advertised claims. Illustrates dubious claims for various products. Describes additional promotions through direct mail ads, catalog sales, person-to-person (multilevel) distributors, telemarketing schemes, and infomercials. Discusses government regulation and suggests ways to strengthen laws.

Government Regulation

Three federal agencies have responsibility for fighting quackery and health frauds. The Postal Service has jurisdiction over products sold by mail. The Federal Trade Commission (FTC) has jurisdiction over advertising of health services and nonprescription products. The U.S. Food and Drug Administration (FDA) has jurisdiction over the labeling of all products marketed with therapeutic claims and also over the advertising of prescription drugs.

State attorneys general have jurisdiction over the marketing of products and services within their respective states. During the past few years, several have formed an alliance for attacking fraudulent nationwide promotions. The New York City Department of Consumer Affairs has also been active, issuing regulations as well as special investigative reports.

Barrett S: The strange case of quackery and the FDA.
Nutrition Forum 1:1–2, October 1984.
Describes how insufficient enforcement action has encouraged the health food industry to market hundreds of food supplements with unapproved therapeutic claims. States that criminal prosecutions could have great deterrent value but the FDA had used very few of them during the previous twenty years. Notes that an FDA staff member has petitioned the agency to use criminal prosecutions routinely. [The petition eventually was denied.]

Sullivan PM et al: Health fraud and the elderly.
Albany, NY, Assembly Republican Task Force on Health Fraud and the Elderly, 1986.
Defines health fraud as "the promotion, for financial gain, of fraudulent or unproven devices, treatments, services, plans or products (including, but not limited to, diets and nutritional supplements) that alter or claim to alter the human condition." Summarizes testimony at legislative hearings from more than thirty health professionals, enforcement agency officials, voluntary health organization representatives, and others interested in consumer protection. Concludes that (1) penalties for false advertising should be increased, (2) commercial use of the title "doctor" should be restricted to individuals with an accredited degree, (3) media outlets should be made accountable for harm resulting from false advertising of unapproved health products, (4) a license should be required to sell health products door-to-door, (5) a health fraud task force should be set up within the state attorney general's office, (6) the FDA should be given authority over intrastate marketing of health products, and (7) the state consumer protection board should establish a public education program on health-care fraud.

Pepper C: Quackery: The need for federal, state, and local response.
Skeptical Inquirer 12:70–74, Fall 1987.
Article by the late Florida Congressman Claude Pepper, whose subcommittee had conducted a major investigation of quackery and health fraud. Mentions a variety of fraudulent products promoted as cures for cancer, arthritis, and other diseases. Discusses the role of federal agencies in combating quackery and explains why they

have failed. Notes that the elderly comprise 12 percent of the population but 40 percent of the victims of quackery. Recommends ways in which federal and state agencies can better fight health fraud.

Barrett S: Quackery and the FDA: A complicated story.
Nutrition Forum 8:41-44, November/December 1991.
Examines the role that the FDA plays in fighting quackery. Notes that the FDA is responsible for enforcement of laws against health fraud, but that for the most part, it is not doing so. Cites examples of weak enforcement. Discusses reasons for this: lack of resources, bureaucratic constraints, and an antiregulatory mood in Washington under the Reagan and Bush Administrations. Urges legislation to strengthen the FDA's ability to attack health fraud effectively.

Barrett S: Federal regulation of quackery: Improvement is needed.
Priorities, pp. 35–36, Fall 1990.
Analyzes strengths and weaknesses of federal laws and programs for combating health frauds. States that the Postal Service has a vigorous program but is hampered by a weak law, that the FTC has a powerful law but insufficient manpower, and the FDA has a powerful law but a weak enforcement program. Suggests legislation that would increase agency resources, increase penalties for law violations, and make agencies more accountable by requiring them to tabulate and inform Congress about what they are doing.

Organizations Promoting "Alternative Methods"

Barrett S: Be wary of the People's Medical Society.
Nutrition Forum 2:81–83, November 1985.
Describes the formation and activities of the People's Medical Society, which attacks the medical profession and encourages the use of "alternative" practices.

Barrett S: The unhealthy alliance: Crusaders for "health freedom."
New York, American Council on Science and Health, 1988.
A detailed report on activities of four organizations that promote questionable health methods: the National Health Federation, the Health Alternatives Legal Foundation, the American Quack Association, and the Coalition for Alternatives in Nutrition and Healthcare. Notes criminal and civil actions taken against some of their leaders. An abbreviated version of this report is published in *Nutrition Today* 23:26-32, July/August 1988.

Raso J: The FAIM symposium: A "complementary medicine" smorgasbord.
Nutrition Forum 8:17-20, May/June, 1991.

Describes a symposium held by the Foundation for the Advancement of Innovative Medicine, a group co-founded by Robert Atkins, MD. Describes the group's purposes, which include "securing the freedom of physicians to offer innovative therapies" and forcing insurance companies to pay for them. Summarizes the presentations of several speakers. Notes that several exhibitors were making unproven claims for their products.

Unorthodox panel considers NIH mandated role in
study of unconventional medical practices.
The Cancer Letter 18:1–3, June 26, 1992.
Describes the initial activities of the National Institutes of Health's Office on Unconventional Medical Practices, which was set up after Congress ordered NIH to foster research into unconventional practices and gave the institutes $2 million to do the job. Describes the formation and first public meeting of an ad hoc advisory panel that included several prominent scientific researchers, but was composed mainly of practitioners and promoters of "alternative" practices. Notes Dr. Stephen Barrett's concern that "the promoters of unproven methods appointed to the panel will trumpet their appointment to the world as evidence that whatever it is they promote is valid. I am also concerned about what the panel's role would be in shaping any report that would be issued under the NIH imprimatur."

Culhane C: New NIH panel exploring 'alternative' medicine
American Medical News 36:10–11, August 3, 1992.
Provides additional information about the NIH Advisory Panel on Unconventional Medical Practices. States that NIH has defined these practices as "diagnostic or therapeutic techniques that traditional scientists consider outside the mainstream of scientific research." Reports optimism from NIH officials that significant research can be generated.

Antiquackery Activities

Several voluntary and professional organizations have shown consistent interest in fighting quackery and health frauds. Some with a broad scope of activity are mentioned below. Publications by groups with a narrower focus appear elsewhere in this book under topics related to their particular focus. (For example, American Cancer Society position papers are discussed in the section on "alternative" cancer treatments.) The addresses and telephone numbers of groups that have published position papers or other antiquackery materials are listed in Appendix 1.

Proceedings, Second National Congress on Medical Quackery.
Chicago, American Medical Association, 1961.

Summarizes speeches by government officials, physicians, and others about enforcement actions, AMA activities, diploma mills, susceptibility to quackery, educational strategies for schools and colleges, and media responsibilities. Co-sponsored by the AMA and the FDA.

O'Donnell WE: Don't sneer at your patient's wonder cure.
Medical Economics 62:77-78, 82, 84, June 24, 1985.
Explores ways in which physicians can respond to patients who claim that alternative treatments they use are working as well as or better than prescribed medicines. Urges physicians not to appear angry, hostile, indifferent, amused, or condescending, but to listen to what their patients are saying. Describes how dialogue between physicians and their patients can help further their relationship.

Monaco GP: The primary care physician: the first line of defense in the battle against health fraud.
Medical Times 114: 43-48, May 1986.
Explores the appeal of unproven methods, especially to desperate patients. Explains how people hear about alternative therapies and why they seek them. Describes how questionable practitioners may attempt to enhance their own credibility by attacking conventional medicine. Advises physicians on how to counsel patients and combat fraudulent practices. Identifies hallmarks of quackery, sources of information on health fraud, and types of government action against dubious practitioners.

Proceedings, Third National Congress on Medical Quackery
Chicago, American Medical Association, 1966.
Summarizes speeches by government officials, physicians, and others about drug and device quackery, nutrition nonsense, obesity cures, antifluoridation campaigns, krebiozen, quackery by physicians, advertising frauds, chiropractic, and dangers of quackery. Co-sponsored by the AMA and the National Health Council.

Health Products & Promotions Information Exchange Network
Washington, DC, National Association of
Consumer Agency Administrators, 1986–1992,
Sourcebook that reports hundreds of state and federal consumer protection activities involving health and nutrition frauds. Updated periodically.

Tyler JI et al: The professional's guide to health & nutrition fraud.
San Francisco, California Medical Association, 1987.
Covers spotting quackery; guidelines for checking advertising claims; food fads, cults and quackery; how to counsel victims; how to speak without legal risk; where to report health frauds; and sources of additional information.

*Holohan TV: Referral by default: The medical
community and unorthodox therapy.*
JAMA 257:1641–1642, 1987.
Suggests that a major factor in the popularity of "alternative" therapies is failure of the scientific community to actively discourage their use.

Barrett S: Fighting quackery: A quick reference guide.
Postgraduate Medicine 81:13, 16, 21, May 15, 1987.
Notes that most quackery victims are unsuspecting and urges physicians to be aware of their patients' use of, or interest in, questionable methods. Suggests that physicians can reduce their patients' susceptibility to quackery by explaining the basis for psychophysiological symptoms and advising patients on the appropriateness of taking vitamin supplements. Suggests safe and effective ways to counter misinformation in the media and to report illegal promotions to government agencies. Also urges doctors to encourage victims of quackery to file lawsuits.

Barrett S: Fighting quackery: Tips for activists.
Nutrition Forum 4:49–52, July 1987.
States that the crucial step in fighting quackery is overcoming any negative feelings about being involved, especially the fear of being sued for libel or slander. States that suits of this type are rare and can be avoided by criticizing ideas rather than individuals. Advises activists not to call anyone a "quack," "fraud," or crook" unless they are willing to defend their name-calling in court. Describes techniques for dealing with the news media, but notes that many effective actions, such as complaining to an enforcement agency or providing background information to a reporter, can be taken without personal exposure. Indicates where to complain and lists sources of additional information.

Dalton R: Quackbusters Inc.: Hot on the heels of medical hucksters.
The Scientist 2:1–3, May 16, 1988.
Describes the history and activities of the National Council Against Health Fraud. Notes the group's educational efforts and its Task Force on Victim Redress, which was set up to help quackery victims sue their victimizers.

Cowart VS: Health fraud's toll: lost hopes, misspent billions.
JAMA 259:3229–3230, 1988.
Reports on matters discussed at the 1988 National Health Fraud Conference. Cites speakers who criticized the FDA for not using criminal prosecution as a primary tool for fighting health frauds. Criticizes immunoaugmentative therapy (IAT), DMSO, vitamin overpromotion, "stress vitamins," "candidiasis hypersensitivity," and unwarranted replacement of mercury-amalgam filings.

Sampson WI: Why quacks befuddle physicians.
California Physician, pp. 16–18, October 1988.
Describes how modern quacks use sophisticated marketing and propaganda techniques to influence public opinion and manipulate government agencies. Notes the use of self-serving dichotomies, such as traditional/nontraditional, orthodox/unorthodox, toxic/nontoxic, synthetic/organic, and establishment/alternative. Notes that quacks claim that there is a "changing paradigm" of healing that cannot be measured by the techniques of "Western medicine." Lists eleven reasons why physicians are not inclined to fight against quackery, including lack of familiarity with particular claims, lack of time to investigate, fear of losing an involved patient, difficulty in persuading patients to stop dubious treatment, and fear of being sued.

Grossmann J: Quack buster.
Hippocrates 2:50-56, November/December 1988.
Focuses on the activities of Dr. Stephen Barrett, a psychiatrist who has increasingly devoted his life to fighting health fraud and quackery. Describes how his investigations of hair analysis and mail frauds had considerable impact. Mentions other leaders in the fight against health fraud. Discusses a variety of dubious products and services and offers tips on how to avoid being quacked.

Nishiwaki R, Bouchard C: Combatting nutrition quackery:
The San Bernardino County Experience.
American Journal of Public Health 79:652–653, 1989.
Reviews efforts by the Department of Public Health in San Bernardino County to combat nutrition quackery in its county. Details their efforts to establish a Nutrition Program to identify nutrition quackery. Mentions assistance by other organizations. Lists activities carried on by the Department's task force on fighting quackery.

Chollar S: Quacks in the system.
New Physician 39:18–21, 23, November 1990.
Describes the antiquackery activities of various individuals and lists sources of help and additional information.

Couzens GS: Quackbusters.
Cooking Light, pp. 30–32, 34, 39, January/February 1992.
Describes the problem of quackery, focusing on the activities of Drs. Stephen Barrett, William Jarvis, and Victor Herbert. Lists twenty tips to avoid being "quacked" and sources of additional information.

Part II: "Alternative" Healing Systems

Acupuncture

Acupuncture has been part of Chinese medicine for thousands of years. Its proponents state that the body's vital energy ("Ch'i" or "Qi") circulates through "meridians" along the surface of the body. They also state that illness and disease result from imbalances or interruptions of Ch'i, which can be corrected by acupuncture. The treatment is applied to "acupuncture points," which are said to be located along the meridians. The existence of meridians or acupuncture points has never been scientifically validated.

Traditional acupuncture, as now practiced, involves the insertion of stainless steel needles into various body areas. Low-frequency current may be applied to the needles to produce greater stimulation. Other procedures used separately or together include: moxibustion (burning of floss or herbs applied to the skin); injection of sterile water, procaine, morphine, vitamins or homeopathic solutions through the inserted needles; applications of laser beams; placement of needles in the external ear (auriculotherapy); and acupressure (use of manual pressure). Some practitioners espouse the traditional Chinese view of health and disease and consider acupuncture and its variations a valid approach to the full gamut of disease. Others reject these trappings and claim (or hope) that acupuncture offers a simple way to achieve pain relief.

Acupuncture was introduced to the United States in about 1825 but generated little interest until President Richard M. Nixon's 1972 visit to China. Since then it has been promoted for the treatment of pain and a wide variety of other problems. Although many articles claiming benefit have been published, the quality of most research studies has been poor. There is no evidence that acupuncture influences the course of any disease.

All states permit acupuncture to be performed—some by physicians only, some by lay acupuncturists under medical supervision, and some by unsupervised laypersons. In 1990 the National Accreditation Commission for Schools and Colleges of Acupuncture and Oriental Medicine was recognized by the U.S. Secretary of Education as an accrediting agency. This recognition is not based upon the scientific validity of what is taught but upon other criteria. Many insurance companies cover acupuncture treatment if performed by a licensed physician, but Medicare and Medicaid generally do not. Acupuncture needles are considered "investigational" devices by the FDA and are not approved for the treatment of any disease.

Critical Literature

Taub A: Quackupuncture?
In Barrett S (ed.): The health robbers, 2nd edition, pp. 257–266.
Philadelphia, George F. Stickley Co., 1980.
Describes acupuncture's history and popularization in the United States in the early 1970s. Describes the author's visit to China to observe acupuncture anesthesia. Reports that patients also received local anesthesia and a narcotic. Describes cases in which complications occurred. Notes the advent of clinics that made glowing promises but offered shoddy care. Concludes that "the mythology of acupuncture has spread rapidly throughout our country. It will be difficult to control. Our best hope is that with time, education and gradual appreciation of its worthlessness, acupuncture will be resisted by the public. Then it will pass beyond us, as have its sister quackeries: purging, leeching, bleeding, et cetera."

AMA Council on Scientific Affairs: Reports of the Council on
Scientific Affairs of the American Medical Association, 1981.
Chicago, American Medical Association, 1982.
Concludes: (1) at this time, it cannot be said that acupuncture has any more certain effect on pain than a placebo or a sham acupuncture (needles inserted at random points rather than at the meridians), (2) acupuncture can produce substantial analgesia in selected patients but the mechanism doesn't operate consistently or reproducibly in the majority of people and does not operate at all in some people, and (3) acupuncture can alleviate pain but provides only temporary relief for patients with chronic pain.

Melzack R, Katz J: Auriculotherapy fails to relieve chronic
pain—a controlled crossover study.
JAMA 251:1041–1043, 1984.
An evaluation of auriculotherapy in 36 patients suffering from chronic pain found that stimulating locations recommended by proponents was no more effective than touching remote points with or without electrical stimulation.

Skrabanek P: Acupuncture: past, present, and future.
In Stalker D, Glymour C (eds.): Examining holistic medicine, pp. 181–196.
Buffalo, Prometheus Books, 1985.
States that "the only development in the last two millennia has been a gradual increase in acupoints, which now exceed two thousand." Notes that acupuncture is effective in some patients with functional and psychosomatic disorders, but so is a placebo.

Vincent CA, Richardson PH: The evaluation of therapeutic acupuncture: concepts and methods.
Pain 24:1–13, 1986.
Describes the core ideas of traditional acupuncture. Notes that their "strangeness" does not preclude the possibility that acupuncture has value. Describes the difficulty in designing valid research protocols. Makes recommendations for future research.

Stryker WS, Gunn RA, Francis DP: Outbreak of hepatitis B associated with acupuncture.
Journal of Family Practice 22(2):155–158, 1986.
Describes the occurrence of acute hepatitis B in six patients who had received acupuncture at a chiropractic clinic where needles had been reused after overnight immersion in benzalkonium chloride. Recommends that needles used for acupuncture either be disposable or be physically cleaned and sterilized by autoclave after each use.

Abrams G: New practitioners getting the point of acupuncture.
Los Angeles Times, pp. 1, 6, September 24, 1986.
Notes that the number of acupuncture schools and practitioners appears to be growing rapidly, especially in California. Discusses the training, licensure, and regulation of acupuncturists and quotes several knowledgeable observers.

Vincent CA, Richardson PH: Acupuncture for some common disorders: a review of evaluative research.
Journal of the Royal College of General Practitioners 37:77–81, February 1987.
Surveys studies on acupuncture's effectiveness in treating asthma, sensorineural deafness and tinnitus, hypertension, psychiatric disorders, obesity, and addiction to cigarettes. Concludes that "the quality of the studies . . . has generally been poor."

McGuire R: Acupuncturists cross needles.
Medical Tribune 30:1, 14, 22, September 14, 1989.
Discusses how lay acupuncturists are lobbying state legislatures to require physicians who wish to perform acupuncture to have the same acupuncture training as non-MD practitioners who are licensed. Notes the existence of courses in acupuncture for physicians. Quotes several critics who regard acupuncture as an unproven technique.

Acupuncture devices by any other name.
FDA Consumer 24:40, June 1990.
Describes how the FDA investigated a purported acupuncture device advertised as

effective against migraine headaches, arthritis, toothache, sciatica, disc problems, nausea, hypertension, bronchitis, vertigo, asthma, gynecological distress, liver and kidney disease, enuresis, and other conditions. An American importer's stock of 955 devices was seized and subsequently destroyed. The investigation was triggered by a complaint from the Alabama Board of Chiropractic Examiners, which had objected to an ad in which the device was referred to as a "natural chiropractic product."

Carlsson J, Augustinsson LE, Blomstrand C, et al: Health status in patients with tension headache treated with acupuncture or physiotherapy. Headache 30:593–599, 1990.
Compares 62 patients who received acupuncture or physiotherapy for the treatment of tension headaches. Overall functioning, mental well-being, and intensity and frequency of headache were assessed before and after treatment. Both groups showed improvement, but the physiotherapy group did significantly better.

Ter Riet, G, Kleijnen J, Knipschild P: A meta-analysis of studies into the effect of acupuncture on addiction. British Journal of General Practice 40:379–382, 1990.
Reviews 22 controlled clinical studies of acupuncture for treating addiction to cigarettes (15 studies), heroin (5 studies), and alcohol (2 studies). Judges that the design of these studies was generally poor. Concludes: "For smoking cessation, the number of studies with negative outcomes exceeded by far the number with positive outcomes. Taking the quality of the studies into account, this negative picture becomes even stronger. For heroin and alcohol addiction, controlled clinical research is both scarce and of low quality. Claims that acupuncture is efficacious as a therapy for these addictions are thus not supported by results from sound clinical research."

Ter Riet G, Kleijnen J, Knipschild P: Acupuncture and chronic pain: A criteria-based meta-analysis. Journal of Clinical Epidemiology 43:1191–1199, 1990.
A technical article discussing the results of research on the methodology of 51 controlled clinical studies on acupuncture's effectiveness in chronic pain management. Concludes that "no studies of high quality seem to exist" and that "the efficacy of acupuncture in the treatment of chronic pain remains doubtful."

Wright RS, Kupperman JL, Liebhaber MI: Bilateral tension pneumothoraces after acupuncture. Western Journal of Medicine 154:102–103, 1991.
Describes how a pregnant woman treated with acupuncture for asthma became extremely short of breath during a session and was hospitalized with bilateral

tension pneumothoraces. States that although acupuncture has been shown to produce bronchodilation, this effect is transitory and less than the result achievable with drugs. Concludes: "Given this knowledge and the untoward effects of acupuncture reported herein, the use of this alternative therapy should be discouraged for the management of asthma. Patients who consider acupuncture for the management of their asthma should be informed of the possibility of life-threatening pneumothorax."

*Hung VC, Mines JS: Eschars and scarring from hot
needle acupuncture treatment.
Journal of the American Academy of Dermatology 24:148–149, 1991.*
Reports the case of a woman treated at a California hospital for injuries suffered from hot needle acupuncture treatment. Her symptoms were not relieved. Notes past instances of contact dermatitis resulting from allergic reactions to contact with an acupuncture needle.

*Sampson W et al: Acupuncture—the position paper
of the National Council Against Health Fraud.
Clinical Journal of Pain 7:162–166, 1991.*
Reviews acupuncture's history, theories, techniques, scientific status, hazards, and legal status. Notes that the greater the benefit claimed in a research report, the worse the experimental design. Observes that "most studies that showed positive effects used too few subjects to be statistically significant. The best designed experiments—those with the highest number of controls on variables—found no difference between acupuncture and control groups." Concludes that: (1) acupuncture is an unproven modality of treatment; (2) its theory and practice are based on primitive and fanciful concepts of health and disease that bear no relationship to present scientific knowledge; (3) research during the past twenty years has not demonstrated that acupuncture is effective against any disease; (4) perceived effects of acupuncture are probably due to a combination of expectation, suggestion, counter-irritation, operant conditioning, and other psychological mechanisms; (5) the use of acupuncture should be restricted to appropriate research settings; (6) insurance companies should not be required by law to cover acupuncture treatment; (7) licensure of lay acupuncturists should be phased out; and (8) consumers who wish to try acupuncture should discuss their situation with a knowledgeable physician who has no commercial interest.

*Butler K: Acupuncture and other wanna-bes.
In Butler K: A consumer's guide to "alternative medicine," pp. 93–146.
Buffalo, Prometheus Books, 1992.*
Calls acupuncture "Mao Tse Tung's hoax." Expresses concern that "acupuncturists

are free to make diagnoses and administer treatment that has no scientific basis. Those who lack medical training are permitted to practice independently in some states and under medical supervision in others." Warns readers never to go to an acupuncturist without consulting a medical doctor to determine the cause of the problem.

Proponent Literature

McRae G: A critical overview of U.S. acupuncture regulation.
Journal of Health Politics 7:163–196, Spring 1982.
Surveys state regulations governing the practice of acupuncture. Notes that some states restrict it to physicians, others allow nonphysicians to perform acupuncture under medical supervision, and others license nonphysician acupuncturists. Notes court cases involving efforts to expand the range of practitioners for acupuncture. Describes FDA regulation of acupuncture equipment. Notes that without licensing laws, acupuncturists will practice illegally. Argues that state laws should be enacted to make acupuncture more readily available and to maintain high standards of practice. [Authors' note: "Alternative" practitioners typically argue that licensing will lead to higher standards and enable responsible practitioners to control abuses. However, the usual result is that licensing becomes touted as an endorsement and is used as a steppingstone to greater privileges.]

Firebrace P: Acupuncture: the illustrated guide.
New York, Harmony Books, 1988.
Provides a comprehensive description of acupuncture's history, theories, and techniques, and the therapeutic claims made for it. Contains a brief section on herbalism and other related practices. Advises how to select an acupuncturist.

Ayurvedic Medicine

Ayurvedic medicine is said by its proponents to date back thousands of years. In the United States it has been promoted by the Maharishi Mahesh Yogi, the Hindu swami who founded the transcendental meditation (TM) movement, and by Deepak Chopra, MD, who practices Ayurvedic medicine in the Boston area and writes and lectures about it.

Proponents of Maharishi Ayur-Veda state the following: The functions of the mind and body are regulated by three physiological principles called "doshas." Everyone is endowed at birth with some value of the doshas, but the proportions vary from person to person and determine the psychophysiological type. There are ten types, derived from combinations of the three doshas. Imbalances of doshas and subdoshas disrupt normal function and are responsible for various disorders. In Ayurvedic "pulse diagnosis," the combinations of doshas and subdoshas are felt as patterns of vibration in the radial artery and alert the practitioner to patterns of imbalance that are responsible for the patient's condition. Once the diagnosis is made, the practitioner prescribes diet, exercise, herbal products, and purification procedures for balancing the patient's doshas. Transcendental meditation is also prescribed.

Critical Literature

Barrett S: My quick tour of Whole Life Expo.
Nutrition Forum 8:7, January/February 1991.
Describes the author's experiences at a health exposition in New York City. After completing a brief questionnaire to determine his "body type," he was informed by a Maharishi Ayur-Veda exhibitor that his "doshas" were imbalanced and was offered a tea to correct this. When the author indicated that his health was good, the exhibitor replied that achieving balance through Ayurvedic measures would prevent future trouble.

Butler K: A consumer's guide to "alternative medicine," pp. 110–119.
Buffalo, Prometheus Books, 1992.
Analyzes the theories of Ayurvedic medicine and the writings of its leading American proponent, Deepak Chopra, MD. Notes its relationship to transcendental meditation (TM). States that some of its recommended practices are universally accepted recommendations for a healthy lifestyle, some are unproven, and some are absurd

and/or dangerous. States that its "body typing" system is so simplistic and absurd that there is no point to attempt to catalog its weaknesses. Challenges Dr. Chopra to demonstrate that levitation (floating above the ground through mental power) can occur, as stated by him and other TM enthusiasts.

Proponent Literature

Lambert C: The Chopra prescriptions.
Harvard Magazine, pp. 24–28, September/October 1989.
Describes the careers and theories of Deepak Chopra. Includes the claim that "skillful pulse diagnosticians can do the Ayurvedic equivalent of a complete clinical workup from the pulse alone."

Franklin D: The Maharishi's medicine man.
In Health 4:78–84, May/June, 1990.
Describes the activities and theories of Deepak Chopra, MD. Includes copy of the questionnaire used to determine "body type." [Note: The article contains comments about Dr. Chopra attributed to Dr. Stephen Barrett, which Dr. Barrett did not make. A letter stating this was published on page 8 of the July/August issue of *In Health*.]

Note: Additional information about Ayurvedic medicine can be found in *JAMA* 265:2633–2637, 266:1741–1750, and 266:1769–1774, 1991.

Chiropractic

Chiropractic traces its foundation to the work of Daniel David Palmer, a grocer and "magnetic healer" who practiced in Davenport, Iowa. In 1895, Palmer concluded that he had restored the hearing of a deaf janitor by "adjusting" a bump on his spine. After further study he theorized that the basic cause of disease was interference with the body's "Innate Intelligence," caused by misaligned spinal bones. The basic treatment advocated by Palmer was adjustment of the spine by hand, which he believed would allow the Innate to effect a cure. He rejected the germ theory and had an aversion to drugs, surgery, and medical diagnosis. The word "chiropractic" was derived from the Greek words *cheir* (hand) and *praktikos* (practice).

Many of today's 45,000+ chiropractors still cling literally to Palmer's idea that spinal misalignments—which they commonly refer to as "subluxations"—are the principal cause of disease. Many others—probably a majority—state that mechanical disturbances of the nervous system impair the body's defenses and are an underlying cause of disease. According to this viewpoint, minor "off-centerings" or "fixations" of the vertebrae can disturb nerve function, lower the body's resistance to germs, and cause or aggravate disease by disturbing nerve impulses to the visceral organs. Some chiropractors maintain that chiropractic deals with the cause of disease while medicine merely deals with the symptoms. Only a small percentage of today's chiropractors have openly disavowed Palmer's theory.

In 1968 a comprehensive study by the U.S. Department of Health, Education, and Welfare concluded that chiropractic education does not prepare its practitioners to make an adequate diagnosis and provide appropriate treatment. Although chiropractic schools have improved considerably since then, they do not provide the depth of diagnostic and therapeutic training that physicians receive. Among other things, the range of ailments seen in patients attending clinics at chiropractic schools is far narrower than that of patients seen at medical school clinics, and chiropractic students receive little or no hospital training. Critics also point out that since much of chiropractic is based on a false premise, neither length of study nor accreditation of its schools can ensure the competence of its practitioners.

Despite their shortcomings, chiropractors are licensed to practice in all fifty states, and most of their schools are now accredited. Their services are partially included under Medicare and covered in most states by private insurance carriers, Blue Shield plans, worker's compensation plans, and Medicaid.

In 1976 five chiropractors filed the first of six antitrust suits charging that the American Medical Association, other professional organizations, and several individual critics had conspired to destroy chiropractic and to illegally deprive chiropractors of access to laboratory, x-ray, and hospital facilities. At various times, most of the defendant groups agreed in out-of-court settlements that their physician members were free to decide for themselves how to deal with chiropractors. In 1987 a federal court judge ruled that even though the AMA's efforts to contain chiropractic were intended to protect the public interest (see reference below), the AMA had engaged in an illegal boycott from 1966 until June 1980, when its principles of medical ethics were revised. The judge issued a permanent injunction forbidding the AMA from restricting, regulating, or impeding the freedom of any AMA member or any institution or hospital to make an individual decision about whether they shall associate with chiropractors, chiropractic students, or chiropractic institutions. This was not an endorsement of chiropractic but was decided on narrow legal grounds. The judge's ruling does not limit the AMA's right to take positions on any issue, including chiropractic, or to express these positions.

Recent research reports that spinal manipulation may be effective for the treatment of low back pain have focused considerable attention on chiropractors. It is important to realize, however, that the terms "chiropractic," and "chiropractic treatment" are ambiguous and are not synonymous with "spinal manipulation." Chiropractic is both a philosophy and a treatment approach. Chiropractic treatment varies and may include a wide variety of dubious measures in addition to appropriate or inappropriate manipulation. Critics believe that the potential usefulness of spinal manipulation may not counterbalance the unscientific philosophy or methods commonly embraced by chiropractors.

History of Chiropractic

Homola S: Bonesetting, chiropractic, and cultism.
Panama City, FL, Critique Books, 1963.
The author, a practicing chiropractor, traces the history of chiropractic and its lack of scientific foundation. Concludes that although manipulation can be a valuable form of treatment, chiropractic faces eventual extinction unless it abandons the theory upon which it was developed. States that "there will be no justification for the existence of chiropractic when an adequate number of medical specialists and medical technicians make scientific manipulation available in a department of medical practice."

Cohen W: Independent practitioners under Medicare: A report to Congress.
Washington, DC, U.S. Department of Health, Education and Welfare, 1968.

Comprehensive study by the U.S. Department of Health, Education, and Welfare, which concluded: "Chiropractic theory and practice are not based upon the body of basic knowledge related to health, disease, and health care that has been widely accepted by the scientific community. Moreover, irrespective of its theory, the scope and quality of chiropractic education do not prepare the practitioners to make an adequate diagnosis and provide appropriate treatment."

Smith RL: At your own risk: the case against chiropractic.
New York, Pocket Books, 1969.
A critical look at chiropractic's development and shortcomings. Includes the author's experiences at a chiropractic practice-building seminar and as a "patient" at chiropractic clinics.

Maynard JE: Healing hands: the story of the Palmer family, discoverers and developers of chiropractic.
Mobile, Al, Jonorm Publishers, 1977.
An "authorized" biography which emphasizes the experiences and theories of Daniel David Palmer (the "discoverer") and his son Bartlett Joshua Palmer (the primary developer).

Getzendanner S: Memorandum opinion and order in Wilk et al v. AMA et al. 671 F Supp 1465, U.S. District Court for the Northern District of Illinois, Eastern Division, September 25, 1987.
Ruling in the antitrust suit that chiropractors filed in 1976 with the hope of preventing the American Medical Association and other medical groups from interfering with what chiropractors do. The judge concluded that during the 1960s "there was a lot of material available to the AMA Committee on Quackery that supported its belief that all chiropractic was unscientific and deleterious." She concluded that the dominant reason for the AMA's antichiropractic campaign was the belief that chiropractic was not in the best interests of patients. However, she ruled that this did not justify attempting to contain and eliminate an entire licensed profession without first demonstrating that a less restrictive campaign could not succeed in protecting the public. The judge also noted that chiropractors still take too many x-rays.

Wardwell WI: Chiropractic: History and evolution of a new profession.
St. Louis, Mosby Year Book, 1992.
Provides a detailed history and political analysis of chiropractic from the viewpoint of a sociologist with a lifelong interest in the subject. Predicts that chiropractors "will most likely evolve slowly into a 'limited medical' status comparable to dentists, podiatrists, optometrists, and psychologists."

Critical Literature

*Modde PJ: Malpractice is an inevitable result of
chiropractic philosophy and training.
Legal Aspects of Medical Practice, pp 20–23, February 1979.*
A former chiropractor's view of hazards he believed were integral to the practice of chiropractic. Presents case histories of several patients who were seriously harmed by failure to diagnose their condition.

*Barrett S: The spine salesmen.
In Barrett S (ed.): The health robbers, 2nd edition, pp. 123–145.
Philadelphia, George F Stickley Co., 1980.*
Comprehensive report on the chiropractic marketplace of the 1970s. Describes how "practice-builders" teach chiropractors how to boost their income. Reports what happened when the author sent people to sixteen chiropractors for a check-up. Provides other information to support the author's conclusion that "going to a chiropractor is a distinct gamble."

*Quigley WH: Chiropractic's monocausal theory of disease.
ACA Journal of Chiropractic 18:52–60, June 1981.*
Reports on a survey in which 1,000 members of the American Chiropractic Association were asked to what extent they believed in the "subluxation" theory. Only 37 of 268 respondents (14 percent) said they "do not believe that the chiropractic subluxation is a significant cause of disease." Asked whether "the chiropractic mono-causal theory is scientifically supported," 12 out of 260 (5 percent) said "completely," 195 (75 percent) said "partially," and 53 (20 percent) said "not at all."

*Brown M: Chiro: How much healing? How much flim-flam?
Quad-City Times, Davenport, IA, December 13, 1981 (special report).*
Presents the findings of a newspaper reporter who conducted a five-month investigation during which he had many bizarre experiences visiting about two dozen chiropractors as a "patient." He reported that each chiropractor said he was a "chiropractic case" and that all but one insisted on obtaining x-ray films before treatment. The reporter also attended a chiropractic convention and a practice-building seminar. He concluded that although "chiropractors clearly perform a valuable service," it is a profession "replete with confusion."

*National Council Against Health Fraud: Position paper on chiropractic.
Loma Linda, CA, 1985.*
Describes a long list of unscientific practices common among chiropractors. Acknowledges that manipulative therapy has value in treating back pain, but

concludes that "a health care delivery system as confused and poorly regulated as is chiropractic constitutes a major consumer health problem." Makes detailed recommendations for consumers, insurance carriers, legislators, basic scientists, educators, attorneys, law enforcement agencies, physicians and other scientific health care providers, and reformist chiropractors.

Moran MC et al: Inspection of chiropractic services under Medicare.
Chicago, U.S. Department of Health and Human Services, 1986.
Reports on an investigation conducted by the Office of the U.S. Inspector General. Concluded that "practice-building courses, popular with many chiropractors, advocate advertising techniques which suggest the universal efficacy of chiropractic treatment for every ailment known to humans." Also concluded that despite evidence of an increased emphasis on science and professionalism in the training and practice of chiropractors, "there also exist patterns of activity and practice which at best appear as overly aggressive marketing—and, in some cases, seem deliberately aimed at misleading patients and the public regarding chiropractic care."

Jarvis WT: Chiropractic: A skeptical view.
Skeptical Inquirer 12:47–55, Fall 1987.
States that "spinal manipulation can be useful, but chiropractic's theoretical basis is a strange and never-demonstrated notion of subluxations." Concludes that "chiropractic's survival and success is undoubtedly due to the reality that there is much more involved in health-care delivery than science" and that "chiropractic and other nonscientific forms of health care will survive until the public demands that scientific justification become a primary justification for legalization and reimbursement."

Kusserow RP: State licensure and discipline of chiropractors.
Washington, D.C., U.S. Department of Health and Human Services, January 1989.
Report by the U.S. Inspector General which notes that the rate of disciplinary actions against chiropractors by state medical boards was higher than that for medical doctors. States that "billing abuses (relating to utilization or to fees) and advertising abuses are the two most common types of violations on which disciplinary actions against chiropractors have been based. Discipline of a chiropractor on the basis of clinical insufficiency is extremely rare." Suggests various ways that regulation of chiropractors could become more effective.

Sanders M: Take it from a D.C.: A lot of chiropractic is a sham.
Medical Economics 67:31–39, September 17, 1990.
Presents the views of a chiropractor who has practiced privately, taught at a chiropractic college, and performed utilization reviews for insurance companies.

Describes how chiropractors use x-rays to "find subluxations that the rest of the community can't." States that the emphasis on "subluxations" tends to make chiropractors overlook serious disease. Notes that he has reviewed hundreds of cases in which chiropractors manipulated patients who had no documented complaints or significant clinical findings.

Barrett S: Views of a chiropractic critic: Your real enemy is yourself!
ACA Journal of Chiropractic. 27:61–64, November 1990.
Reports the author's views of unscientific and unethical practices that the author believes are still common among chiropractors. Adapted from a speech he delivered in 1988 to the American Chiropractic Association's House of Delegates.

Chiropractic: Still not recommended.
In Barrett S et al: Health schemes, scams, and frauds, pp. 158–185.
New York, Consumer Reports Books, 1990.
In a lengthy report, Consumers Union concludes that "chiropractic is still a significant hazard to many patients. Current licensing laws lend an aura of legitimacy to unscientific practices and . . . . allow persons with limited qualifications to practice second-rate medicine under another name." The report advises people to avoid chiropractic care but provides guidelines for people who decide to use it.

How to win patients and influence people.
Consumer Reports Health Letter 3:11, 1991.
Describes methods taught by two chiropractic practice-builders. One published a book suggesting hundreds of ways to attract new patients, such as having oneself paged in public places. The other taught how to recruit "research" volunteers and convert them into "lifetime patients," even if they have no symptoms. Reports criticism of these techniques by chiropractic officials.

Barrett S: Don't let chiropractors fool you.
Priorities, pp. 36–38, Spring 1992.
Interprets three recent events that chiropractors have used to promote themselves. Explains that the AMA antitrust ruling was decided on legal grounds rather than the merits of chiropractic. Notes that a study published in the *British Medical Journal* [described below] compared chiropractic and hospital outpatient treatment in patients who underwent careful medical screening, which is not what takes place when patients consult chiropractors in their offices. Notes that the RAND report, which concluded that manipulation may be effective for treating low-back pain, was not an endorsement of chiropractic because very little of the research on which the conclusion was based was done by chiropractors. Also notes the bizarre experiences reported by two investigators who visited many chiropractic offices for "checkups."

Fultz O: Chiropractic: What can it do for you?
American Health 11:41–44, April 1992.
Describes the experience of a reporter who—by coincidence—had visited a chiropractor for a checkup shortly before he was invited to write an article about chiropractic. The reporter was given an eight-page report and told he had six "subluxations" that could wreak havoc on his health unless corrected. The chiropractor advised a series of about fifty visits costing $50 each, followed by "maintenance" visits every one to four weeks. An American Chiropractic Association official who reviewed the reporter's experience said it was one of the worst he had ever encountered, but a leader of the National Association for Chiropractic Medicine (a reformist group) said it was "typical of the way many chiropractors treat patients."

Homola, Samuel. Seeking a common denominator.
in the use of spinal manipulation.
Chiropractic Technique 4:61–63, May 1992.
The author, a leading advocate for chiropractic reform, suggests that chiropractors confine their treatment to musculoskeletal disorders, stop claiming that spinal manipulation is effective in "restoring and maintaining health," and stop performing unnecessary spinal manipulations on healthy, symptom-free patients.

Coletti RE: The manipulators.
Florida Trend 35:32–36, June 1992.
Citing many examples of overutilization, a reporter concludes that "workers' compensation is fraught with abuse, but no other players in the system rile business more than the chiropractors."

Alexander A: Claim-filing advisers tread thin line.
Asbury Park Press 113:A1, A6, October 6, 1992.
Describes how several chiropractic practice-management consultants teach chiropractors how to recruit people for long-term treatment of their "subluxations."

Chiropractors and Nutrition

"Nutrition" against disease: A close look at a chiropractic seminar.
Nutrition Forum 5:25–28, April 1988.
Reports on a seminar sponsored by a company that markets nutritional products to chiropractors. Written by a prominent investigative reporter who gained entrance by pretending to be a chiropractor. Describes a manual distributed at the seminar which lists the company's products for the treatment of epilepsy, heart disease,

diabetes, kidney failure, and more than 100 other health problems. Also described how the seminar's leader offered to help chiropractors engage in "creative billing" of insurance companies. Suggests that such activities deserve more attention from federal regulatory agencies.

Newman CF, Downes NJ, Tseng RY et al: Nutrition-related backgrounds and counseling practices of doctors of chiropractic.
Journal of the American Dietetic Association 89:939–943, 1989.
Reports on a survey of 438 members of the San Francisco Bay Area Chiropractic Society. Of the 100 who responded, 60 percent said that they routinely provide nutrition information to their patients, 38 percent said they provide it on request, 60 percent claimed that they treat patients for nutritional deficiencies, 19 percent said they use hair analysis, and 9 percent indicated that they use "applied kinesiology" for nutritional assessment. [Neither hair analysis nor applied kinesiology are valid for nutritional assessment of patients.]

Barrett S: Chiropractors and nutrition: The supplement underground.
Nutrition Forum 9:25–28, July/August 1992.
Describes how many companies market "dietary supplement" products to chiropractors with therapeutic claims that would be illegal on product labels. States that although use of these products poses considerable danger to consumers, government enforcement agencies have been reluctant to explore it. Sidebar on page 28 contains an interview with the chairman of the American Chiropractic Association's Council on Nutrition.

Studies of Spinal Manipulation

Crelin E: A scientific test of the chiropractic theory.
American Scientist 61:574–580, 1973.
D.D. Palmer's "subluxation" theory was tested by a prominent anatomist who collected the spines of six people within 3 to 6 hours after their death. Using instruments to twist their spines, he observed the spinal nerves and the opening through which they passed. No nerve compression took place regardless of the force applied.

Goldstein M (ed): The research status of spinal manipulative therapy, monograph 15, 1975.
National Institute of Neurological and Communicative Disorders and Stroke.
Proceedings of an interdisciplinary workshop attended by physicians, chiropractors, physiologists, and others interested in manipulative therapy. Many participants felt

that manipulative therapy was valuable for treating back pain, but no evidence was presented that manipulation was useful for treating disorders of internal organs. Participants noted that precise definitions of the terms such as "subluxation" would be necessary for meaningful research to take place.

Meade TW et al: Low back pain of mechanical origin: Randomised comparison of chiropractic and hospital outpatient treatment.
British Medical Journal 300:1431–1437, 1990.
Reports on a study of 741 patients between the ages of 18 and 65 who lacked signs of spinal nerve root compression, infectious disease, or other conditions that required medical intervention. Found that chiropractic treatment spanned up to 30 weeks (vs. 12 weeks for hospital-based treatment) and cost about 50 percent more. The outcome was measured by a self-administered questionnaire about pain intensity, not a clinical evaluation. Patients with no prior history of back pain showed no difference in outcomes. Among patients with such a history, those in the chiropractic treatment group scored significantly better than those in the hospital-based group at 6-, 12-, and 24-month follow-up intervals. Report concludes that "For patients with low back pain in whom manipulation is not contraindicated, chiropractic almost certainly confers worthwhile, long-term benefit in comparison with hospital outpatient management . . . . mainly in those with chronic or severe pain."

Smidt GL: Research study analysis.
Journal of Orthopaedic and Sports Physical Therapy 13:288–291, 1991.
[Additional commentaries pp. 292–299]
Points out serious methodological shortcomings in the British Medical Journal study of manipulation for back pain. Followed by commentaries from an orthopedist and three physical therapists.

Assendelft WJJ, Bouter LM, Kessels AGH: Effectiveness of chiropractic and physiotherapy in the treatment of low back pain: A critical discussion of the British randomized clinical trial.
Journal of Manipulative and Physiological Therapeutics 14:281–286, 1991.
Describes methodological defects in the British Medical Journal study and concludes that "it is premature to draw conclusions about the long-term effectiveness of chiropractic based on this study alone."

Does anything work for back pain? Physicians don't have the answer. Do chiropractors?
Consumer Reports on Health 4:9–11, 1992.
Provides guidelines for self-care of back pain but indicates when immediate medical

attention is warranted. Describes various medical measures, but provides guidelines for people considering spinal manipulation. States that if manipulation is going to work, it generally begins to work quickly—so if manipulation does not help after a few weeks, another approach should be tried. States that there is no convincing evidence of any benefit from a prolonged program of "maintenance" manipulations after the patient's pain has disappeared.

Shekelle PG et al: The appropriateness of spinal manipulation for low-back pain. Part I: Project overview and literature review. Santa Monica, Calif., 1991, RAND.
An interdisciplinary panel that reviewed 67 articles and 9 books published between 1955 and 1989 concluded that data from 22 controlled studies support the use of manipulation for acute low-back pain in patients showing no signs of lower-limb nerve root involvement. Most of the studies were performed by physicians (not chiropractors). The panelists also noted: (1) it is not clear how many, if any, manipulations are necessary after a patient has become pain-free; and (2) there has been no systematic study of the frequency of complications from spinal manipulation for low-back pain. Although the risk appears small when compared to the large number of manipulations performed, no firm conclusions may be drawn because there are few data in the scientific literature.

Assendelft WJJ, Koes BW, Van Der Heijden GJMG, et al: The efficacy of chiropractic manipulation for back pain: Blinded review of relevant randomized clinical trials. Journal of Manipulative and Physiological Therapeutics 15:487–494, 1992.
Notes how the authors located five randomized trials of spinal manipulation (RCTs) performed by chiropractors and published in medical or chiropractic literature between 1966 and 1990. Reports that blinded evaluation of the studies' methodology yielded scores ranging from 20 to 48 out of a possible 100. Concludes: "Although the small number of chiropractic RCTs and the poor general methodological quality preclude the drawing of strong conclusions, chiropractic seems to be an effective treatment of back pain. However, studies with better methodology are clearly needed.... In addition, more effort should be made to establish long-term follow-up."

Proponent Literature

Palmer DD: Text-Book of the science, art, and philosophy of chiropractic. Portland, OR, Portland Printing House, 1910.
Comprehensive report of the theories and experiences of chiropractic's founder.

Wilk CA: Chiropractic speaks out: a reply to medical propaganda, bigotry and ignorance.
Park Ridge, IL, Wilk Publishing Co., 1973.
Written by the chiropractor who later became the lead plaintiff in the antitrust suit against the American Medical Association and other medical organizations. States that it was "written to show that organized medicine is placing a vicious and cruel restraint upon the public by dissuading many people from chiropractic care." Provides the author's viewpoint about the development, advantages, and recognition of chiropractic and the "confusion" he believed was involved in antichiropractic views. States that health care "cannot be the finest unless chiropractic is placed into proper perspective within the healing arts."

Sportelli L: Introduction to chiropractic, 9th edition.
Palmerton, PA, 1989.
A prominent chiropractor's view of what chiropractic offers patients. States that "regular spinal adjustments are a part of your body's defense against illness."

Haldeman S (ed): Principles and practice of chiropractic.
New York, Appleton & Lange, 1992.
Describes the history, philosophy, and modern clinical practice of chiropractic from the viewpoint of leading chiropractic educators.

A study of chiropractic worldwide. Facts Bulletin Vol. 4, 1992.
Arlington, VA, Foundation for the Advancement of
Chiropractic Tenets and Science, 1992.
A compendium of facts and figures about chiropractic's legal status and educational institutions.

Sweere JJ (ed.) et al: Chiropractic family practice: A clinical manual.
Gaithersburg, MD, Aspen Publishers, Inc., 1992.
A comprehensive reference book covering many aspects of clinical practice plus a few sections on chiropractic history and other nonclinical topics. Includes discussions of "chiropractic cardiology" and the role of acupuncture, Chinese medicine, "nutritional therapy," and applied kinesiology ("strictly provisional") as adjuncts to chiropractic care. Chapter on chiropractic care in hospitals states that "undeniably, chiropractic belongs everywhere there is any disease, and especially where the sickest patients are being housed and are in need of all the clinical help they can obtain. . . . Health care in the hospital is too important to be left to any one profession."

Christian Science

Christian Science is a religious denomination founded in 1866 by Mary Baker Eddy. She was a patient and follower of a "magnetic-healer," Phineas Parkhurst Quimby, who promoted a number of mind-cure approaches in the latter part of the nineteenth century. Later, following a serious accident, she allegedly was healed after reading one of the New Testament healing miracles. She devoted the rest of her life to spreading the doctrines of Christian Science, which may have been influenced considerably by Quimby's ideas.

Devout Christian Scientists reject scientific medicine in favor of Christian Science practitioners who utilize spiritual healing. They contend that illness is an illusion caused by faulty beliefs, and that prayer heals by replacing bad thoughts with good ones. Christian Science practitioners try to argue the sick thoughts out of the person's mind. Consultations can take place in person, by telephone, or even by mail. Individuals may also be able to attain correct beliefs by themselves through prayer or mental concentration. "You can Heal," a pamphlet of the Christian Science Publishing Society, states that "every student of Christian Science has the God-given ability to heal the sick." Two weeks of class instruction are required to become a practitioner.

The weekly magazine *Christian Science Sentinel* publishes several "testimonies" in each issue. To be considered for publication, an account must be "verified" by three individuals who "can vouch for the integrity of the testifier or know of the healing." During the past two years, believers have claimed that prayer has brought about recovery from anemia, arthritis, blood poisoning, corns, deafness, defective speech, multiple sclerosis, skin rashes, total body paralysis, visual difficulties, and various injuries. Most of these accounts contain few details, and many of the diagnoses were made without medical consultation.

Christian Science appears to be on the decline. Between January 1976 and February 1991, the number of churches listed in *The Christian Science Journal* decreased from 1,780 to 1,450, and the number of practitioners dropped from 4,302 to 2,237.

Critical Literature

Swan R: Faith healing, Christian Science, and the medical care of children. New England Journal of Medicine 309: 1639-1641, 1983.

Gives a brief history of the Christian Science church's efforts to secure recognition of its practitioners as healers on the same basis as medical doctors. Describes the church's efforts to secure passage of religious exemption laws to protect members from charges of child neglect. Reviews state laws impacting on Christian Science. Describes how the church pressures its members to shun medical care. Warns that "neither parents nor their counselors should be allowed to deny children medical care in the name of religion."

Larrabee J, Johnson P: States take on power of prayer.
USA Today, pp. 1, 2A, May 2, 1988.
Reviews the case of two Christian Science couples who lost children to treatable diseases after relying on Christian Science practitioners for healing. Discusses the debate over whether Christian Science parents should be allowed to have their children treated by Christian Science spiritual healers.

Novotny T, Jennings, CE, Doran M, March C, et al: Measles outbreaks in religious groups exempt from immunization laws.
Public Health Reports 103:49-54, January-February, 1988.
Discusses efforts by public health officials to control outbreaks of measles at a Christian Science college and a Christian Science camp. Describes quarantine procedures utilized to contain the outbreaks. Notes reluctance of Christian Scientists and some other denominations to accept immunization and conventional medical care, and advises public health officials to attempt to establish working relationships with leaders of churches and other facilities affiliated with these groups.

Oppenheim EB: Summary judgment.
Western Journal of Medicine 151: p. 681, 1989
Describes a physician's encounter with a patient who is a Christian Scientist. The patient had a growth on her nose that probably was cancerous. The anecdote brings out the clash between the beliefs of Christian Science and scientific medicine.

Simpson WF: Comparative longevity in a college cohort of Christian Scientists.
JAMA 262: 1657-1658, 1989.
Compares longevity of alumni of Principia College, a Christian Science college at Elsah, Illinois, with alumni of the University of Kansas in Lawrence, Kansas. Concludes that Principia College alumni had a higher death rate than those who had attended the university even though Christian Scientists are forbidden to use tobacco or alcoholic beverages.

Dolnick E: Murder by faith.
In Health 4:58–65, January/February 1990.

Provides a vivid picture of the trial of two Christian Science parents following the death of their daughter from medically untreated diabetes.

Swan R, Nartonis DK, Simpson WF [Letters to the editor]: Comparative longevity of Christian Scientists.
JAMA 263:1634, 1990.
In correspondence about the previous article, Dr. Swan notes that it refuted claims that the Christian Science Church had data showing that its methods are twice as effective as medical science at healing children. Dr. Nartonis, a church official, claimed that Dr. Simpson's interpretations of the his data were incorrect. Dr. Simpson indicated why Dr. Nartonis was incorrect.

Brahams D: Medicine and the law, religious beliefs and parental duty.
Lancet 336:107-108, July 14, 1990.
Discusses the case of David and Ginger Twitchell, a Christian Science couple from Boston, who were convicted of involuntary manslaughter and reckless disregard for their child's health. The couple relied on prayer and did not call a physician to care for their young son who died of a treatable bowel obstruction. Reviews interpretations of the laws of Massachusetts and the United Kingdom regarding religious exemptions on spiritual healing.

Margolick D: In child deaths, a test for Christian Science.
The New York Times, pp. 1A, 11A, August 6, 1990.
Notes the criminal conviction of Christian Science parents whose 2-year-old boy died from medically untreated bowel obstruction. Describes five other cases in which criminal prosecutions followed the death of a child from meningitis, cancer, or diabetes. Outlines the pertinent legal doctrines and the arguments made by prosecutors and Church representatives.

Skolnick A: Christian scientists claim healing efficacy equal if not superior to that of medicine.
JAMA 264:1379-1381, 1990.
Notes current efforts by the Christian Science church to secure religious exemption legislation to protect church members from prosecution for failure to obtain medical care to treat their sick children, and legislation to recognize Christian Science healing as equal to conventional medical care. Describes qualifications of Christian Science practitioners and standards of care in Christian Science nursing homes. Reviews claims of Christian Science healers, noting refusals to back up claims or reveal the identity of "doctors who allegedly write in to substantiate remarkable healing claims." Notes that Christian Scientists consider medical treatment to be sinful; hence, many would rather die than submit to it.

*Swan R: The law's response when religious beliefs
against medical care impact on children.
Sioux City, IA, CHILD, Inc., 1990.*
Describes how Christian Science practitioners and other faith healers won religious exemptions from medical licensing requirements, provided they conduct themselves in certain ways. Describes the legal basis for religious immunity from parental requirements to provide immunization and general medical care, which exist in almost all states. States that the prospects for changing this situation are poor.

*Skolnick A: Religious exemptions to child neglect laws still
being passed despite convictions of parents.
JAMA 264:1226, 1229, 1233, 1990.*
Reviews efforts by the Christian Science church to secure religious exemptions to child neglect laws and to assist parents being prosecuted for failure to seek medical treatment for their children. Notes discrepancies in the church's instructions regarding medical care in the United States, Great Britain, and Canada.

*1990 American Medical Association Policy Compendium, p. 45, 1990.
Chicago, American Medical Association, 1990.*
Reports the American Medical Association's position on the repeal of religious exemptions in child abuse and medical practice statutes. Reaffirms existing policy articulated in the American Medical Association Board of Trustees Report JJ (I-86) supporting repeal of the religious exemption from state child abuse statutes. Recognizes that constitutional barriers may exist with regard to elimination of the religious exemption from state medical practice acts. Encourages state medical associations that are aware of problems with respect to spiritual healing practitioners in their areas to investigate such situations and pursue all solutions, including legislation where appropriate, to address such matters.

*Gevitz, Norman. Christian Science healing and the health care of children.
Perspectives in Biology and Medicine 34:421-438, 1991.*
Explores the history of Christian Science and its doctrines regarding medical care. Discusses the denomination's success in gaining insurance coverage for its practitioners and religious exemptions from laws on child neglect. Describes efforts by critics to eliminate such exemptions and to prosecute parents who fail to provide medical care for their children. Notes the church's erosion of membership as younger members fail to retain the beliefs of their parents.

*Simpson W: Comparative mortality of two college groups, 1945–1983.
Mortality and Morbidity Weekly Report 40:579–582, 1991.*
Compares longevity of alumni of Principia College, a Christian Science college at

Elsah, Illinois, with alumni of Loma Linda University, which has a predominantly Seventh-day Adventist student population. Concludes that Principia College alumni had a much higher death rate than those who had attended the university. Both religious groups proscribe alcohol and tobacco; the Seventh-day Adventists also tend to eat little or no meat.

Kase LM: Swan's way: One woman's crusade against spiritual healing.
American Health 11:16, 18–19, July/August 1992.
Relates the story of Rita Swan, whose 16-month-old son died of meningitis under the care of two Christian Science practitioners in 1977. Describes how she left the church and founded CHILD, Inc., an organization working for legal reforms to protect children from inappropriate treatment by faith healers. States that since 1982 there have been 25 convictions of parents who let their child die as a result of rigid religious dogma.

Proponent Literature

Talbot NA: The position of the Christian Science Church.
New England Journal of Medicine 309: 1641-1644, 1983.
Describes the Christian Science view of healing. Claims that Christian Scientists "would not have relied on Christian Science for healing . . . if this healing were only a myth." Discusses testimonials obtained over the years attesting to healing by Christian Science practitioners. Notes recognition of Christian Science practitioners by health insurance companies. Reviews Christian Science doctrines regarding the use of prayer versus medical treatment.

Committee on Publication: An empirical analysis of medical evidence in Christian Science testimonies of healing 1969-1988.
Boston, The First Church of Christ Scientist, April 1989.
Claims that Christian Scientists do not denigrate medical care or those who choose it, but see its "intense focus on the body . . . as often reinforcing disease." Claims that since 1900, some 53,900 testimonies of healing have been published in the denomination's periodicals. Admits that such testimonies are "manifestly religious rather than medical documents," but claims that many of the conditions were "authoritatively diagnosed."

Faith Healing

The notion that prayer, divine intervention, or the ministrations of an individual healer can cure illness has been popular throughout history. Miraculous recoveries have been attributed to a myriad of techniques commonly lumped together as "faith healing." Although many people believe that faith healing is effective against organic disease, there is no scientific evidence to support this belief. Faith in a healer may lead to a lessening of psychosomatic symptoms, but the potential value of this must be weighed against several risks: (1) not being helped can make people depressed, (2) using a healer instead of effective medical care can be disastrous, and (3) substantial sums of money can be lost.

Physicians find no fault with patients who turn to religion as a means of moral and mental support while continuing with effective medical care. However, most physicians do not approve of the activities of self-proclaimed faith healers or state laws protecting parents who fail to secure medical attention for their children, especially in cases of serious illness or injury. This latter subject is discussed further in the section on Christian Science.

Critical Literature

Rose L: Faith healing.
Baltimore, 1971, Penguin Books.
Describes how the author, a British psychiatrist, investigated hundreds of alleged faith-healing cures by communicating with healers and patients throughout the world. He sent each correspondent a questionnaire and sought corroborating information from physicians. After nearly twenty years, he concluded "I have yet to find one 'miracle cure'; and without that (or, alternatively, massive statistics which others must provide) I cannot be convinced of the efficacy of what is commonly termed faith healing."

Nolen W: Healing—A doctor in search of a miracle.
New York, 1974, Random House.
Describes how the author, who considered himself a religious man, spent two years tracking down individuals who had sought the services of Kathryn Kuhlman, Norbu Chen, and Philippino "psychic surgeons." Reports that he was unable to find a single person who had been cured of an organic disease. Concludes that healers sometimes provide compassion or relieve a person's symptoms, but that reliance on a healer for the treatment of organic disease can have tragic results.

*Sholes J: Give me that prime-time religion: An insider's
report on the Oral Roberts Evangelistic Association.*
New York, Hawthorn Books, 1979.
Exposes the ways in which the author believes that Oral Roberts and his organization mislead and exploit people.

Kinsolving L: The miracle merchants.
In Barrett S (ed.): The health robbers, 2nd edition, pp. 220–230.
Philadelphia, George F. Stickley Co., 1980.
Describes the activities of Oral Roberts, Kathryn Kuhlman, Reverend Ike, and Christian Science. States that faith healers don't know their limitations and rarely try to distinguish between people they may be able to help and those that are beyond their ability. Notes that many people with serious disease have died as a result of abandoning effective medical care after being "healed." Notes that when "healing" fails, people may feel depressed and unworthy. Also notes that money spent for a fruitless experience is another negative factor.

Bernstein E: Lourdes.
In 1982 Medical and Health Annual, pp. 129–147.
Chicago, Encyclopedia Britannica, 1982.
Examines the history of the shrine at Lourdes and the way that alleged "miracles" have been evaluated. Describes how independent specialists reviewed an alleged cure of organic hemiplegia and concluded that the diagnosis had been wrong. Notes that as medical knowledge grew, "miraculous cures" waned. Concludes that Lourdes is not a miracle mill but still might provide spiritual benefit to its visitors.

Brand P, Yancey P: A surgeon's view of divine healing.
Christianity Today, pp. 14–21, November 25, 1983.
Presents the views of a Christian physician who says he shares the same goals as the faith healers on television but differs enormously in his technique and style. Critiques current faith-healing beliefs and practices that are widespread within the fundamentalist Christian community. Questions the extreme faith-healing perspective and cites medical claims that are both dubious and dangerous. Describes needless deaths and unsuccessful attempts to raise the dead. Discusses the power of the mind to control pain, relieve symptoms, work thorough suggestion, produce conversion disorders, and deal effectively with stress. Also covers the negative psychological effects of healing failures. States that faith can help a chronic disease sufferer cope with life (heal the spirit), which is blessing enough.

Frame R: Indiana grand jury indicts a faith-healing preacher.
Christianity Today 28:38–39, November 23, 1984.

News report on the indictment of fundamentalist Christian preacher Hobart Freeman and two members of his sect on charges stemming from the death of a child due to failure to receive medical care. Notes that other members of the group had already been convicted of similar charges due to the death of children. Describes the career and teachings of Freeman, who rejected all medical care, immunization, insurance, and even safety measures such as the use of seat belts.

Spence C, Danielson TS: The Faith Assembly, a follow-up study of faith healing and mortality.
Indiana Medicine 86:238–240, 1987.
Notes that between 1975 and 1982 the infant and childbirth-related death rates for members of the Faith Assembly were much higher than those of the general population. Notes that since the death of the sect's founder (due to a treatable disease), members have softened their views on medical treatment and lowered their infant and maternal death rates.

Pankratz L: Magician accuses faith healers of hoax.
Journal of Religion and Health 26:115–124, Summer, 1987.
Describes activities of magicians, psychics, spiritualists, and faith healers. Notes the difference between deceiving people for entertainment and exploiting them for personal gain. Focuses on anti-fraud efforts of Harry Houdini and James Randi.

Tierney J: Fleecing the flock.
Discover 18:50–58, November 1987.
Describes how faith healer Peter Popoff used trickery to persuade people that he received messages about them from God when the information actually was broadcast from Popoff's wife offstage to a receiver in his ear. Describes how this technique was exposed by magician James Randi, who had recorded the broadcast messages and played them on "The Tonight Show." Notes, however, that some people are so eager to believe in faith healing that they find ways to rationalize away evidence of deception.

American Academy of Pediatrics, Committee on Bioethics: Religious exemptions from child abuse statutes.
Pediatrics 81:169–171, 1988.
Position paper cites examples and notes that children sometimes die or become disabled due to the failure to receive medical treatment because of religious beliefs of their parents. Explores the conflict between religious liberty and parental freedom versus the rights of children to be safe from harm. Notes that some groups have secured passage of state laws allowing religious exemptions that protect parents from prosecution under laws against child abuse when they fail to seek medical

attention for their children. Argues for repeal of such laws and urges members of the organization to work for repeal.

Randi J: The healing touch: Gift or gimmick?
In 1988 Medical and Health Annual, pp. 151–161.
Chicago, Encyclopedia Britannica, 1988.
States that although the author has diligently sought evidence of any genuine healing by faith, he has not been provided with a single example. Explains the trickery involved in "calling out" members of their audience and having "healed" individuals rise and walk away from wheelchairs (in which the healers' staff placed them before the performance). States that the risks of being exploited by the healer are greater than the likelihood of temporary symptom reduction due to a placebo effect.

Barnhart J: Faith healers in a naturalistic context.
The Humanist 48:5–7, 36, September/October 1988.
Describes methods of W.V. Grant, noting how some people attending his services participate in deception by behaving as though they have been healed. Explores the evolution of the beliefs of Calvinists and Pentecostals regarding the role of God and of evil in the world. Discusses "positive reinforcement" which the newer faith healing communities offer their followers.

Alexander D: A closer look at today's faith healers.
The Humanist 48:8–12, 38, September/October 1988.
Examines the theory and methods of faith healers, particularly traveling and television preachers. Focuses on the activities of Charles and Frances Hunter, a husband-and-wife team of traveling evangelists who hold healing services at which they collect large sums of money. Describes training sessions they hold for healers, which feature a combination of diet fads, chiropractic theory, and instructions in various prayers and incantations. States that fundraising methods, financial accountability, and supernatural healing claims of faith healers deserve close investigation. Speculates that if faith healers were required to disclose how their money is spent, the public might become disillusioned.

King DE, Sobal J, DeForge BR: Family practice patients'
experiences and beliefs in faith healing.
Journal of Family Practice 27:505–508, 1988.
Describes a survey of patients attending a rural North Carolina clinic. Reports on their attitudes toward faith healing and the extent of their participation in faith-healing activities. Notes that 58 percent did not believe in faith healing, but 29 percent felt it could help when physicians could not. States that the higher the person's level of education, the less likely the person was to accept faith healing.

Suggests that physicians consider what role faith may have in their patients' treatment.

Emery CE: Are they really cured?
Providence Sunday Journal Magazine, January 15, 1989.
Describes how the author attended one of Father DiOrio's services and recorded the names of nine people who had been blessed during the service and nine others who had been proclaimed cured. DiOrio's organization offered ten more cases that supposedly provided irrefutable proof of the priest's ability to cure. During a six-month investigation, the author found no evidence that any of these 28 individuals had been helped.

Randi J: The faith healers.
Buffalo, Prometheus Books, 1989.
Describes criteria by which the effectiveness of faith healing should be judged: (1) the ailment must be one that normally doesn't recover without treatment, (2) there must not have been any medical treatment that would be expected to influence the ailment, and (3) both diagnosis and recovery must be demonstrable by detailed medical evidence. Describes the author's extensive efforts to locate cases that can meet these criteria and his extensive efforts to expose the frauds perpetrated by evangelistic healers. Concludes that faith healing cannot influence the outcome of organic disease and does far more psychological harm than good. Urges the Internal Revenue Service and law enforcement authorities to pay more attention to evangelistic healers who accrue large sums of money.

Brenneman RJ: Deadly blessings: Faith healing on trial.
Buffalo, NY, Prometheus Books, 1990.
Describes the criminal prosecutions of three practitioners of "alternative healing": a Christian Scientist, a psychic surgeon, and a "New Age" psychotherapist who used LSD and other psychedelic drugs. Examines why people choose such treatment, whether the state should intervene, the tragedies that can arise from misplaced belief, and the law's response to such tragedies.

Barrett S: Faith healing.
Priorities, pp. 32–34, Spring 1990.
Describes some of the experiences and observations of Dr. Louis Rose, Dr. William Nolen, James Randi, and reporter Eugene Emery, Jr., each of whom conducted follow-up investigations of people purported to be healed. Describes how the author observed W.V. Grant "lengthen" the leg of a confederate to cure his "limp" and how the author saw Grant push an elderly woman off her feet to create the illusion that she had been "slain in the spirit." Describes the author's survey of Christian Science

testimonials and the basis on which they were "verified." Expresses hope that more reporters will do follow-up studies of people claimed to have been "healed."

Witmer J, Zimmerman M: Intercessory prayer as medical treatment? An inquiry. Skeptical Inquirer 15:177–180, Winter 1991.
Reports that a thorough search of the scientific literature found only three controlled examinations of the effects of prayer by third parties on people who were unaware of the prayers. Of these, one (described below) claimed benefit but was poorly designed, while the others found no benefit and were well designed. Surprised by the small number of published studies, the authors asked 38 journal editors whether they had ever received but rejected a manuscript on the subject of intercessory prayer. They also asked the editors to ask their readers whether they knew of any such study, published or unpublished. No editor or reader responded affirmatively.

King DE, Sobal J, Haggerty Jesse III, et al: Experiences and attitudes about faith healing among family physicians. Journal of Family Practice 35:158–162, 1992.
Tabulates the responses from 594 physicians in seven states who were polled by mail. About half said they were aware of at least one patient in their practice who had had a faith-healing experience. Fifty-five percent agreed and 20 percent disagreed that reliance on faith healers often leads to serious medical problems. Thirty-nine percent said that faith healers are "quacks." However, 44 percent thought that physicians and faith healers can work together to cure some patients, and 23 percent believed that faith healers divinely heal some people whom physicians cannot help.

Proponent Literature

Byrd RC: Positive therapeutic effects of intercessory prayer in a coronary care unit population. Southern Medical Journal 81:826–829, 1988.
Reports on a double-blind study of patients admitted to the coronary care unit at a San Francisco Hospital to determine the effects of prayer by others on the outcome of hospitalization. Concludes that the results show benefit for those in the prayer group. [Note: The above report by Witmer and Zimmerman states that the method of tabulating results was statistically flawed and that the protocol was not double-blind. The biggest problem was that complications that were interrelated were scored separately and therefore given too much weight. The average length of hospital stay, which was not subject to this type of scoring error, was identical for the treatment and control groups.]

Folk (Traditional) Medicine

Webster's New Collegiate Dictionary defines folk medicine as "traditional medicine as practiced nonprofessionally by people isolated from modern medical services and involving especially the use of vegetable remedies on an empirical basis." Folk medicine, even when known to be erroneous, is not generally considered to be quackery so long as it is not done for gain. Thus self-treatment, family home treatment, neighborly medical advice, and the noncommercial activities of folk healers should not be labeled as such.

Folk medicine and quackery are closely connected because folk medicine often provides a basis for commercial exploitation. For example, herbs long gathered for personal use have been packaged and promoted by modern entrepreneurs, and practitioners who once served their neighbors voluntarily or for gratuities may market themselves outside their traditional communities.

Shamans and Indian medicine men have become popular among New Age devotees and advertise in slick New Age publications. The notorious "psychic surgeons" of the Philippines and Brazil are marketed as traditional healers who possess special, mystical powers. Traditional medicine is largely primitive medicine, which assumes that supernatural forces are responsible for both the cause and cure of disease. Even herbal remedies may be said to harbor either good or evil spirits, so that believers can explain failures or successes in supernatural terms.

Some articles in this section offer insight into the reasons why people engage in folk practices. Some articles note the importance of recognizing when a folk belief may interfere with the ability or willingness of a patient to cooperate with or respond to scientific treatment. Other articles illustrate how folk medicine is related to quackery and how folk practices can be dangerous.

Descriptive Literature

Hand WD: American folk medicine.
Berkeley, University of California Press, 1976.
A collection of twenty-six papers presented at the 1973 UCLA Conference of American Folk Medicine. Covers history of folk medicine and miscellaneous practices among a number of cultural groups including American Indians, Spanish Americans, French Canadians, Pennsylvania Germans, Amish, Black Americans, Utah Mormons, Jamaicans, and inhabitants of southwest Texas.

Finkler K: The nonsharing of medical knowledge among spiritualist healers and their patients: A contribution to the study of intra-cultural diversity and practitioner-patients relationship.
Medical Anthropology 8:195–209, Summer 1984.
Questions the homogeneity of even simple primitive societies and explores diversity and individuality. Notes that healers and patients don't always share etiologic explanations, but agreement is not essential for compliance. States that some spiritualist healers are dualists with a view that corresponds more closely to Cartesian mind/body dichotomy than to traditional holistic concepts.

Buckman R: Catfish man of the woods: Alternative medicine, Appalachian style.
Canadian Medical Association Journal 142:1298–1303, 1990.
Describes a visit by a film crew to interview a West Virginia folk healer whose "office" was a shack in the woods. Described how he examined two women (with "an immense amount of groping" in the chest region), said they had kidney disease, and prescribed herbs for them.

Avery C: Native American medicine: Traditional healing.
JAMA 265:2271, 2273, 1991.
Notes that traditional Native American medicine is in widespread use. Discusses the theory behind healing rituals, noting the close relationship between religion and medicine among Native Americans. Describes some of the rituals and other methods of Native American medicine. Urges physicians to use an integrated approach to practice among Native Americans, combining aspects of traditional and western medicine.

Chee VE: Medicine men.
JAMA 265:2276, 1991.
Describes how an elderly Navajo woman with a shoulder dislocation had her first medical experience at a clinic. After the shoulder was replaced, she was "treated" by the tribal medicine man who administered herbs and conducted an hour-long ceremony.

Tauber AI: On pigeons, physicians and placebos.
Journal of the Royal Society of Medicine 84:328–331, 1991.
Discusses the popularity of various forms of folk medicine, even in a city like Boston. Mentions a range of specific folk remedies and describes several. Discusses the issue of patient acceptance of physician advice. Notes that folk remedies sometimes produce a placebo effect, but argues against using unproven methods even for the placebo effect since this would be a sham.

Folk Medicine and Quackery

Smith, NL: Why are Mormons so susceptible to medical & nutritional quackery?
Journal Collegium Aesculapium, pp. 1–15, December 1983.
Describes how the Mormon Word of Wisdom and other early Mormon teachings are exploited by purveyors of cancer quackery, herbalism, nutritional faddism, iridology and so forth. States that quacks have mastered the art of medicine—the ability to engender trust, hope and faith—but disdain the science of medicine as man-made. Cites harm caused by unscientific medicine and reveals that the Mormon Church officially disclaims health fads allegedly justified by Church documents.

Young JH: Folk into fake.
Western Folklore, 44:225–239, 1985.
Notes that folk medicine has served as a key source of commercialized proprietary medicines. Notes that throughout history, many outright quacks have perverted traditional remedies. States that folk medicine, patent medicine, and scientific medicine have all been open-ended evolving systems that, at any given time, have included some therapeutic practices that are centuries old and others of recent origin.. States that all have practices that become obsolete over time, and each influences the others. Points out that scientific medicine discards inferior therapies as science advances, but folk medicine and quackery continues to use these as long as a demand persists. Shows how the success of popular remedies, such as Lydia E. Pinkham's Vegetable Compound and Hadacol, illustrate these points.

Corchado A: Folk healers stay popular with poor in rural Southwest.
The Wall Street Journal, p. 1, January 4, 1989.
Notes the wide popularity of curanderos among the poor, especially more recent immigrants from Mexico. Describes some folk medicines and rituals. Notes that state laws against practicing medicine without a license are rarely enforced against folk healers.

Potential Harm

Poma PA: A dangerous folk therapy.
Journal of the National Medical Association 76:387–389, 1984.
Focuses on the use of azarcón or greta, lead-based folk remedies to treat "empacho," a gastrointestinal syndrome common among Hispanic populations. Urges additional screening of children to detect lead poisoning, especially migrant children.

*Boyd EL, Shimp LA, Hackney MJ: Home remedies and the
black elderly—a reference manual for health care providers.
Ann Arbor, University of Michigan, 1984.*
Discusses trends in usage and the detrimental effects of folk remedies. Provides a compendium of home remedy information for professional reference. Includes ingredients and the known uses of substances listed.

*Ripley GD: Mexican-American folk remedies: their place in health care.
Texas Medicine 82:41–44, November 1986.*
Reviews theories behind Mexican-American folk medicine, noting the strong influence of Spanish-Moorish medicine at the time of the conquest of Mexico by the Spaniards. Notes the reliance on religion to some extent. Discusses the case of a Mexican-American woman who was given conventional treatment for diabetes, but who also turned to a popular folk medicine for her diabetes. Mentions reports of lead poisoning and other serious illnesses resulting from folk treatment. Lists illnesses for which lead-based household remedies are prescribed. Urges physicians to learn how culture-related beliefs and practices can affect treatment outcome.

*Adams, WR: Economic factors influencing the use of folk remedies.
Texas Medicine 82:32–33, December 1986.*
Replies to the above article, noting that many patients continue to use folk remedies because they are less expensive. Discusses the relationship of the extended family to the healing process among Mexican-Americans. Notes that the family attempts to reduce expenses as long as the patient is ill, and thus dilutes Western-style medicines or uses folk medicines instead.

*Marsh WW, Hentges K: Mexican folk remedies and conventional medical care.
American Family Physician 37:257–262, March 1988.*
Describes a survey which found that half of the Hispanic families in West Texas used folk medicine. Lists common folk illnesses and their alleged causes and symptoms. Notes potential hazards of some folk remedies, but states that compliance with scientific treatment may be enhanced by incorporating a family's harmless folk practices into the medical plan. Advises doctors to ask patients why they think they became ill and what they have done to treat the problem.

*Cone LA, Boughton WH, Cone LA, et al: Rattlesnake capsule-induced
Salmonella arizonae bacteremia.
Western Journal of Medicine 153:315–316, 1990.*
Reports on two cases of *Salmonella arizonae* caused by ingestion of folk remedies contaminated by the organism. Discusses the use of rattlesnake meat or powder in

Mexican folk medicine to treat cancer, diabetes, and other diseases and ailments. Notes that others have reported three cases of this infection in patients with AIDS.

De Smet PAGM: Is there any danger in using traditional remedies? Journal of Ethnopharmacology 32:43–50, 1991.
States that "it is well established that all sorts of vegetable, animal, and mineral remedies used in a traditional setting are capable of producing serious adverse reactions." Reviews examples of individuals who suffered fatal consequences as a result of ingesting azarcón powder, rattlesnake meat, herbal teas, and other folk medicines. Discusses the hazards of using these and other folk medicines, some of which are worse than the disease they are alleged to cure. Notes that some folk remedies, such as feverfew, have therapeutic benefits, while others may have psychosocial effects. Urges education of consumers and native healers to reduce harmful folk-medicine practices.

Herbs

Webster's New Collegiate Dictionary defines an herb as "a plant or plant part valued for its medicinal, savory, or aromatic qualities." Herbalism is common to all types of traditional folk medicine systems. It has strong roots in Judeo-Christianity based upon the Biblical tree of life, which is said to possess the ability to sustain eternal life. Many herbalists cite Biblical references to promote their status.

Herbs also have a long and honored history in medicine and pharmacology. Willow bark yielded salicin (the source of aspirin), foxglove was the source of digitalis, and snakeroot was the source of reserpine. Herbs continue to be the sources of new drugs such as the cancer remedy taxol from the pacific yew tree. However, the value of natural herbs can be exaggerated when pointing to their modern scientifically-established uses. Most herbs for which effectiveness was demonstrated years ago have been replaced by synthetic compounds that are more effective.

The difference between responsible herbalism (pharmacognosy) and quackery is that the former is founded upon science and adheres to ethical guidelines. Responsible people acknowledge the potential harm of herbs, while quacks imply that because herbs are natural, they are automatically safe. Pharmacognosists are careful to accurately identify their specimens, while pseudoherbalists often work with misidentified plants. Medicines derived from herbs must have their doses standardized to assure that patients will get the same amounts of the active ingredients time after time. Raw, crude herbs can vary manyfold in strength, making their use like Russian roulette.

Herbs are used by folk healers, health food stores, herbalists, naturopaths, and other types of "alternative practitioners." Some are prescribed at clinics devoted to the cure of specific diseases such as cancer. Some people also use herbs on their own initiative to maintain health, prevent specific diseases, and to treat disease or ailments. Herbs may be obtained in various forms ranging from the plants themselves grown in gardens or harvested in the wild to processed herbal products such as pills. Critics have noted that many of the conditions for which herbs are recommended are not suitable for self-treatment and that with safe and effective medicines available, treatment with herbs rarely makes sense. The most practical sources of reliable information on herbs are the writings of Varro E. Tyler, PhD, author of *The Honest Herbal* (discussed below), and *The Lawrence Review of Natural Products*, a newsletter described in Appendix 2.

Unfortunately, the FDA has permitted herbal products to be marketed as "foods" as long as no therapeutic claims are directly made for them. This ignores the reality that an herb such as *Cascara sagrata* is a laxative whether it says so on the label or not. This has led to a brisk market in pharmacologically active herbs sold as over-the-counter medicines. The OTC herbal business amounts to over $1 billion a year. Regular OTC drugs must be accurately labeled, standardized, and proved to be safe and effective. Herbal preparations escape such regulation. Such a double standard is not in the public's best interest.

Critical Literature

Toxic reactions to plant products sold in health food stores.
The Medical Letter 21:29–31, April 6, 1979.
Identifies and discusses about thirty herbal tea ingredients that can cause toxic effects, including some that are potentially lethal.

Hogan RP III: Hemorrhagic diathesis caused by drinking an herbal tea.
JAMA 249:2679–2680, 1983.
Describes the case of a 25-year-old woman whose blood clotting ability decreased after she had been drinking a "seasonal tonic" for about two months. Notes that the fact that the woman had been using herbal teas was not revealed during the initial history-taking.

Larkin T: Herbs are often more toxic than magical.
FDA Consumer 17:4–10, October 1983.
Warns consumers not to assume that herbs are safe simply because they are still marketed. Lists twenty-eight plant products that the FDA says are too toxic to be used in foods.

Herbs hazardous to your health.
American Pharmacy NS24:20–21, March 1984.
Lists herbs that are hazardous to human health, explaining why they are dangerous. Notes that these herbs are sometimes included in so-called natural medicines, diet aids, and herbal teas. Urges pharmacists to be aware of the danger posed by these herbs.

Tyler VE: Perspective on herbal medicine.
Nutrition Forum 1:11, November 1984.
Suggests that reawakening of interest in herbal medicine is related to disillusionment

with the medical establishment and the "back-to-nature" philosophy that is popular worldwide. Notes that the literature promoting herbs is not only extremely unreliable, but ignores the toxic nature of various plant constituents.

Tyler VE: Pau d'arco.
Nutrition Forum 2:8, January 1985.
States that pau d'arco tea is probably the most popular herbal cancer "cure" of recent times. Discusses some inaccurate statements made by some of its promoters. Notes that an active ingredient, lapachol, does possess some anticancer properties but is too toxic for practical use.

Farnsworth NR, Akerele O, Bingel AS, et al: Medicinal plants in therapy.
Bulletin of the World Health Organization 63:965–981, 1985.
Reports that about 80 percent of the world's population relies on traditional healing, a major part of which involves the use of plants, while populations in developed countries use many drugs that have been derived from plants. Describes the difficulties involved in evaluating the use of plants to treat specific diseases. Lists sources, traditional uses, and therapeutic indications of many plant-derived drugs and in-vitro bioassays for determining useful drug effects or improvement of health.

Tyler VE: More herb research needed.
Nutrition Forum 3:48, June 1986.
States that little clinical research on herbs is done in the United States because the cost of obtaining FDA approval is high and the likelihood of patent protection is very low. Thus little of the information reaching the public is based on scientific sources.

Saxe TG: Toxicity of medicinal herbal preparations.
American Family Physician 35:135–142, May 1987.
States that toxicity of herbs is related to dose, duration of use, coexisting disease, improper identification, manner of preparation, contaminants, and interactions with other active compounds or drugs. Discusses the adverse effects of aloe, ginseng, pokeweed, may apple, cohosh, periwinkle, pennyroyal, sassafras, lobelia, goldenseal, wild garlic, wild onion, bloodroot, castor bean, black cherry, chamomile, alfalfa, wormwood, nutmeg, morning glory, and calamus. Suggests that physicians ask directly about the use of herbs and herbal teas when taking a history.

Miller RW: Can herbs really heal?
FDA Consumer 21:32–34, June 1987.
Discusses FDA regulation of herbal products. Notes that herbal remedies that work generally do so only on minor diseases. Describes how the National Cancer Institute's Natural Products Branch follows up on folklore claims and screens plants,

marine organisms, and microorganisms that might contain some anticancer chemical.

Gazella JG, Pinto JT: Herbs: Use and abuse.
Current Concepts and Perspectives in Nutrition 6:1–20, July 1987.
States that most of the world's plants are poorly classified, largely untested, and therefore remain obscure for practical use. Notes that herbal preparations often have considerable batch-to-batch variability. Lists the toxicities and potential use of seventy-five common herbal preparations.

Baldwin CA, Anderson LA, Phillipson JD: What pharmacists should know about feverfew.
The Pharmaceutical Journal 239:237–238, August 29, 1987.
States that feverfew has been demonstrated effective in preventing migraine headaches and has also been used traditionally for treating arthritis, toothache, menstrual pains, and other ailments. Discusses dosage, side effects and conditions precluding use.

Tyler VE: Book review of Health From God's Garden, *by Maria Treben.*
Nutrition Forum 5:52, July/August 1988.
States that "the world's best-selling herbal author has compiled 128 more pages of fairy tales for her vast audience of natural-medicine enthusiasts who value fantasy and hope more highly than facts." Notes that the book is little more than a rearrangement of the author's *Health from God's Pharmacy* [1980], which had sold more than 4 million copies. States that the author seems oblivious to modern scientific and clinical findings about the adverse effects of many herbs.

Klein AD, Penneys NS: Aloe vera.
Journal of the American Academy of Dermatology 18:714–719, 1988.
Reviews the use of aloe vera to treat burns, frostbite, and other body tissue injuries. Explains chemical composition of the leaves and their healing and cosmetic properties. Discusses the case of a woman who used aloe vera successfully to treat severe radiation dermatitis. Notes complications associated with aloe vera.

Bailey CJ, Day C: Traditional plant medicines as treatments for diabetes.
Diabetes Care 12:553–564, 1989.
Notes that more than 400 plants have been recorded as treatments for diabetes, but only a few have received scientific evaluation to assess their effectiveness. States that hypoglycemic action from some treatments has been confirmed in animal models and in non-insulin-dependent diabetics. Describes proven effects and known toxicity of several herbs and herbal derivatives. Concludes that traditional treatments are

unlikely to lead to a substitute for insulin, but may provide valuable clues for the development of new oral hypoglycemic agents.

Tyler VE: False tenets of paraherbalism.
Nutrition Forum 6:41–44, November/December 1989.
Differentiates between true herbalism (pharmacognosy), involving the scientific testing and ethical marketing of herbs, and paraherbalism, which the author describes as a pseudoscience blindly accepting untested information on plants. Notes how paraherbalists promote toxic herbs without mentioning their side effects. Lists and refutes ten erroneous tenets embraced by paraherbalists. One is the ancient belief ("Doctrine of Signatures") that the form and shape of a drug source determine its therapeutic virtue.

Ball AL: Herbal tonics now share drugstore shelves with Dristan.
Vogue 180:454–458, September 1990.
Warns against the indiscriminate use of herbal remedies. Lists some herbs such as aloe gel and peppermint that can be helpful and others that are hazardous such as comfrey, ginseng, sassafras, and licorice. Describes the variety of herbal products available in stores selling health foods and oriental herbs. Discusses the lack of interest in herbs on the part of drug companies and the enthusiasm for them on the part of herbalists, but notes that some herbalists avoid stores that sell herbs on the grounds that the products they sell are often worthless.

Huxtable RJ: The harmful potential of herbal and other plant products.
Drug Safety 5(Supplement 1):126–136, 1990.
Discusses some harmful effects of using herbal and other plant products, especially those containing pyrrolizidine compounds. Notes dangerous and sometimes fatal results of misidentifying plants and using plants known to be toxic. Examines problems of variability in chemical composition of herbs depending on where they are harvested and stored. Notes hazards caused by differences in names from country to country. Explores risks posed to various population groups by use of herbal preparations. Suggests regulatory measures.

Winship KA: Toxicity of comfrey.
Adverse Drug Reactions & Toxicological Reviews 101:47–59, 1991.
Reviews the medicinal use of comfrey, an herb also fed to livestock. Discusses the plant's chemical makeup and metabolism in animals. Notes that comfrey is carcinogenic, toxic to the liver, and can cause fetal malformations. Notes that despite comfrey's hazards, many people assume that since it is natural, it is safe. Urges doctors to be aware of their patients' use of herbs.

Snider S: Beware the unknown brew, herbal teas and toxicity.
FDA Consumer 25:30–33, May 1991.
Discusses the toxicity of some herbal teas, especially comfrey, lobelia, and sassafras, all of which have been linked to serious diseases. Advises consumers to use moderation in drinking herbal teas considered safe, because large doses can be toxic. Notes the cases of individuals who have suffered ill effects from drinking herbal teas known to be toxic or from misidentifying teas or drinking teas derived from plants to which they were allergic. Discusses the regulatory status of herbs.

Haines JD: Sassafras tea and diaphoresis.
Postgraduate Medicine 90:75–76, September 15, 1991.
Reports on the case of an elderly woman who visited a physician's office complaining of hot flashes much like those experienced during menopause. Notes that the symptoms promptly disappeared after she stopped drinking sassafras tea, which she had started drinking as a tonic on the advice of a family member. Discusses the historic use of sassafras in medicine and in popular drinks, including sassafras tea and root beer. Notes that the FDA banned its use in food in 1960 after discovering that its major chemical component was carcinogenic. Even so, sassafras continues to be sold in health food stores.

Lakey J: Parents get 2-year terms.
Toronto Star, pp. A1, A4, July 25, 1990.
Brent B: Third trial in starvation charges.
Toronto Star, pp. A1, A5, March 3, 1992.
Part of a lengthy series of articles describing the case of Sonia and Khachadour Atikian, who were charged with failing to provide the necessities of life after their 17-month-old daughter had died of malnutrition and pneumonia. The couple was tried three times. The first trial resulted in conviction but was overturned on appeal. The second trial ended with a hung jury. The third trial was ended by the judge when it was discovered that the prosecution had concealed information about a phone call made by Mrs. Atikian shortly before the child died. During the proceedings the Atikians testified that they had been following the advice of an "herbalist" who had promised them a "superbaby" if they adhered to his diet regimen of fruit, rice, and tea. The prosecution noted that the child had weighed only eleven pounds at the time of death, that her body was withered, her skull half-bald, and her skin so covered with rashes and open sores that it looked like the child had been splashed with acid. The Atikians testified that they had trusted the herbalist and had honestly believed they were doing the right thing for their daughter. Their lawyer urged that the government set up a royal commission or an inquest "to deal with the problem of lethal quackery this trial exposed."

Tyler VE: Book review of Earl Mindell's Herb Bible.
Nutrition Forum 9:40, September/October 1992.
States that the book is filled with unproven and inaccurate statements about the usefulness of herbs. Notes that the author recommends several herbs that are toxic. Concludes: "As a sales tool for health food stores, it undoubtedly will do well. As "bible," it fails miserably. Why do you suppose a major publisher is willing to put its imprint on such a book?"

Tyler VE: The honest herbal, 3rd edition.
Binghamton, NY, Haworth Press, 1992.
Provides an authoritative, referenced analysis of the reputed and actual therapeutic properties of more than one hundred herbs and related substances. Notes that herbs possess no magical or mystical properties, and like other drugs, must be administered in proper doses for appropriate periods of time to produce their benefits. Notes that practically all writings promoting herbs to the public "recommend large numbers of herbs for the treatment of a variety of ailments based on hearsay, folklore, and tradition; in fact, the only criterion which seems to be avoided is scientific evidence." Notes that in many instances, even poisonous herbs are recommended. Warns that consumers generally "are less likely to receive good value for money spent in the field of herbal medicine than in almost any other."

"Holistic Medicine"

The word "holistic" has become a marketing term for homeopathy, chelation therapy, clinical ecology, acupuncture, stress reduction, nutritional therapy, and many other "alternative" methods discussed in this book. Some of these methods have found limited acceptance by scientific medicine, but most are not accepted. Victor Herbert, MD, JD, characterizes holistic medicine as "not a distinct concept but rather a melange of banalities, truisms, exaggerations, and falsehoods, overlaid with disparagement not only of scientific conclusions but of logical reasoning itself." According to proponent's rhetoric, holistic practitioners seek to treat the whole person by considering emotional factors and lifestyle as well as the patient's disease. Competent physicians have always done so, but holistic advocates present this approach as something new.

"New Age" medicine—covered elsewhere in this book—resembles "holistic" medicine in its emphasis on healing the spirit and its acceptance of "alternative" methods. However, New Age practices appear more focused on mental, spiritual, and ethereal fantasies.

Critical Literature

Sampson WI: Wolves in sheep's clothing.
In Barrett S (ed.): The health robbers, 2nd edition, pp. 281–290.
Philadelphia, George F. Stickley Co., 1980.
Identifies and criticizes five themes that appear central to the philosophy of holistic medicine: (1) individuals have primary responsibility for their health. Physicians don't treat patients as much as teach them how to remain healthy; (2) general measures, such as "reducing stress" and "correcting imbalances," can make people far less susceptible to disease; (3) medicine is too rigid and impersonal; (4) medicine is just one healing system among many; and (5) "alternative" approaches, though indefinable, unendorsable and unproven, should be promoted vigorously. Describes the origins and purposes of the American Holistic Medical Association. Notes that holistic proponents promote and use a wide variety of "alternative" practices that have no scientific basis. Concludes: "At one time in the past, the holistic label had a valuable and specific meaning. Today, however, it is a banner around which all manner of questionable practitioners are rallying. It appears to me that the concept of holism has been irretrievably corrupted by confused practitioners

and promoters of quackery. The word 'holistic' and its associated slogans should therefore be abandoned by scientific practitioners."

Anonymous: A visit to a holistic health center.
Environmental Nutrition 5:5–6, August 1982.
Reports the experience of a dietitian who visited a holistic health center in New York City. Notes that the first procedure was registration and payment of the $250 fee, which included the cost of a hair analysis, saliva test, shiatsu evaluation, a computerized diet and health history analysis, and the usual physical examination and urinalysis. Notes that the diet and health survey form seemed defective because many commonly consumed foods were not listed, and that the health history form listed various symptoms ranging from constipation to excessive fatigue. Notes that she received an extensive computer analysis that associated each symptom with a disease state or nutritional deficiency. States that many nutritional supplements were prescribed, including vitamin C even though the computer analysis said that her vitamin C intake was already six times the RDA and more than three times the clinic's recommended level. Describes how a shiatsu specialist diagnosed a hiatal hernia and "tilted pelvis," which, if ignored could cause serious endocrine, renal, gynecological, and intestinal problems. Notes that reading about all the possible diseases associated with supposed vitamin and mineral imbalances "might well scare the average patient into following a very expensive treatment regimen to prevent or cure conditions he may not be at the slightest risk of developing."

Glymour C, Stalker D: Engineers, cranks, physicians, magicians.
New England Journal of Medicine 308:960–964, 1983.
Describes "holistic medicine" as a social movement that ties together an odd jumble of people who require the abandonment of scientific methods and rational thinking to establish their claims. Notes that "chiropractors, iridologists, reflexologists, tongue diagnosers, zone therapists, and many others all claim to treat or diagnose the whole from some anatomical part. Of course, they differ about which part, but that does not seem to bother either them or the editors of holistic books."

Vanderpool HY: The holistic hodgepodge: A critical analysis
of holistic medicine and health in America today.
Journal of Family Practice 19:773-781, 1984.
States that the so-called "holistic movement" actually encompasses four different approaches to medicine and health, each with its own theoretical perspective, historical background, and set of therapeutic operations. Describes what he calls: (1) the "biopsychosocial approach," which includes scientific diagnosis and therapy; (2) "whole-person medical care," which emphasizes the patient's inner feelings, perceptions, and beliefs; (3) "high-level healthiness," which emphasizes

preventive care; and (4) "unconventional and esoteric diagnosis and healing," which includes philosophies and practices contrary to those of scientific medicine. Notes that the first three approaches are scientifically based and are not new to American medicine, while the fourth includes some methods that merit serious exploration and others that are patently outlandish. Suggests that the term "holistic" be abandoned for more descriptive categories like those he lists.

Stalker D, Glymour C (eds.): Examining holistic medicine.
Buffalo, Prometheus Books, 1985.
A devastating exposé of "holistic" propaganda and practices. Covers acupuncture, homeopathy, chiropractic, mental imagery, therapeutic touch, vitamin C therapy for cancer, iridology, hazards of herbal medicine, inappropriate use of biofeedback, holistic nursing, and holistic psychotherapies.

Goldstein MS, Sutherland C, Jaffe DT, et al: Holistic physicians and family practitioners: Similarities, differences and implications for health policy.
Social Science and Medicine 26:853–861, 1988.
Reports on a study comparing 340 members of the American Holistic Medical Association with a 142 family practitioners (FPs) in California. Notes that while 81 percent of FPs were board-certified, only 45 percent of the AHMA members were certified. Tabulates the percentages of both groups that use any of twenty-five healing techniques, including meditation/relaxation (used by 86 percent of AHMA members and 70 percent of FPs), nutritional supplements (83 vs. 53 percent), acupuncture (69 vs. 51 percent), chiropractic manipulation 72 vs. 51 percent), homeopathy (42 vs. 8 percent), psychic diagnosis and healing (30 vs. 4 percent), applied kinesiology (35 vs. 8 percent), polarity therapy (21 vs. 1 percent), reflexology (23 vs. 2 percent), and iridology (13 vs. 1 percent). Concludes that many physicians not identified as "holistic" are engaged in practices that can be considered deviant, but that it is not possible to be certain that the FPs surveyed are representative of FPs throughout the United States. [Additional details of the study are available in Goldstein MS, Jaffe DT, Sutherland C, et al: Holistic physicians: implications for the study of the medical profession, *Journal of Health and Social Behavior* 28:103–119, 1987.]

Copeland C: Deception at a New Age clinic.
Journal of Christian Nursing 6:5–7, Spring 1989.
Describes how a woman was drawn to a leading "holistic practitioner" [identified by a fictitious name]. His initial recommendations appeared logical and effective, and he was very attentive to her concerns. She remained with him for about sixteen years. At first she was diagnosed with hypoglycemia. Later she was told she had hypothyroidism and was treated with thyroid hormone. Then she developed a

"stubborn case" of iron-deficiency anemia that was treated with very high oral doses of iron and several vitamins plus injections containing iron, liver extract, and vitamin B_{12}. She also developed persistent constipation with bouts of abdominal pain. When additional symptoms developed, she sought help elsewhere and learned that all of the previous diagnoses had been incorrect and that her symptoms were due to iron and vitamin poisoning, thyroid hormone overdose, a grapefruit-sized ovarian cyst, and endometriosis (which, undiagnosed, had prevented her from bearing children). The woman complained to the state licensing board, which concluded that her care had been inadequate, but which permitted the doctor to remain in practice.

Wassersug JD: Keep That holistic 'care' and send him a surgeon, please. American Medical News 34:34–35, July 22, 1991.
Relates the experience of a physician in Boca Raton, Florida, who visited The Holistic Physical Injury Center for treatment of an injured ankle when his trusted orthopedist was away on vacation. Describes how the clinic nutritionist checked to be sure he didn't injure his ankle because of some nutritional imbalance and a former high-school basketball coach and a social worker both advised how he could become more wholesome. Describes his contact with the physician, who noted that the ankle was very tender. States that after two weeks of [unspecified] holistic treatment, his ankle, which he kept wrapped in an elastic bandage, was as sore as ever. Notes that when his orthopedist returned from vacation, he diagnosed a fracture that needed open surgical reduction. Also notes that a clinic ad and two staff members said "We care for you."

Homeopathy

Homeopathy originated in Europe in the late eighteenth century when Samuel Hahnemann, a German physician, began formulating its basic principles. Hahnemann was justifiably distressed about bloodletting, leeching, purging, and other medical procedures of his day that did far more harm than good. Instead, he developed his "law of similars"—that the symptoms of disease can be cured by substances that produce similar symptoms in healthy people. The word "homeopathy" is derived from the Greek words *homeo* (similar) and *pathos* (suffering or disease).

Hahnemann also concluded that diseases represent a disturbance in the body's ability to heal itself (a disturbance of "vital force") and that only a small stimulus is needed to begin the healing process. In line with this—and to avoid toxic side effects—he experimented to see how little medication could be given and still cause a healing response. At first he used small doses of accepted medications. But later he used enormous dilutions and concluded that the smaller the dose, the more powerful the effect—a principle he called the "law of infinitesimals."

Hahnemann and his early followers conducted "provings" in which they administered herbs, minerals and other substances to healthy people, including themselves, and kept detailed records of what they observed. Later these records were compiled into lengthy reference books called *materia medica*, which are used to match a patient's symptoms with a "corresponding" drug.

Homeopathic remedies are made from minerals, botanical substances, zoological substances, and several other sources. The remedies are prepared by multiple dilutions of 1 to 10 or 1 to 100. According to the laws of chemistry, there is a limit to the dilution that can be made without losing the original substance altogether. This limit, called Avogadro's number, corresponds to homeopathic potencies of 1 part in 10^{24}. Hahnemann himself realized there is virtually no chance that even one molecule of original substance would remain after extreme dilutions. But he said that the vigorous shaking or pulverizing with each step of dilution leaves behind a spirit-like essence which cures by reviving the body's "vital force." Hahnemann's theories have never been accepted by scientifically oriented physicians, who charge that homeopathic remedies are placebos.

Despite this fact, homeopathic remedies were given legal status by the 1938 Federal Food, Drug, and Cosmetic Act, which was shepherded through Congress by a Senator who was also a homeopathic physician. One provision of this law recognized as drugs all substances included in the *Homeopathic Pharmacopeia of the United States*. Now in its ninth edition, this book lists more than 1,000 substances and the historical basis for their inclusion: not modern scientific testing, but homeopathic "provings" conducted as long as 150 years ago. Although it could do so, the FDA does not require that homeopathic drugs be proven effective for their intended use.

In most states, homeopathy can be practiced by any physician or other practitioner whose license includes the ability to prescribe drugs. Three states—Arizona, Nevada and Connecticut—have separate homeopathic licensing boards. The Nevada situation is notable because some of its practitioners acquired licenses as homeopaths after other states revoked their medical license for cancer quackery. The 1990 directory of the National Center for Homeopathy lists about 350 licensed practitioners, approximately half of them physicians and the rest mostly dentists, veterinarians, nurses, chiropractors and naturopaths. Some of the physicians use only homeopathic methods while others use conventional treatments as well. Homeopathic remedies can also be purchased from health food stores, a few pharmacies, mail-order companies and person-to-person (multilevel) distributors.

During 1988 the FDA issued guidelines stating that "homeopathic drugs cannot be offered without prescription for such serious conditions as cancer, AIDS, or any other requiring diagnosis and treatment by a licensed practitioner. Nonprescription homeopathics may be sold only for self-limiting conditions recognizable by consumers." The guidelines caution, however, that compliance with the standards set forth in the *Homeopathic Pharmacopeia* does not establish that a product is safe and effective.

Some published studies have concluded that homeopathic remedies were more effective than placebos. Critics respond, however, that almost all such studies are flawed and that the few that appear well-designed are insignificant compared to the drastic revision of chemistry that would be needed to make homeopathy conceivable.

History of Homeopathy

Holmes OW: Homeopathy and its kindred delusions [original date 1842]. In Stalker D, Glymour C (eds.): Examining holistic medicine, pp. 221–243. Buffalo, Prometheus Books, 1985.
Text of two lectures delivered by Oliver Wendell Holmes ridiculing homeopathy during its early days in America. Demonstrates that even at a time when knowledge

of disease processes and pharmacology were primitive, it was possble to show why the theories of homeopathy's founder were absurd.

Fishbein M: The rise and fall of homeopathy.
In Fishbein M: The medical follies, pp. 29–43.
New York, Boni & Liveright, 1925.
Describes how homeopathy arose at a time when scientific medicine had little to offer patients. Explains how some of Hahnemann's theories evolved because he did not have the benefit of modern knowledge of the causes of disease. Notes that "Hahnemann seems to have known practically nothing of, or to have been unwilling to recognize, the existence of those definite changes in the human body that are associated with disease, and that are now included in the science of pathology. To him disease was chiefly a matter of spirit."

Kaufman M: Homeopathy in America.
Baltimore, Johns Hopkins Press, 1971.
Traces the history of homeopathy from its foundation until the late 1960s. Notes that at the turn of the twentieth century, homeopathy had 14,000 practitioners and 22 schools in the United States alone. But as medical science and medical education advanced and medical schools raised their standards, homeopathy could not compete and declined sharply, particularly in America, where its schools either closed or converted to modern methods.

Gorman J: Take a little deadly nightshade and you'll feel better.
New York Times Magazine 7:23, 26–28, 73, August 30, 1992.
Describes the history of homeopathy and current marketing of homeopathic remedies in the United States. Describes what happened when the author asked two prominent medical editors to review three of the reports most often cited by homeopaths as evidence that their remedies are effective. Both editors found the reports unimpressive but said they would welcome research that is more carefully designed.

Critical Literature

Webb EC, et al: Report of the Committee of Inquiry into Chiropractic,
Osteopathy, Homoeopathy and Naturopathy, pp. 101–115.
Canberra, Australian Government Publishing Service, 1977.
Describes and debunks several lines of propaganda that homeopaths use to claim that there is scientific support for their theories. Notes that "there is not one example in the whole area of pharmacology in which simple dilution of a drug

enhances the response it produces any more than diluting a dye can produce a deeper hue, or adding less sugar can make food sweeter."

Avina RL, Schneiderman, LJ: Why patients choose homeopathy.
Western Journal of Medicine 128:366–369, 1978.
Reports that interviews with 100 homeopathic patients in the San Francisco Bay area revealed that most were young, white, well-educated, and had white-collar jobs, and that most had previously tried mainstream medical care and found it unsatisfactory. The majority were simultaneously involved in other nontraditional health-care activities.

Rados B: Riding the coattails of homeopathy's revival.
FDA Consumer 19:30–34, March 1985.
Notes the revival of homeopathy in recent decades in response to an interest in "natural" cures. Describes an FDA survey which found that many companies were marketing over-the-counter products for the treatment of serious disease. Describes FDA regulatory actions against two such companies. Expresses concern about unlicensed, untrained practitioners who call themselves homeopaths to profit from homeopathy's popularity.

Proceedings of the AMA House of Delegates, December 7–10, 1986, pp. 52–54.
Chicago, American Medical Association, 1986.
Notes a resolution asking that the American Medical Association urge the FDA to cease official recognition of the *Homeopathic Pharmacopoeia*, the list of standard drugs used by homeopathic practitioners. Gives a brief history of the publication and of homeopathy. Lists basic tenets of homeopathy and allopathic views regarding them. Discusses current status of homeopathic remedies. Concludes that the FDA lacks legal authority to cease recognition of the *Homeopathic Pharmacopoeia*. Notes that since a few states still license homeopathic physicians, a standard of drug identity is essential to the practice of homeopathy; hence the American Medical Association's Board of Trustees felt it was undesirable to attempt to amend the law to withdraw recognition.

Scofield AM: Experimental research in homeopathy—a critical review.
British Homeopathic Journal 73:161–180, 73:211–226, 1984.
Thoroughly reviews published homeopathic research and concludes: "Despite a great deal of experimental and clinical work there is only a little scientific evidence to suggest that homeopathy is effective. This is because of bad design, execution, reporting or failure to repeat promising experimental work and not necessarily because of the inefficacy of the system which has yet to be properly tested on a large enough scale . . . It is hardly surprising in view of the quality of much of the

experimental work as well as its philosophical framework, that this system of medicine is not accepted by the medical and scientific community at large." Recommends that controlled experiments be done to test homeopathy further.

Morice A: Adulterated "homeopathic" cure for asthma.
Lancet, pp. 862–863, April 12, 1986.
Reports a case of asthma that responded strikingly to Dumcap, a "homeopathic" remedy that later was found to contain effective amounts of steroid drugs.

Kerr HD, Yarborough GW: Pancreatitis following
ingestion of a homeopathic preparation.
New England Journal of Medicine 314:1642–1643, 1986.
Describes how a 34-year-old man was treated by a chiropractor with "BHI Regeneration Tablets," a mixture of 19 ingredients promoted for the treatment of cancer (according to its package insert). After taking 16 tablets rapidly as directed, he experienced severe epigastric pain and nausea that persisted for two days and were accompanied by repeated vomiting.

Homeopathic remedies—These 19th-century medicines offer
safety, even charm. But efficacy is another matter.
Consumer Reports 52:60–62, January 1987.
Reviews the development of homeopathy and the theory behind it, noting scientific objections based on Avogadro's law. Notes the revival of homeopathy in recent years, accompanied by a growing number of untrained practitioners calling themselves homeopaths and the marketing of products, alleged to be homeopathic, for the treatment of serious illnesses. Notes that the FDA, which previously had ignored homeopathy, had stopped one company from marketing anticancer tablets and other alleged remedies for serious diseases. Reports that about half the faculty members from 49 U.S. pharmacy schools responding to a survey felt that homeopathic remedies should be completely removed from the marketplace. Notes the view of scientific medicine that homeopathic remedies are no more than placebos. Concludes: "Any system of medicine embracing the use of such remedies involves a potential danger to patients whether the prescribers are M.D.s, other licensed practitioners, or outright quacks. Ineffective drugs are dangerous drugs when used to treat serious or life-threatening disease. Moreover, even though homeopathic drugs are essentially nontoxic, self-medication can still be hazardous. Using them for a serious illness or undiagnosed pain instead of obtaining proper medical attention could prove harmful or even fatal."

Barrett S: Homeopathy: Is it medicine?
Nutrition Forum 4:1–6, January 1987.

Briefly reviews the history and theories of homeopathy. Explains the preparation and composition of homeopathic remedies. Describes the proliferation of homeopathic remedies marketed with a wide variety of unproven claims. Notes that the FDA has not required homeopathic remedies to be proved effective in order to remain on the market. States that if the agency required such proof, homeopathy would face extinction in the United States. Sidebar describes how a leading homeopathic practitioner takes a history and selects remedies to treat his patients.

Hayslett J: Rx for Nevada: Trick or treatment.
Las Vegas Review Journal, March 1–8, 1987.
An 8-part investigative report on homeopathy and related practices in Nevada. Exposes how homeopaths achieved licensure in Nevada and how false credentials were used to gain licenses for four practitioners, one of whom was later convicted of killing a woman with a drug overdose. Describes the attitudes of patients, the use of remedies and devices that lack FDA approval, and the future of homeopathy in Nevada as envisioned by its proponents.

van Ulsen J, Stolz E, van Joost T: Chromate dermatitis from a homeopathic drug.
Contact Dermatitis 18:56–57, 1988.
Reports a case of a patient with known allergy to a chromium compound whose condition worsened when he was given a homeopathic remedy containing only 10 micrograms of the chromium compound.

Maddox J, Randi J, Stewart WE: "High-dilution" experiments a delusion.
Nature 334:287–290, 1988.
Describes how the editor of *Nature* and two other investigators visited the laboratory to evaluate the methods used in an experiment reported in an earlier issue of the journal [333:816–818, 1988]. The original report concluded that a solution of an antiserum diluted so many times that no molecule of the original substance remained was still able to trigger a release of histamine from certain cells. When the investigators added better controls to the handling of the specimens, the experimentors could not reproduce the original result. The investigators concluded that the design of the original experiment was not valid because it did not prevent observer bias from influencing the collection of data.

Furnham A, Smith C: Choosing alternative medicine: A comparison of the beliefs of patients visiting a general practitioner and a homeopath.
Social Science and Medicine 26:685–689, 1988.
Discusses a study of 87 patients comparing the reasons why some chose to visit a general practitioner and others chose a homeopathic physician. Reports that the

homeopathic patients were more critical of conventional medicine and that they tended to be sicker and more psychologically disturbed. Notes, however, that there are several possible explanations for these findings and that the population studied was too limited to draw general conclusions about the people who consult "alternative" practitioners.

Beaven DW: Alternative medicine a cruel hoax—your money and your life? New Zealand Medical Journal 102:416–417, 1989.
States that "the fundamental difference between orthodox and alternative methods is largely whether one accepts the inheritance of 20th century principles or whether one wishes, out of personal belief or unsatisfactory previous experiences, to rely solely on the placebo effect." Discusses hazards of utilizing alternative medicine, focusing on homeopathy. Argues that alternative practitioners may neglect important symptoms, thus denying their patients effective therapy. Discusses recent research in homeopathy, noting flaws. Urges better education in science in the schools and more effective exposure and prosecution of fraudulent and unproven medical practices. Argues that the media need qualified medical reporters to expose fraudulent health practices.

Hill C, Doyon F: Review of randomized trials of homeopathy. Review of Epidemiology 38:139–142, 1990.
Analyzes forty published randomized trials in which the results of homeopathic treatment are compared to those of a standard treatment, a placebo, or no treatment. Notes that all but three of the trials had major flaws in their design and that only one of the three well-designed studies had reported a positive result. Concludes that there is no evidence that homeopathic treatment has any more value than that of a placebo. Suggests that additional large-scale randomized trials "may imply costs out of proportion to their usefulness" and are unlikely to produce results that will modify the opinons of physicians or patients toward homeopathy.

Kleijnen J, Knipschild P, ter Riet G: Clinical trials of homeopathy. British Medical Journal 302: 316–323, 1991.
Analyzes the quality of 96 articles covering 107 controlled trials of homeopathy's effectiveness in treating various health problems. Discusses the possible influence of "publication bias," in which "alternative" publications are more likely to publish positive results, regular journals may be more likely to publish negative results, and some investigators may not submit negative results for publication. Concludes that most of the published trials were not well-designed, but that enough positive results have been reported to warrant additional research. Suggests ways that future experiments can be improved.

Court backs board's right to revoke license.
American Medical News 34:24, May 27, 1991.
Describes how the North Carolina Supreme Court backed up the state medical board's decision to revoke the license of George A. Guess, MD, unless he stopped practicing homeopathy. The board had ruled that homeopathic practice constituted unethical conduct. Although no one at the board's hearing had testified that Guess's homeopathic treatment had ever harmed a patient, the Supreme Court reasoned that a general risk of endangering the public is inherent in any practice that fails to conform to "acceptable and prevailing" medical standards.

Proponent Literature

Baker, WP: Introduction to homeopathy and homeotherapeutics.
In The Homeopathic Pharmacopeia of the United States, 8th Edition, First Supplement, pp. 32–34.
Washington, DC, Homeopathic Pharmacopeal Convention of the United States, 1982.
Describes the principle of similars and the way a homeopathic physician approaches the diagnosis and treatment of patients. Claims that, "Homeopathic drugs are safe, effective and compatible with all types of medical, surgical, psychological, physical and nutritional therapy. Since sensitivity reaction seldom occurs, Homeotherapeutics is the safest method of treating infants, children, elderly patients, and individuals who have an allergic diathesis or history of previous drug reactions, whether iatrogenic or from poisoning."

Hahnemann S: Organon of medicine (English translation).
Los Angeles, J.P. Tarcher, Inc., 1982.
Details the thoughts and experiences of homeopathy's founder.

Ullman D: Homeopathy: medicine for the 21st century.
North Atlantic Books, Berkeley, CA, 1988.
Presents the views of America's most active homeopathic publicist. Covers the history, theories, and scope of homeopathy, and tells where to get additional information. Claims that "the homeopathic physician prescribes a single medicine at a time that will stimulate the person's immune and defense capacities and bring about an overall improvement in that person's health." Predicts that homeopathic medicines will become the treatment of choice in viral conditions and that their increased use will sharply reduce the amount of iatrogenic (doctor-induced) disease. Predicts that homeopathy will (1) be used to heal a wide assortment of acute and chronic conditions, (2) help physicians and scientists to better understand the nature of healing" and (3) offer scientific medicine a large number

of new remedies. Also predicts that "alternative" medicine will no longer be considered "alternative," but will be an integral part of a comprehensive health-care system.

Swayne JMD: Survey of the use of homeopathic medicine in the UK health system. Journal of the Royal College of General Practitioners 39:503–506, 1989.
Discusses a survey of 73 homeopathic physicians in the United Kingdom. Reports that 2,507 (35 percent) of 7,218 consultations resulted in 3,032 homeopathic prescriptions being issued. Estimates that the prescribers represented about 11 percent of the doctors actively using homeopathic medicine, the total number of prescriptions issued in the United Kingdom each year probably exceeds 750,000. Concludes that this figure "represents a level of clinical activity that needs to be taken seriously and examined carefully."

King FJ Jr: Ryan itis: A homeopathic case study. Digest of Chiropractic Economics 34:46–47, June 1992.
Case report written by a chiropractor whose biographical sketch states that he founded and directs a homeopathic manufacturing company "dedicated to the marriage of homeopathy and chiropractic." States that during his first visit, "Mr. Itis" completed a Personal Health History Worksheet indicating that he had "very severe" hay fever, allergies to dust, mold, and animals, frequent sinusitis, constant postnasal drip; "severe" frequent cough, cold hands and feet, skipped heart beats; and "moderate" unhealthy skin, insomnia, abdominal bloat, and slowness in healing skin sores. States that chiropractic examination revealed various "subluxations" [see chiropractic section of this book] that were confirmed by x-ray examination. Notes that the patient's liver was slightly swollen and moderately tender and his intestines were tender. Notes that the patient "responded positively" to sublingual muscle-testing and leg-length tests using the author's homeopathic Allergy-Hayfever and Liver Detox & Drainage formulas. Notes that blood, urine, and saliva profiles were also performed. Describes treatment with spinal manipulation and homeopathic remedies. States that the patient improved considerably within two days and continued to improve over a nine-month period, after which he was scheduled for a "three-month maintenance checkup." Provides an "itemized bill" that includes: $75 for the initial examination; $350 for two sets of blood, urine, and saliva tests; $165 for x-rays; $67.28 for homeopathic remedies; $100 for ten "minimal" office visits (seven of which took five minutes each); and $25 for chiropractic manipulations made during those visits. Concludes: "On the business side of the case, the total bill was $1007.20 over 11 visits. . . . As the doctor I spent an estimated total of 107 minutes on this case, which calculates to $9.41/minute or $564.79/hour for my services. My total expenses in lab tests were $64.24. During the 11 visits with this patient he referred seven new patients with many diverse conditions."

Iridology

Iridology, also called "iridiagnosis," is based on the belief that each area of the body is represented by a corresponding area in the iris of the eye. According to this viewpoint, states of health and disease can be diagnosed from the color, texture, and location of various pigment flecks in the eye. Iridology practitioners claim to diagnose "imbalances" that can be treated with vitamins, minerals, herbs, and similar products. They may also claim that the eye markings can reveal a complete history of past illnesses as well as previous treatment. Iridologists have developed many charts mapping the areas in each eye that supposedly correspond to specific parts of the body.

Proponents of iridology attribute its development to Ignatz von Peczely, a Hungarian physician who, during his childhood, had accidentally broken the leg of an owl and noticed a black stripe in the lower part of the owl's eye. (Non-adherents suggest that von Peczely may have developed his theory to pass time while he was imprisoned after the 1848 Hungarian revolution.) After his release from prison, he allegedly saved the life of his mother with homeopathic remedies, recalled the incident of the owl's eye, and began studying the eyes of his patients. The birth of iridology is said to have taken place in about 1861. Iridology was imported to the United States in 1904 by Dr. Henry Lane, who wrote *Iridology, the Diagnosis of the Eye*.

For several decades the leading proponent of iridology in the United States has been Bernard Jensen, DC, whose many publications include two volumes entitled *The Science and Practice of Iridology*. Most practitioners are chiropractors and naturopaths, but laypersons who do "nutrition counseling" also are involved.

Critical Literature

Simon A, Worthen DM, Mitas JA: An evaluation of iridology.
JAMA 242:1385–1389, 1979.
Describes how Bernard Jensen, DC, and two other practitioners examined photographs of the eyes of 143 persons in an attempt to determine which ones had kidney impairments. The iridologists showed no statistically significant ability to detect which patients had kidney disease and which did not.

Report F: Evaluation of iridology.
Proceedings of the AMA House of Delegates, p. 197, June 7–11, 1981.

Observes that the charts used by iridologists resemble those used in phrenology in which protuberances of the skull were related to the mental faculties and the character of the individual. Concludes that "iridology has not yet been established as having any merit as a diagnostic technique."

Worrall RS: Iridology: Diagnosis or delusion.
Skeptical Inquirer 7:23–35, Spring 1983.
Discusses the appeal of iridology as a means of diagnosing disease. Mentions the origins of iridology with Dr. Ignatz von Peczely and its current promotion in the United States by chiropractor Bernard Jensen. Describes the rationale behind iridology and includes several charts illustrating the theory. Notes that there are many different iridology charts that disagree with each other about the location and interpretation of various iris signs. Notes that two recent studies had found iridology ineffective as a diagnostic tool. Mentions two examples of misdiagnosis by iridologists. Concludes that iridology is a pseudoscience with no clinical value.

Knipschild P: Looking for gall bladder disease in the patient's iris.
British Medical Journal 297:1578–1581, 1988.
Reports on an experiment in which five leading iridologists were asked to examine stereo color slides of the right iris of 78 people, half of whom had gall bladder disease, presented in a random order. None of the iridologists could distinguish between the patients with gall bladder disease and the people who were healthy. Nor did they agree with each other about which was which. Concludes that iridology is not a useful diagnostic aid.

Knipschild P: Changing belief in iridology after an empirical study.
British Medical Journal 299:491–492, 1989.
Reports on a study of how the above report influenced 78 authors of articles published in scientific and "alternative" journals. Reports that the opinions about iridology among those who already had strong views either way did not change, but that two-thirds of those who had been undecided did not believe in iridology after reading the paper.

Emery CE Jr: Iridology: Do the eyes have it?
Nutrition Forum 6:4–5, January/February 1989.
Describes how three iridologists in Rhode Island were unable to live up to their claimed diagnostic ability. One told the reporter (who never drank coffee) that he had "caffeine spots from too much coffee." Another said (incorrectly) that he had cardiovascular problems. That one and a third iridologist were unable to identify the health problems of several people by looking at photographs of their eyes. They also

failed to notice anything amiss when shown a photograph of a glass eye against a black background.

Proponent Literature

Jensen B: Iridology simplified.
Escondido, CA, Iridologists International, 1980.
Booklet by the leading American practitioner describes the origin, theories, and practices of iridology. Contains several iridology charts and many color photographs claimed to show significant markings in the iris. Claims that "Nature has provided us with a miniature television screen showing the most remote parts of the body by way of nerve reflex responses." Also claims that "iridology points out where the inherent weaknesses are; and what is needed nutritionally to strengthen them. When the organs and tissues are given the correct minerals, vitamins, nerve strength and rest, healing takes place."

Jensen B: Iridology: Science and practice in the healing arts, Volume II.
Escondido, CA, Bernard Jensen, 1982.
A 600-page compendium covering all aspects of iridology, illustrated with dozens of charts and hundreds of vivid color photographs.

Natural Hygiene

Natural Hygiene is a philosophy of health and "natural living" stemming from the nineteenth-century beliefs that intestinal toxicity causes a wide variety of maladies. Its followers denounce most medical treatment and advocate eating a raw food diet of vegetables, fruits, and nuts. They also advocate periodic fasting and "food combining" (avoiding food combinations it considers detrimental). *Health Science*, the magazine of the American Natural Hygiene Society (ANHS), states that the Natural Hygiene movement was founded during the 1830s by Sylvester Graham, but declined until "resuscitated" from "almost dead" by naturopath Herbert M. Shelton [1895–1985]. ANHS was founded in 1948 by Shelton and several associates and is now headquartered in Tampa, Florida. The group has about 6500 members and has been active in promoting certification of "organic foods" and opposing compulsory immunization, fluoridation, and food irradiation. *Health Science* lists twenty practitioners on its "professional referral list." Most are chiropractors, but a few hold medical, osteopathic or naturopathic degrees.

Several advocates of Natural Hygiene have produced best-selling books. *The Beverly Hills Diet* [Macmillan Publishing Co., 1981], by Judy Mazel, advocates eating just fruit for the first ten days, then adding other types of foods in various combinations. *Fit for Life*, by Harvey and Marilyn Diamond [Warner Books, 1985], claims that the body has three natural cycles: appropriation (eating and digesting) from noon to 8 p.m., assimilation (absorption and use) from 8 p.m. to 4 a.m., and elimination (of body wastes) from 4 a.m. to noon. The book calls for eating fruit only in the morning and mostly vegetables during the rest of the day. A third book, *Unlimited Power* [Ballantine Books, 1986], by Anthony Robbins, confines similar misinformation to a single chapter. Robbins is known best for his advocacy of firewalking and other techniques said to build self-confidence.

Critical Publications

Mirkin GB, Shore RN: The Beverly Hills Diet: Dangers of the newest weight-loss fad. JAMA 246:2235–2237, 1981.
Labels the book's theories about weight gain "nutrition nonsense." Lists and debunks eighteen scientifically inaccurate statements from the book. Describes three cases of severe diarrhea, muscle weakness, and dizziness caused by the diet. Warns that the diet can cause hypovolemic shock, potassium deficiency, and arrhythmia.

Brown LJ, Swenerton H, Simms LS: Fit For Life (book reviews)
Journal of Nutrition Education, 18:136–138, 1986.
Separate reviews by three nutrition educators summarize and rebut many of the major points in the book. They also describe the diet as nutritionally unbalanced and warn that following it could increase the risk of developing osteoporosis and other health problems.

Kenney JJ: Fit for life: Some notes on the book and its roots.
Nutrition Forum, 3:57–59, August 1986.
Describes the success of *Fit For Life*, which became the fastest-selling diet book in U.S. history. Provides background information on Natural Hygiene and the activities of co-founder Herbert Shelton. States that *Fit for Life* was also based on the theories of John H. Tilden, MD, author of *Toxemia Explained* [1926], who said that incompletely digested food causes accumulation of toxic waste material, which causes overweight. Notes that Harvey Diamond's "PhD degree" was obtained at the American College of Life Science, which was operating without authorization from the Texas Commissioner of Higher Education. Notes that Texas authorities had obtained an injunction forbidding the operator of the school from using the word "college" or granting academic credits or degrees.

Moll L: Between the lines of Fit for Life.
Vegetarian Times, pp. 39–40, 42–43, September 1986.
Describes how talk-show publicity built *Fit for Life* into a best seller. Quotes criticisms by several experts, one of whom did a computer analysis and concluded that the diet is low in zinc, calcium, and vitamins D and B_{12} and marginal in iron. Describes the authors' plans to produce a sequel, make videos, and establish a chain of "Fit for Life" restaurants.

Power L: Food combining: Fit for laughs.
Shape 6:38, January 1987.
Criticizes the bogus credentials used by the book's authors. Explains why their contention that weight gain results from foods rotting in the intestine is invalid.

Raso J: Natural hygiene: Still alive and dangerous.
Nutrition Forum 7:33–36, September/October 1990.
Describes the history and philosophy of Natural Hygiene, including its advocacy of fasting, even for children. Mentions a court case in which a jury awarded $800,000 to the survivors of a man who died while undergoing a distilled water 30-day fast at a facility run by Herbert Shelton. Describes the activities at a 1990 conference attended by the author. Concludes that "Natural Hygiene is dangerous because it trivializes nutrient needs, encourages prolonged fasting, and discourages medical

interventions almost across the board. While its recommended diet has two admirable characteristics (low fat content and high fiber content), its proscription of both dairy products and supplements in its primarily raw food diet is an invitation to osteoporosis."

Naturopathy

Naturopathy—sometimes referred to as "natural medicine"—is said to be based on the healing power of nature. Naturopaths claim to remove the underlying causes of disease and to stimulate the body's natural healing processes. They state that diseases are the body's effort to defend itself and that cures result from increasing the patient's "vital force" by ridding the body of waste products and "toxins."

Most naturopaths believe that virtually all diseases are within the scope of their practice. They offer treatment at their offices and at spas where patients may reside for several weeks. Their current methods include fasting, "natural food" diets, vitamins, herbs, homeopathy, tissue minerals, cell salts, manipulation, massage, exercise, colonic enemas, acupuncture, "Chinese medicine," natural childbirth, minor surgery, and applications of water, heat, cold, air, sunlight and electricity. Radiation may be used for diagnosis but not for treatment. Although naturopaths claim that they stress prevention of disease, they tend to oppose immunization procedures.

The term "naturopathy" was coined in 1895 by John Scheel, a practitioner in New York City, to describe his methods of health care. In 1902, he sold rights to the term to Benedict Lust, who had come to the United States in 1892 to promote hydrotherapy. Lust was largely responsible for naturopathy's growth in this country.

Before 1961 the doctor of naturopathy (ND) degree could be obtained at a few chiropractic schools; now it is available only from two full-time schools of naturopathy and a few correspondence schools. In 1987 the U.S. Secretary of Education approved the Council on Naturopathic Medical Education as an accrediting agency for the full-time schools. The leading naturopathic institution, Bastyr College in Seattle, has also received full accreditation from the Northwest Association of Schools. As with acupuncture and chiropractic schools, accreditation is not based upon the scientific validity of what is taught but upon other criteria.

Naturopaths are licensed as independent practitioners in seven states and the District of Columbia, and may legally practice in a few others as well. The American Association of Naturopathic Physicians has about 400 members. The total number of practitioners is unknown but includes chiropractors and acupuncturists who practice naturopathy. Bastyr College offers degrees in naturopathy, acupuncture, nutrition and Oriental medicine. During the past two years, it has also teamed with the National Nutritional Foods Association to produce educational programs for "health food" retailers.

History of Naturopathy

Gort EH, Coburn D: Naturopathy in Canada: Changing relationships to medicine, chiropractic and the state.
Social Science and Medicine 26:1061–1072, 1988.
Traces the history of naturopathy in the United States and Canada.

Baer HA: The potential rejuvenation of American naturopathy as a consequence of the holistic health movement.
Medical Anthropology 13:369–383, 1992.
Provides a detailed history of naturopathy, tracing its rise, near-extinction, and recent rejuvenation. Suggests that the future of naturopathy remains tenuous.

Critical Literature

Cohen WJ: Independent practitioners under Medicare: A report to Congress, pp. 126–145.
Washington, DC, Department of Health, Education, and Welfare, 1968.
Briefly describes the history of naturopathy in the United States. Describes naturopathic philosophy, practices, and education, as gathered from materials submitted to the Department of HEW. Notes that some naturopaths include iridiagnosis [iridology] in their examination of patients. Concludes: "Naturopathic theory and practice are not based upon the body of basic knowledge related to health, disease, and health care which has been widely accepted by the scientific community. Moreover, irrespective of its theory, the scope and quality of naturopathic education do not prepare the practitioner to make an adequate diagnosis and provide appropriate treatment."

Shapiro B: A visit to a naturopathic clinic.
The Gazette, Montreal, p. 25, April 20, 1972.
Describes a reporter's visit to a naturopath selected at random from the Yellow Pages. A second reporter, posing as a patient, told the naturopath she had chronic fatigue (false), diabetes since childhood (true), and a breast lump. The naturopath performed a perfunctory physical examination, said the woman had liver and kidney disease, advised various dietary changes, sold "Vitaminex" products from a firm he owned, and said all the woman's problems would disappear in time if she followed his instructions to the letter. The naturopath did not examine the woman's alleged breast lump but said it was due to magnesium deficiency.

Webb EC, et al: Report of the Committee of Inquiry into Chiropractic, Osteopathy, Homoeopathy and Naturopathy, pp. 69–99.

Australian Government Publishing Service, April 1977.
Reports that "although the syllabuses of naturopathic schools were reasonable in their coverage of basic biomedical sciences on paper, the actual instruction bore little resemblance to the documented course." Describes the use of herbalism, Bach flower remedies, reflexology, iridology, acupuncture, tissue salts (the rationale for which the Committee said was based on "pure imagination"). Concludes that naturopaths should not be licensed because licensing "may give a form of official imprimatur to practices which the Committee considers to be unscientific and, at best, of marginal efficacy."

Sovereign AE: Naturopathic services.
Canadian Medical Association Journal 142:708, 1990.
Letter to the editor describes the case of a young boy who was having mood swings, school problems, and behavioral problems. Notes that the boy was previously treated by a naturopath who prescribed a restrictive diet and a large number of pills containing vitamins and other substances at a cost of $100 per month. Complains that the pills are unscientific and possibly harmful and that going to the naturopath delayed successful conventional treatment. Argues that much of naturopathy is unscientific and that government should address these concerns before allowing naturopathy to play an expanded role in medicine.

Bogus degrees in the news.
Nutrition Forum 7:32, July/August 1990.
Reports on a scandal involving Kurt Donsbach and several other individuals who obtained naturopathic licenses by submitting altered photocopies of a chiropractic diploma as their "naturopathic" diplomas.

Proponent Literature

Pizzorno JE: What is a naturopathic physician?
Let's Live 2:64–65, February 1988.
Written by the president of Bastyr College. Describes how an 18-month-old child with chronic ear infections was treated with dietary manipulation at the school's clinic. Briefly reviews the philosophy and training of naturopaths. States that naturopaths have begun organizing to lobby for licensure in several states.

Pizzorno JE, Murray MT: A textbook of natural medicine.
Seattle, John Bastyr College Publications, 1985–1991.
Currently the largest collection of information about naturopathy and its methods. Covers naturopathic philosophy, history, diagnostic procedures, therapeutic modalities, and naturopathic viewpoints and treatment approaches to a large

number of health problems. Intended primarily for practitioners. Updated periodically.

Pizzorno JE, Murray MT: Encyclopedia of natural medicine.
Rocklin, CA, 1990, Prima Publishing, 1990.
Comprehensive handbook intended primarily for laypersons. Discusses naturopathic principles and gives naturopathic advice for the treatment of more than sixty health problems.

"New Age" and Occult Practices

The 1988 Guide to New Age Living defines New Age thinking as "a form of utopianism, the desire to create a better society, a 'new age' in which humanity lives in harmony with the cosmos." According to this source, the movement's elements include such things as "human potential, holistic health, recycling, organic foods, grassroots activism, practical spirituality, meditation, ecology, appropriate technology, feminism, and progressive politics." *Time* magazine describes the New Age movement as a "cornucopia of beliefs, fads [and] rituals" to which some followers subscribe and others do not.

One of the prominent New Age modalities is "trance-channeling," which can be defined as the communication of information to or through a live person (the medium or channel) from a source purported to be from another dimension or reality. One well-known practitioner is J.Z. Knight, who claims that a 35,000-year-old man named Ramtha uses her body to speak words of wisdom. Another is actress Shirley MacLaine, who claims that channeling provides useful information about "past lives."

J. Gordon Melton, director of the Institute for the Study of American Religion and author of the *New Age Encyclopedia*, states that it is easier to understand the New Age in terms of its ideals and goals rather than a set of beliefs to which it gives assent. "The central vision," he says, "is one of radical transformation. On an individual level that experience is very personal and mystical. It involves an awakening of a new reality of self—such as a discovery of psychic abilities, the experience of a physical or psychological healing, the emergence of new potentials within oneself, an intimate experience within a community, or the acceptance of a new picture of the universe."

The extent to which occult beliefs and practices influence the mental and physical health of Americans may be considerable. Yet, for the most part, the popular press has treated occult events as novelties without attempting to determine whether they actually help or harm people. The publishing industry has promoted and exploited the situation by producing hundreds of books extolling occult claims, but only a few that examine them critically. The major source of critical information is the network of experts affiliated with the Committee for the Scientific Investigation of Claims of the Paranormal (CSICOP), which publishes a quarterly magazine, *Skeptical Inquirer*, and a quarterly newsletter, *Skeptical Briefs*.

Descriptive Literature

Levine A, Kyle C, Dworkin P: Mystics on main street, while skeptics cast doubts, psychics count dollars.
U.S. News & World Report 102:67–69, February 9, 1987.
States that the popularity of the New Age movement is growing despite critics' skepticism, particularly among business and professional people. Notes claims of cures by alternative healers. Discusses the hiring of New Age gurus to help improve corporate performance. Reports criticism voiced by scientific and religious leaders. Notes examples of mental breakdowns, suicides, and other harmful effects sparked by some New Age promotions.

Friedrich O, Cronin M, Riley M, et al: New age harmonies.
Time 130:62–66, 69, 72, December 7, 1987.
Describes the "New Age" as "a whole cornucopia of beliefs, fads [and] rituals" to which some followers subscribe and others do not. Notes that the beliefs include crystal healing (said to help the body balance and realign its "energy fields"), therapeutic touch, healing through mental imagery, pendulum power, and dozens of others. Discusses the role of Shirley MacLaine in popularizing various aspects of the New Age movement. Mentions criticism of the New Age movement by mainstream religion. Notes the popularity of other unorthodox movements throughout American history.

Melton JG: New Age encyclopedia.
Detroit, Gale Research Inc., 1990.
Provides more than 300 factual accounts of the people, organizations, practices, and philosophies related to New Age activities. States that by the mid-1980s, the New Age movement became a significant social-religious force in Western culture, representing "more than just another subgroup within the larger occult-metaphysical community in America." States that the movement is centered on "personal transformation" from orthodox modes of thought, poverty, illness, boredom, purposelessness, and/or hopelessness to one of "new openness and new egalitarian relationships with a sense of abundance, regained vitality and health, excitement, intensity, new meaning, and a new future." States that participants have either had or are seeking such an experience. Observes that the New Age and holistic health movements share ideology and are intertwined.

Gallup GH Jr, Newport F: Belief in paranormal phenomena among adult Americans.
Skeptical Inquirer 15:137–146, Winter 1991.
Describes the findings of a Gallup Mirror of America survey of 1,236 adults

conducted in June 1990. Reports that the following percentages of people said they believed in: the Devil (55 percent), extrasensory perception (55 percent), possession by the Devil (49 percent), spiritual or psychic healing (49 percent), mental telepathy (36 percent), clairvoyance (26 percent), astrology (25 percent), ghosts (25 percent), reincarnation (21 percent), channeling (11 percent), and pyramid power (4 percent). Also reports that 25 percent of those surveyed believed they had been able to heal their body using their own mental power alone. States that only 29 percent of those polled said they had heard of the New Age movement and that most of these felt unfavorably about it.

Critical Literature

Keene ML: The psychic mafia.
New York, St. Martin's Press, 1976.
Written by a former professional psychic. Describes how some American psychics exchange information with each other about clients but pretend to derive this information by psychic means.

Jerome LE: Astrology disproved.
Buffalo, Prometheus Books, 1977.
Details the theories and practices of astrology from ancient times through the mid-1970s. Describes various reasons why people believe in it.

Bainbridge WS: Biorhythms: evaluating a pseudoscience.
Skeptical Inquirer 2:40–56, Spring/Summer 1978.
Describes and debunks the theory that behavior is characterized by three innate cycles said to begin at the moment of birth, oscillate predictably throughout life, and influence an individual's strength, endurance, energy, resistance, mood, and self-confidence. Describes various tests, performed by the author, which showed that events predicted by biorhythm calculations did not differ from what would be expected by chance. Notes that students have readily accepted "biorhythm calculations" that the author actually derived by flipping a coin.

Gauquelin M: Dreams and illusions of astrology.
Buffalo, Prometheus Books, 1979.
Notes that astrologers and their adherents are convinced that the position of the planets in the heavens at the time and place of their birth is a factor that strongly influences a person's destiny. Describes how astrologers ply their trade and ways in which their pronouncements have been tested.

Hyman R: Occult healing.
In Barrett S (ed.): The health robbers, 2nd edition, pp. 26–34.
Philadelphia, George F. Stickley Co., 1980.
Critically examines several approaches to healing that involve use of a supposed force or technique that is unrecognized by medical science. Discusses several ways that people are misled into believing in unorthodox methods. Worries that America's educational system is not preparing students to be prudent consumers.

Watkins AJ, Bickel WS: A study of the Kirlian effect.
Skeptical Inquirer 10:244-257, Spring 1986.
Explains the physical basis of Kirlian photography, which is done by applying a high-voltage, high-frequency discharge across a grounded object placed on a sheet of film laying in the high-voltage plane. Notes that this produces a glowing discharge of that appears to the eye as a purple-blue fuzzy light called an aura. Observes that since the 1970s, claims have been made that the aura of human body parts such as fingers and toes communicate information about the physical, psychological, and psychic state of the individual. Notes that proponents claim that the photographic image provides information about the person's "life-force," "life-energy," or "bioplasma." States that the image is actually determined by the moistness of the fingers, how hard they are pressed on the photographic plate, sensitivity of the photographic film, exposure and development times, and seventeen other variables. According to Kurt Butler's book, *A Consumer's Guide to "Alternative Medicine"* [Prometheus Books, 1992], some practitioners claim that auras reveal current diseases, latent diseases, (including incipient cancer and "organ weaknesses"), nutritional deficiencies, drug abuse, and mental disorders that can be treated or prevented with vitamins, acupuncture, homeopathy, and other measures.

Kurtz P et al: CSICOP on trans-channelers.
The Pseudoscientific Monitor, p 4, November 1987.
Notes that the Committee for the Scientific Investigation of Claims of the Paranormal (CSICOP) has offered to test trance-channelers under laboratory conditions but has had no takers. States that it is "surprising that trance-channelers have been allowed to make uncorroborated and unverified claims, charge people hundreds or thousands of dollars for public and private audiences, and offer advice on business and personal matters without providing evidence that they indeed have contact with discarnate beings." States that many people have been harmed by such practices. Suggests that the public be extremely cautious about these claims.

Gordon H: Channeling through the new age.
Buffalo, Prometheus Books, 1988.

Describes and debunks the "teachings" of Shirley MacLaine and other "channelers," some of whom claim to be able to contact prehistoric entities who provide advice through them. States that there have always been alleged psychics, mediums, fortune-tellers, prognosticators, astrologers, and other "faddists who adopt every way-out innovation"—the big difference now is that major publishing houses, entertainers, and the TV networks are participating in a big way.

Basil R (ed.): Not necessarily the new age: Critical essays.
Buffalo, Prometheus Books, 1988.
Contains a history of the New Age movement and critical discussions of karma, reincarnation, past-life regression, out-of-body experiences, channeling, UFO-abductions, and many other New Age practices and events. States that "in the past few years, the New Age movement has grown from a fervently supported countercultural underground to yet one more social force blanched into uniform inanity by the mass media. . . . In short, what used to be called 'the occult'—which means *hidden*—is occult no longer. This has encouraged millions to check out nontraditional spiritual beliefs and alternative healing practices, but too, too few to critically examine these beliefs and practices."

Lawrence GM: Crystals
Skeptical Inquirer 13:397–400, Summer 1989.
Notes that quartz has two unique properties that can be explained by quantum physics but is falsely alleged to have additional ones. States that typical New Age mystics use scientific terms like harmonics, vibration, resonance, bonding, and electromagnetic field to manipulate their audiences and claim that crystals are capable of producing healing. Cites one proponent who promises "clearing away negative attitudes, centering personal energies, enhancing communications, promoting healing, opening the heart to love and courage, simplifying decisionmaking, balancing the spirit, focusing the mind, tapping into psychic powers, and using chakras and colors." States that some proponents even promise to help people with cancer, AIDS, and other dire diseases "if treated early enough." Describes the author's experience in confronting a "healer" who glibly evaded various questions.

Frazier K: Time-Life's descent into the New Age.
Skeptical Inquirer 13:412–415, Summer 1989.
Critiques the "Mysteries of the Unknown" series published by Time-Life Books, which is said to be the most successful series in the company's history. Notes that Time-Life Books normally does an excellent job to ensure that its science books are scientifically respectable and "could have helped a confused public sort through the

bewildering array of paranormal claims that everywhere assault the mind." Notes that although the editors are quite well-informed, the books "exhibit a determined reluctance to openly criticize what deserves criticism and an equal determination to provide a sympathetic hearing to the defenders of paranormal explanations."

Cold reading: How to convince strangers that you know all about them.
In Hyman R: The elusive quarry: A scientific appraisal
of psychical research, pp. 402–419.
Buffalo, Prometheus Books, 1989.
Describes "cold reading" as a procedure by which a "reader" is able to persuade a client whom he or she has never met before that the reader knows all about the client's personality and problems. Notes that this can be accomplished with highly general statements that can fit any individual or with statements based on cues picked up by observing the client in person. Describes how people tend to give credit to things that seem to fit, but forget about things that do not. Lists thirteen tactics that can make someone a successful character reader.

Bloch BW: Cosmic confidence.
Health 22:70–73, 84, December 1990/January 1991.
Describes the author's experience in a "self-empowerment" class in which participants are told that changes begin when people acknowledge that their thoughts create everything that occurs in their life. Describes the teaching of "guided visualization, a form of self-hypnosis used to construct a distinct image of how you would like things to be." States that one cosmic consultant charges $15,000 per group for four-day brainstorming sessions in which company executives "explore their belief systems, examine their goals, and discover ways to transcend their limits." Quotes a psychoanalyst who says that the personal growth approach to solving problems not only sidesteps the real issues but is likely to cause a good deal of harm—and that the best ways to improve productivity are better capital investment and employment of people who already know how to solve problems.

Raso J: The Legacies of Edgar Cayce.
Nutrition Forum 8:1–4, January/February 1991.
Describes the activities of Edgar Cayce (1877–1945), who is alleged to have conducted over 14,000 "psychic readings" between 1910 and his death. Notes that he gained nationwide renown for diagnosing illnesses and prescribing dietary remedies while in a self-induced hypnotic state. Describes various activities of Cayce's followers who offer courses, conferences, books, mail-order remedies, and "holistic" medical care.

City skips rock healing course.
Chicago Tribune, Part 1, p. 3, March 15, 1992.
Describes how officials in Hollister, California, cancelled a city-sponsored course that was claimed to teach people how to heal serious illnesses by holding rocks. States that after state medical board officials called the practices involved "illegal" and "quackery," the city manager expressed concern about liability if someone were hurt as a result of what was taught in the class. Notes that the would-be teacher, a clerk in a rock shop, said that she tells patients to hold rocks in their hands for twenty minutes, four times a day, or to soak the rocks in water and drink the water—and that the healing comes from electromagnetic properties in the rocks and "resonating vibrations in the human body."

Barrett S: Can "psychic astrology" solve your problems?
Skeptical Briefs 2:5, May 1992.
Describes how "psychic astrologer" Irene Hughes mailed a computer-generated solicitation offering to help the recipient with "a serious personal problem . . . eating away at you." Notes that Ms. Hughes said she knew of the problem because she was "concentrating" on the recipient at that very moment. States that the letter's recipient was not an actual person but a name assumed by a reporter whose name is circulating on "sucker lists."

Part III:
Major Diseases

Questionable Cancer Treatment

The American Cancer Society defines questionable methods as "lifestyle practices, clinical tests, or therapeutic modalities that are promoted for *general* use for the prevention, diagnosis, or treatment of cancer and which are, on the basis of careful review by scientists and/or clinicians, not deemed to have real evidence of value." Today's questionable methods include biological products, bogus devices, herbal concoctions, dietary approaches, megavitamin therapies, mental imagery, faith healing, and "psychic surgery." Use of these approaches can divert people from effective treatment and cause physical, emotional, and financial harm. Every year, thousands of American cancer patients turn to such treatments. Many do so when conventional treatments appear to offer no hope, but others are lured by the seductive promises that the treatments are "natural" and "non-toxic" (i.e., without side effects) and that they "work." Many patients find unconventional methods appealing because they are explained in commonsense terms that seem plausible and offer an opportunity to play an active role in fighting their disease.

General Information About Cancer

Hubbard SM, Henney JE, DeVita VT Jr: A computer data base for information on cancer treatment.
New England Journal of Medicine 316:315–318, 1987.
Describes the Physician Data Query (PDQ) system, a computer data base developed to make current information on cancer treatment widely available to the medical community. The computer system provides information about state-of-the art cancer treatment, which is updated monthly by an editorial board. It also enables clinicians to locate clinical trials and to retrieve information on specialists for consultation or referral.

National Cancer Institute: What are clinical trials all about?
NIH Publication No. 90-706.
Washington, DC, U.S. Government Printing Office, 1989.
Provides information on the nature of clinical trials (true alternatives to proven treatment) and how patients can attempt to enroll in them.

Boring CC, Squires TS, Tong T: Cancer statistics 1992.
Ca – A Cancer Journal for Clinicians 42:19–38, 1992.

Provides facts and figures on the incidence, death rates, and survival rates for cancers. Indicates how survival rates have increased for certain cancers.

Characteristics of Questionable Methods

Janssen WF: Cancer quackery: Past and present.
FDA Consumer 11:27–32, July/August 1977.
Provides history of cancer quackery and advice to patients with cancer.

Faw C, Ballentine R, Ballentine L, et al: Unproved cancer remedies: a survey of use in pediatric outpatients.
JAMA 238:1536–1538, 1977.
Describes study which found that 27 of 69 patients (39 percent) had tried, considered, or received recommendations for an unproven remedy.

Wood CG, Pressley BM: The cruellest killers: An update.
In Barrett S (ed): The health robbers, 2nd edition, pp. 108–122.
Philadelphia, 1980, George F Stickley Co.
Provides an excellent overview of cancer quackery through the late 1970s.

Shils ME, Hermann MG: Unproved dietary claims in the treatment of patients with cancer.
Bulletin of the New York Academy of Medicine 58:323–340, 1982.
Explores the reasons why alternative cancer treatments are available and why cancer patients seek them out. Compares procedures used in conventional medicine with those used by alternative practitioners. Examines several theories about cancer that are common among purveyors of unproven therapies and explains why they are erroneous. Discusses methods and costs of Gerson Therapy, the William D. Kelley "Non-Specific Metabolic Therapy," the Paavo Airola vitamin treatment, the Leo Roy system of enemas (fasts, dietary supplements and special diets), the macrobiotic diet, laetrile, the Adelle Davis diet, and the E.T. Krebs diet. Offers suggestions on how health professionals should deal with patients who choose unorthodox treatment.

Patients on unproved cancer therapy told how to make insurance companies pay.
Medical World News, p. 131, June 7, 1982.
Describes how patients treated by Lawrence Burton, MD, were given a guide telling them how to pressure insurance companies in the U.S. to pay for his unproven treatment. Notes concern by a leading health lawyer that patients could be misled into thinking that their chances for reimbursement are good—which they are not.

The lawyer also notes that insurance companies that settle too many contested claims out-of-court may expose themselves to unexpected liability for other claims.

Unproven methods of cancer management.
New York, American Cancer Society, 1982.
Provides detailed information on the techniques used to promote unproven methods.

American Society of Clinical Oncology Subcommittee on Unorthodox Therapies: Ineffective cancer therapy: a guide for the layperson.
Journal of Clinical Oncology 1:154–163, 1983.
Discusses the appeal of popular unproven cancer remedies and reviews the claims made for the Hoxsey herbal tonic, krebiozen, laetrile, iscador, and immunoaugmentive therapy (IAT). Notes some similarities in promotion of these remedies, including (1) reliance on unproven theories, (2) claims for painless, nontoxic treatment that can prolong life or be used as a preventive, (3) insistence that only a special practitioner can administer their treatment, (4) reliance on the popular press in promoting their treatment, (5) attacks on the medical and scientific establishment, and (6) demands for "freedom of choice" in medical treatment.

Eidinger RN, Schapira DV: Cancer patients' insight into their treatment, prognosis, and unconventional treatments.
Cancer 53:2736–2740, 1984.
Describes a Canadian study in which 190 patients with metastatic cancer were interviewed to determine their insight into their disease, treatment, and prognosis, and whether they felt guilty or became more religious. The authors also examined the feelings of 315 cancer patients toward unconventional therapies. Discusses results of the study, noting considerable interest in alternative forms of cancer treatment among the latter group. Mentions some alternatives of which patients were aware, including laetrile, special diets, and vitamins. Concludes that most patients, despite increased efforts to provide them with adequate information, still are not well-informed on the nature of their disease, their treatment, and whether alternatives might work for them.

Cassileth BR, Lusk EJ, Strouse TB, et al: Contemporary unorthodox treatments in cancer medicine.
Annals of Internal Medicine 101:105–112, 1984.
Presents a study of cancer patients who were diagnosed through conventional means. The group included 282 who used orthodox therapy alone, 325 who received both conventional and alternative treatments, and 53 who relied on unconventional treatment alone. The unorthodox methods included "metabolic"

treatment, diet, megavitamins, imagery, spiritual healing, and immune therapy. The article reports on usage according to practitioner and notes that most patients were treated by physicians who used alternative methods. The article reports that, in general, the patients were educated people who wished to take an active role in their care. The patients were attracted to alternative therapies that reflected social emphasis on personal responsibility, the environment, and nutrition and that avoided perceived defects of conventional medicine; hence, the interest in natural, nontoxic alternative regimens. It compares attitudes of groups of patients toward conventional and unorthodox medical care and attitudes of practitioners on both sides.

Thompson R: The sad allure of cancer quackery.
FDA Consumer 19:36, 38, May 1985.
Describes a series of quack cancer operations run by James Gordon Keller and his associates at various locations in the United States and Mexico until the Mexican clinic was closed and some of Keller's associates and employees arrested. At the time of the article, Keller and his brother were armed fugitives. The article describes Keller as an extreme example of the larger issue of cancer patients seeking treatment from alternative practitioners. [Keller eventually was brought to trial and sentenced to prison for wire fraud.]

Markman M: Medical complications of "alternative" cancer therapy.
New England Journal of Medicine 312:1640, 1985.
Letter to the editor from a San Diego physician who reports on four patients who required hospitalization after undergoing supposedly "nontoxic" treatments at Mexican cancer clinics. One developed chemical phlebitis following intravenous ozone therapy, and three developed life-threatening infections following coffee enemas.

Kreiger L: Plethora of miracle cures touted at
annual reunion of "medical rebellion."
American Medical News 28:3, 31–34, August 9, 1985.
Reports on a conference of practitioners of alternative cancer remedies. Quotes several practitioners, promoters, and advocates of alternative treatment on the merits of alternative and conventional medicine in the treatment of cancer. Describes several unorthodox cancer remedies, nutritional regimes, ozone therapy, live cell injections, laetrile, and vaccine injections at the Livingston-Wheeler Medical Clinic.

Kreiger L: Unorthodox clinics flourishing in Tijuana.
American Medical News 28:3, 25–30, August 9, 1985.

Discusses the popularity of several alternative cancer clinics located in Tijuana, Mexico. Describes the Hoxsey treatment at the Bio-Medical Center, the Gerson Therapy Hospital, the Manner Clinic, the Centro Medico Del Mar run by Dr. Edward Contreras, and American Biologics Hospital run by Dr. Rodrigo Rodriguez, which utilizes live-cell therapy. Quotes the views of practitioners at each clinic on the merits of their approach.

Ross WE: Unconventional cancer therapy.
Comprehensive Therapy 11:37–43, September 1985.
Summarizes common characteristics of unconventional cancer therapies. Discusses laetrile, high-dosage vitamin C, macrobiotic diets, mental imagery (the Simonton method), immunoaugmentative therapy (IAT) and the Greek Cancer Cure.

Shaving chemotherapy: 'killing patients with kindness.'
Medical World News, pp. 24–25, April 28, 1986.
Describes a warning by former NCI Director Vincent DeVita that administering less than state-of-the-art chemotherapy dosages (to decrease side effects) to potentially curable patients is "throwing away the cure rate."

Durant JR. Judging the alternative cancer treatments.
Washington Post, Health Section, p. 6, May 7, 1986.
Suggests that most people who choose unproven cancer treatments do so out of fear of the orthodox treatment and because unorthodox practitioners appear to offer a more personal approach to treating the patient. Also notes that some cancers are incurable at present, leading people to try anything out of desperation. Lists ten criteria for judging claims of new, unproven cancer treatments.

Stokes S: Cancer quackery: A continuing problem.
Journal of the Tennessee Medical Association 79:415–421, 1986.
Traces the history of cancer quackery in the twentieth century, giving a brief description and history of major cancer remedies, including the Koch treatment, the Hoxsey treatment, Krebiozen, laetrile, and immunoaugmentive therapy (IAT). Offers suggestions on how the public can recognize unproven methods of treating cancer, noting differences between scientific medicine and unorthodox practitioners in their approaches to investigation of a therapy, publication of findings, and diagnosis and treatment of disease. Advises physicians on how to counsel patients to avoid such treatments. Discusses the importance of psychosocial questions regarding unproven methods.

Herbert V: Unproven (questionable) dietary and nutritional methods in cancer prevention and treatment. Cancer 58:1930–1941, 1986.

Defines unproven and questionable treatments. Explains the peer-review process for judging treatments. Discusses the problem of health fraud and the methods that quacks use to promote their products. Suggests ways of recognizing fraudulent claims and identifying quacks. Discusses the hazards of unproven methods, focusing on nutritional and metabolic therapies, macrobiotic diets, laetrile, and immunoaugmentive therapy (IAT). Mentions several practitioners who were sued or subjected to government enforcement action. Includes the executive summary from the report on quackery of the Subcommittee on Health and Long-Term Care of the Select Committee on Aging, U.S. House of Representatives.

Jarvis WT: Helping your patients deal with questionable cancer treatments. Ca – A Cancer Journal for Clinicians 36:293–301, 1986. [Also published separately as a booklet.]
Notes that promoters of unproven cancer treatment methods take advantage of misconceptions about cancer to convince patients to use their remedies. Provides factual responses to fourteen commonly held myths and fallacies about cancer and its treatment.

Brigden M: Unorthodox therapy and your patient. Postgraduate Medicine 81:271–280, 1987.
Notes that over 50 percent of patients undergoing conventional cancer treatment simultaneously resort to unconventional treatments, often at an early stage. Discusses reasons for the popularity of alternative therapy with special mention of "commonsense" conclusions about disease and the ability of a patient to control disease. Lists a six-element "formula for promoting unorthodox therapy." Notes how proponents rely on anecdotal data and state that they are "too busy treating patients" to gather statistical evidence by which their method could actually be evaluated. Offers suggestions to physicians on how to recognize and combat alternative therapies.

Clinical Oncology Group: New Zealand cancer patients and alternative medicine. New Zealand Medical Journal 100:110–113, February 25, 1987.
Reports on a survey of 148 cancer patients in New Zealand who said they had been advised to use various "alternative" approaches. The most common approaches were diet, vitamins, and herbs. Discusses how the patients learned of these approaches and why those who followed them had elected to do so. Notes that most learned of alternative therapy from friends (52 percent) or family (20 percent) and had not been pressured in making their choice. Most were also satisfied with conventional medicine and accepted alternative therapy only as a supplement to orthodox medicine.

Goldman B: A cure for cancer quackery needed, conference told.
Canadian Medical Association Journal 136:1295–1296, 1987.
Summarizes discussion of quackery and treatment of cancer at a conference of the Canadian Cancer Society. Offers tips for spotting quacks and helping patients cope with their cancer. Urges oncologists to take chances and follow hunches in their treatment of cancer as they may discover new remedies that work.

Hurst J: Hope sold at clinics of Tijuana.
Los Angeles Times, October 22, 1987.
Describes the facilities and claims made for the treatment at several clinics offering "alternative" treatments for cancer and arthritis. Follows up on three former patients. One died of a treatable disease, another had intestinal obstruction misdiagnosed as "candidiasis," and the third was a child whose cancer was probably cured by conventional radiation therapy, but whose mother credited his treatment at a Mexican clinic.

Hurst J: Paying for the unorthodox treatments in Tijuana.
Los Angeles Times, October 23, 1987.
Describes how an agency attempted to secure payment from insurance companies by submitting what an insurance executive described as "misleading:" claim forms for "alternative" treatments. Describes how one woman received payments covering two weeks when she was no longer at the clinic. Describes how a reporter sent one of the clinics blood samples from himself, a cat , and a chicken, and was told that he had an "aggressive cancer," a liver inflammation, a "prelymphomic condition," and "latent" cancer.

Kill KA: Unproven cancer therapies.
American Pharmacy NS28:18–22, February 1988.
Notes that the word "unproven" is considered by some to be a euphemism for quackery. Advises pharmacists and other health care practitioners who deal with cancer patients to be aware of unproven treatments for cancer and suggests ways in which pharmacists can counsel such patients. Discusses the promotion of unproven methods and the reasons patients resort to them. Lists, but does not examine, 63 examples of unproven cancer treatments and offers 11 tips on how to recognize an unproven therapy. Describes hazards of unconventional treatments.

Cassileth BR, Brown H:. Unorthodox cancer medicine.
Ca – A Cancer Journal for Clinicians 38:176–186, 1988.
Explores why people choose unorthodox cancer treatments, noting the interest people have in controlling their own medical treatment. Notes that many forms of

cancer are still not curable, hence their victims are willing to try anything that might work. Mentions major unorthodox treatments of the nineteenth and twentieth centuries. Surveys a range of current unproven therapies, including metabolic therapy, special diets, megavitamins, and mental imagery. Offers suggestions to physicians for helping patients who go to "alternative" practitioners.

Danielson KJ, Stewart DE, Lippert GP: Unconventional cancer remedies.
Canadian Medical Association Journal 138:1005–1011, 1988.
Explores factors influencing people to choose unproven methods for treatment of cancer. Briefly describes some treatments. Notes the similar interest in unproven methods on the part of patients with AIDS. Mentions risks involved in using alternative treatments. Notes that unproven cancer treatments share four characteristics: promise, pseudoscience, profit, and philosophy. Offers suggestions to physicians for helping patients who choose to utilize alternative medical services.

The promise of a cure: how far will people go?
Coping 2:10–15, Summer, 1988.
Explores the debate over the use of alternative cancer therapies and describes treatments at cancer clinics in Tijuana, Mexico and elsewhere. Mentions the Gerson clinic, the Hoxsey clinic, immunoaugmentive therapy (IAT). Quotes opinions by practitioners, patients, mainstream critics, and advocates.

An element of faddism: NCI researcher investigates cure claims.
Coping 2:16, Summer, 1988.
Notes that many alternative cancer therapies parallel advances in scientific medicine. Describes the interest in device-oriented treatments in the 1940s and 1950s when mainstream medicine relied on radiation therapy, and the popularity of krebiozen and then laetrile in the 1960s and 1970s when chemotherapy became the accepted treatment in conventional medicine. Briefly describes the Hoxsey treatment, krebiozen, laetrile, immunoaugmentive therapy (IAT), antineoplastons, and metabolic therapies.

Mogadam M: Cancer and nutritional misconceptions: A perspective.
American Journal of Gastroenterology 88:1346–1351, 1988.
Argues that studies have shown little or no association between diet and risk of cancer. Surveys claims by nutritionists and faddists regarding cancer risk or prevention due to intake of fat and red meat, fiber, vegetables and fruits, caffeine, Vitamins C and E, calcium, gene dysregulation, and high energy intake diets. Concludes that most of the claims are misleading and urges that people follow a sensible diet to maintain weight at or just below the ideal body weight.

Cassileth BR: The social implications of questionable cancer therapies.
Ca – A Cancer Journal for Clinicians 39:311–316, 1989.
Surveys the history of alternative theories of healing, especially as they relate to cancer. Discusses the appeal of current versions of alternative medicine with their reliance on self-control of one's own health and treatment. Notes the belief that individuals control their own destiny and can heal themselves if they have a will to live. Questions this belief in the face of scientific evidence regarding disease and its treatment and the survival of those with a disease.

Sikora K: Complementary medicine and cancer treatment.
The Practitioner 233:1285–1286, 1989.
Reports on the use of twelve types of alternative or complementary medical treatments as an adjunct to conventional therapies by oncologists at the Royal Postgraduate Medical School's Hammersmith Hospital in London. Describes the use of counseling, information centers, group support, relaxation, and visualization as means of helping patients cope with chemotherapy and radiation therapy. Provides no data on effectiveness.

Lowenthal RM: Can cancer be cured by meditation and "natural therapy"?
A critical review of the book You Can Conquer Cancer *by Ian Gawler.*
Medical Journal of Australia 151:710–715, 1989.
Reviews a book which argues that cancer can be cured by meditation. The reviewer agrees that meditation may offer some benefits to patients but argues that there is no scientific evidence that meditation or any other psychological factor will affect survival in cases of cancer. Notes inconsistency in popular claims that survival is increased in those who are hostile to the disease when the aim of meditation is to help patients become adjusted to the disease and less hostile. Also notes inconsistencies in the author's claims regarding his own treatment for cancer and for those who follow his recommendations. Mentions some hazards of some of the author's recommended approaches.

Read MH, St. Jeor S, Seymour K, et al: Supplementation
practices of a group of patients with cancer.
Journal of the American Dietetic Association 90:278–279, 1990.
Describes a study of 32 cancer patients who were interviewed regarding their use of dietary supplements or herbs. Reports that 24 of them were using vitamin/mineral supplements and 21 were using herbs. Concludes that use of such products may be higher among cancer patients than among the general population. Suggests that dietitians question cancer patients about their use of supplements because they have no proven effectiveness and might be harmful.

Baginal FS, Easton DF, Harris E, et al: Survival of patients with breast cancer attending Bristol Cancer Help Center.
Lancet 336:606–610, 1990.
Describes a study of patients with breast cancer at the Bristol Cancer Help Center, an "alternative" medical center that offered counseling, "healing," a vegetarian diet, homeopathy, acupuncture, and various other therapies said to enhance quality of life and to help develop a positive attitude toward cancer. Reports that patients at the Bristol Center had significantly lower survival and metastasis-free survival than matched control patients treated at conventional hospitals.

Tobias J: Surely a natural cancer remedy can't be dangerous—can it?
British Medical Journal 301:613, 1990.
Comments further on the above study, noting that he has seen patients who have lost substantial amounts of weight on the restrictive diet. Labels as arrogant the attitude of "alternative" proponents who insist that an unproven diet has central importance in their treatment approach.

Richmond C: Report on UK cancer survival rates raises questions about alternative medicine.
Canadian Medical Association Journal 143:922–923, 1990.
Discusses the popularity of the Bristol Cancer Help Center, which uses "alternative" methods, including a strict vegetarian diet, to treat cancer. Reports on the abovementioned study, which found that the clinic's patients fared much less well than those who used conventional methods. Notes reactions to the study by the clinic's staff and by conventional physicians.

Gelband H et al: Unconventional cancer treatments.
Washington, DC, U.S. Government Printing Office, 1990.
By far the most comprehensive study of "alternative" cancer treatments ever published. Contains detailed analyses backed by almost 1,000 references. Indicates that proponents rarely if ever collect analyzable follow-up data on their patients. Copies [GPO stock number 052-003-01207-3] can be obtained for $14 from the Superintendent of Documents, Government Printing Office, Washington, DC 20402.

Fintor L: OTA Report disputes success of unconventional cancer therapies.
Journal of the National Cancer Institute 82:1668–1669, 1990.
Reports on a study of unconventional cancer therapies by the congressional Office of Technology Assessment (OTA). They report that claims made by proponents of even the most promising treatments are far more extravagant than the evidence supports. Discusses the debate over the report's fairness and its proposal for allocation of

funds to study unconventional cancer therapies. Notes that Lawrence Burton, an alternative practitioner whose practice is based in the Bahamas and who promoted immunoaugmentive therapy (IAT), refused to cooperate with the investigation study team.

Barrett S, Cassileth BR: Dubious cancer treatment: A report on "alternative" methods and the patients and practitioners who use them.
Tampa, FL, American Cancer Society, Florida Division, 1991.
Updates information presented at a 1977 seminar sponsored by the American Cancer Society. Covers how treatments are proven, promotion of dubious treatments, reasons for their use, ethical considerations, historical trends, dubious credentials of certain promoters, Mexican cancer clinics, immuno-augmentative therapy, mental imagery, perspective on vitamin C, how quackery harms, legal and insurance issues, and the need for more antiquackery action.

Cassileth BR: Counseling the cancer patient who wants to try unorthodox or questionable therapies.
Primary Care & Cancer, pp. 53–60, September 1991.
Describes why patients turn to unorthodox methods and suggests that counseling be based on the reasons for their interest in the method(s) under consideration.

Questionable cancer practices in Tijuana and other Mexican border clinics.
Ca – A Cancer Journal for Clinicians 41:310–319, 1991.
Summarizes questionable therapies used at Mexican border clinics that cater to clients from the United States. Notes that most use some form of "metabolic therapy." Describes the variations used by each clinic as well as some dubious diagnostic methods. Discusses hazards and strongly urges avoidance of these clinics.

Hunter M: Alternative dietary therapies in cancer patients.
Recent Results in Cancer Research 121:293–295, 1991.
Lists various types of dietary regimes used in treatment of cancer and disadvantages associated with them. Explains how some such diets may achieve modest success due to the placebo effect. Argues that alternative diets are not nutritional therapy, but a form of psychotherapy.

Gelb L: Unproven cancer treatments: help or hoax?
FDA Consumer 26:10–15, March 1992.
Debunks the concepts of freedom of choice and the "gambler's fallacy," which suggest that terminally ill patients have nothing to lose by trying unproven treatments. Describes the difference between responsible experimentation and patient exploitation.

Lerner IJ, Kennedy BJ: The prevalence of questionable methods of cancer treatment in the United States.
Ca – A Cancer Journal for Clinicians 42:181–191, 1992.
Reports that 452 (9 percent) of 5047 cancer patients identified through a telephone survey had used questionable treatments. Notes that 49 percent of these had used "mind therapies" (mental imagery, hypnosis, or psychic therapy) and 38 percent had used diets.

Questionable methods of cancer management.
Atlanta, 1992, American Cancer Society.
Discusses the types, hazards, and promotion of questionable methods and presents various strategies for combatting them. Indicates how patients are misled into thinking that questionable treatments are safe and effective.

Cornacchia HJ, Barrett S: Cancer.
In Cornacchia HJ, Barrett S: Consumer health: A guide to intelligent decisions., 5th edition, pp. 388–408.
St. Louis, Mosby Year Book, 1993.
Presents an overview of unconventional methods of cancer treatment with summaries of today's prevalent methods.

American Cancer Society: Questionable methods of cancer management: Questionable "nutritional" therapies in the treatment of cancer.
Ca – A Cancer Journal for Clinicians (in press).
Notes that although dietary measures may be helpful in preventing certain cancers, no scientific evidence indicates that any dietary approach is appropriate as a primary treatment for cancer. Describes the questionable nature of treatment with high-dosage vitamin C, pau d'arco tea, the Gerson diet, Hoxsey herbal therapy, the macrobiotic diet, Manner metabolic therapy, and Kelly metabolic therapy. Some of these involve a diet that is nutritionally inadequate. Some involve potentially toxic doses of vitamins and/or other substances. Some are quite expensive. All pose the risk that patients who use them will abandon effective treatment.

Diet and Cancer Prevention

Although it has been found that diet may play a role in the prevention of certain cancers, supplementation with vitamins, minerals, or fiber should not be regarded as a substitute for eating an adequate diet. Nor should any dietary regimen be relied upon as a primary means of attempting to *treat* cancer.

NAS Committee on Diet, Nutrition, and Cancer: Diet, nutrition, and cancer.
Washington, D.C., 1982, National Academy of Sciences.
Examines evidence relating diet to cancer and makes "interim recommendations" to limit fat consumption, consume a diet with plenty of whole-grain cereals and fruits and vegetables, especially those rich in vitamin C and beta-carotene. But cautions that since it is not known which dietary factors, if any, might be helpful, supplementation with individual nutrients is not advisable.

Ballentine C: On cabbages and cancer.
FDA Consumer 18:29–30, April 1984.
Reports on action taken by the FDA against PharmTech Research, a firm that sold Daily Greens, a dietary supplement product containing dehydrated vegetables and various nutrients. The FDA seized supplies of the product, which was promoted as a preventive against cancer, and ordered the company to cease misrepresentations of the product. The FTC and the Pennsylvania Department of health also took regulatory action. The product was advertised with claims that it was based on recommendations of the National Academy of Sciences' report on diet and cancer. However, as noted above, the report recommended against taking supplements of these nutrients because it was not known which components, if any, of the diet might be effective.

American Cancer Society guidelines on diet, nutrition, and cancer.
Ca – A Cancer Journal for Clinicians 41: 334–338, 1991.
Updates the Society's recommendations for a total dietary pattern for reducing cancer risk: (1) maintain a desirable body weight; (2) eat a varied diet; (3) include a variety of both vegetables and fruits in the daily diet; (4) eat more high-fiber foods, such as whole grains, cereals, legumes, vegetables and fruits; (5) cut down on total fat intake; (6) limit consumption of alcoholic beverages, if you drink at all; and (7) limit consumption of salt-cured, smoked, and nitrite-preserved foods. Also addresses a variety of items that have received much attention but do not warrant firm recommendations at this time: food additives ("at most only a small contribution to increased cancer risk"); vitamin E (more research needed); selenium (supplement use not recommended); artificial sweeteners; coffee (no indication that moderate use of caffeine is unsafe); serum cholesterol (any link with cancer remains inconclusive); and cooking meat at high temperatures (animal tests demonstrate that frying, broiling, and grilling produce substances that can cause cancer and DNA damage in experimental animals).

Kritchevsky D: Diet and cancer.
Ca – A Cancer Journal for Clinicians 41:328–333, 1991.

Notes that dietary fibers have value beyond their possible role in preventing colon cancer and discourages the use of fiber supplements. Emphasizes that "a high-fiber diet is not merely a low-fiber diet with fiber added. . . . All components of diets containing fiber-rich foods are important."

Antineoplastons

In the late 1960s, Stanislaw R. Burzynski, MD, PhD, developed a theory that a naturally occurring and continuously functioning biochemical system in the body, distinct from the immune system, could "correct" cancer cells by means of "special chemicals that reprogram misdirected cells." He called these chemicals antineoplastons and said they were naturally occurring peptides and amino acid derivatives that inhibit the growth of malignant cells while leaving normal cells unaffected. He developed a course of treatment for cancer based on antineoplastons, which he originally extracted from urine and later manufactured in his laboratory. His facility, the Burzynski Research Institute, is located in Houston, Texas. He and his colleagues at the institute have published more than 100 papers in which they report on animal and biochemical studies of antineoplastons, as well as their use in cancer patients. At a seminar in 1990 Dr. Burzynski announced that he had begun treating patients with AIDS. In 1992, the Texas Attorney General filed suit to stop the Burzynski Institute from selling, distributing, or advertising antineoplastons in Texas. The case is still pending.

Antineoplastons.
Atlanta, 1982, American Cancer Society.
Describes Dr. Burzynski's background and claims. States that the American Cancer Society does not have evidence that treatment with antineoplastons results in objective benefit to cancer patients. Urges individuals afflicted with cancer not to participate in treatment with antineoplastons.

Stanislaw Burzynski: Antineoplastons.
In Gelband H et al: Unconventional cancer treatments, pp. 91–97.
Washington, D.C., U.S. Government Printing Office, 1990.
Summarizes Dr. Burzynski's theories and research reports. Describes tests done by the National Cancer Institute in 1983 and 1985 that found no antitumor effect of three of Burzynski's antineoplastons. Discusses an evaluation by Canadian health officials who visited the Burzynski Institute and reported no evidence of benefit among 16 patients whom they reviewed. Discusses a study by the Canadian Bureau of Prescription Drugs, which found no objective benefit among 36 cases reported to it. Concludes that there is insufficient information to judge whether the treatment is likely to benefit cancer patients.

Green S: 'Antineoplastons': An unproved cancer therapy.
JAMA 267:2924–2928, 1992.
Provides detailed information and raises many questions about Dr. Burzynski's background, credentials, theories, research, and published reports. Concludes that "none of Dr. Burzynski's publications between 1964 and 1990 contain objective experimental evidence supporting the postulate that a naturally occurring antineoplastic biochemical surveillance system exists in humans." Also concludes that antineoplastons are not peptides and that "none of the independent tests carried out with antineoplastons in experimental tumor systems have shown anticancer activity."

Gerson Cancer Therapy

The Gerson cancer treatment was developed by Dr. Max Gerson, a German-born physician who moved to the United States where he offered his treatment until his death in 1959. During his lifetime, he and his treatment were the subject of much controversy. In 1977, his daughter, Charlotte Gerson Straus, along with Norman Fritz, co-founded the Gerson Institute, in Bonita, California, which then established a clinic in Tijuana, Mexico. The clinic treats about 600 patients yearly. Imitators have spread the Gerson therapy to other countries.

The theory of the Gerson treatment is that cancer can only be cured if toxins are eliminated from the body. The treatment utilizes coffee enemas to help "detoxify" the system. Patients must follow a strict special diet for several years and avoid all meat, fish, dairy products, nuts, berries, drinking water, coffee, salt, oil, and all foods that are bottled, canned, preserved, or frozen. Various other treatments, including laetrile, have been added in recent years.

Scientific medicine considers the Gerson treatment as unproven and sometimes dangerous. Dr. Gerson himself reported some deaths due to liver damage. Deaths have also been reported due to the coffee enemas administered in the Tijuana clinic. The clinic's use of raw calf liver juice in its treatment has led to infections with *Campylobacter fetus,* an organism living in the intestinal tract of cattle and sheep. Several such infections have proved fatal. The National Cancer Institute analyzed Dr. Gerson's book *A Cancer Therapy: Results of Fifty Cases* concluded in 1959 that most of the cases failed to meet the criteria (such as histologic verification of cancer) for proper evaluation of a cancer case.

Lowell J: The Gerson Clinic.
Nutrition Forum 3:9–12, February 1986.
Describes the author's visit to the Gerson clinic and promotional activities of clinic

publicists. Discusses the components and hazards of the treatment. Notes lack of laboratory and other diagnostic facilities at the clinic. Notes that although promoters claim high cure rates, they actually have no organized system for following patients after they leave the clinic.

Unproven methods of cancer management, Gerson method.
Ca – A Cancer Journal for Clinicians 40:252–256, 1990.
Reviews the theory behind the Gerson regime. Describes dietary restrictions and utilization of coffee, castor oil and other enemas. Describes daily medications such as royal jelly and sometimes laetrile. Notes side effects of treatment. Describes career of Dr. Max Gerson and establishment of the Gerson Institute and the clinic by his daughter, Charlotte Gerson Straus. Reviews efforts to evaluate the Gerson therapy. Discusses instances of serious illness and death resulting from treatment at the Gerson clinic.

Reed A, James N, Sikora K: Mexico: juices, coffee enemas, and cancer.
Lancet 336:677–678, 1990.
Reports on a study of the Gerson regimen by three British researchers. Mentions the vegetarian diet and coffee enemas prescribed by the clinic. Lists various numbers of patients by type of cancer and clinical course. Notes that there was little objective evidence that the Gerson therapy is effective in treating cancer, but that patients felt a high control over their health and thus have more self-confidence. Argues that these approaches suggest ways in which oncologists can help desperate cancer patients manage their cancer.

The Gerson treatment.
In Gelband H et al: Unconventional cancer treatments, pp. 44–51.
Washington, DC, U.S. Government Printing Office, 1990.
Surveys the history of the Gerson therapy, including a brief biographical sketch of Dr. Gerson. Describes the treatment and the theory behind it. Notes claims of effectiveness. Reviews studies of the therapy undertaken by various researchers. Notes the hazards of coffee enemas and of Campylobacter infections attributed to the clinic's use of raw calf liver juice [no longer used].

Greek Cancer Cure

The principal proponent of the Greek Cancer Cure was microbiologist Dr. Hariton-Tzannis Alivizatos, of Athens, Greece, who died in 1991. The same treatment is allegedly used at the Hospital Del Mar in Tijuana, Mexico, although Dr. Alivizatos denied any connection with that institution. Dr. Alivizatos used a blood test that he claimed would diagnose the location and extent of a person's cancer. Treatment then consisted of a serum injected daily into the patient's body for six to thirty days. Dr. Alivizatos claimed that the serum boosted the body's natural immune system and helped rid the body of cancer. He advised patients to follow a diet low in salts and acids, to limit their physical activities, and to avoid certain drugs such as aspirin and laxatives. He further advised them to discontinue all chemotherapy and radiation programs before beginning his treatment.

Dr. Alivizatos was in trouble with regulatory officials in Greece on several occasions. For a time, he lost his license to practice medicine in Greece due to failure to submit his serum to the government for testing. He regained it when he submitted the substance. The Greek government asked him not to use the serum because they could not establish that it was effective against cancer. His license was again suspended in 1983 for two years following an investigation by the Hellenic Medical Association. Following his suspension, he resumed treating cancer patients. The American Cancer Society and the National Cancer Institute asked Dr. Alivizatos several times to submit information on how his treatment worked, but he never replied. He also refused to divulge the composition of his blood test or the serum that he injected into patients.

Seattle surgeon Ross Fox, MD, who was president of the Washington division of the American Cancer Society, traveled to Greece posing as a cancer patient in order to investigate the treatment. He managed to obtain some serum samples that later were analyzed at the University of Washington. The serum turned out to be nicotinic acid (niacin), a B-vitamin. Although Dr. Alivizatos claimed to cure most of his patients, many died within a few months after returning home.

Chazottes M: Exposed! Greek quack duped many cancer victims.
The Medical Post (Toronto), p. 38, July 23, 1985.
Describes how Dr. Fox posed as a cancer patient to gain admittance to Dr. Alivizatos's clinic, where he secured samples of the serum. Mentions several patients who were at the clinic in various stages of terminal cancer, some of whom would have benefitted from treatment by an oncologist.

Dugan WM Jr: Cancer corner.
Indiana Medicine 81:1046, 1988.
Notes the popularity of the Greek Cancer Cure and the lack of evidence that it was effective. Identifies three reasons why patients develop false beliefs in questionable methods. Offers tips on how physicians can help cancer patients who are thinking of trying an unproven method.

Cancer treatments questioned, man loses wife weeks after cure told.
The Dispatch (Cookeville, Tennessee) 26:1–2, January 15, 1989.
Relates the experience of a retired couple from Cookeville who traveled to Greece for treatment of the woman's lung cancer. Discusses the wife's treatment by Dr. Alivizatos and his use of blood tests to diagnose cancer and monitor progress. Describes how two other patients were told that they were cured but actually remained very ill.

Unproven methods of cancer management, Greek Cancer Cure.
Ca – A Cancer Journal for Clinicians 40:368–371, 1990.
Describes the methods used by Dr. Alivizatos in treating cancer patients. Discusses efforts by Greek medical officials to curtail his activities. Notes the lack of medical literature supporting the effectiveness of his treatment. Warns against using the Greek Cancer Cure as a treatment for cancer or any other disease.

Loschiavo SR: The danger of unrecognized cancer treatment clinics.
Journal of the National Cancer Institute 83:212–213, 1991.
Letter to the editor by the father of a deceased cancer patient. Describes his son's treatment by Dr. Alivizatos' clinic and the suffering that preceded the son's death. Warns cancer victims to avoid clinics offering unproven methods of fighting cancer.

Hoxsey Cancer Treatment

The Hoxsey cancer treatment is an herbal treatment developed by the late Harry Hoxsey. It was offered at clinics in the United States from 1924 until repeated clashes with the Food and Drug Administration (FDA) led Hoxsey to close his main clinic in Dallas in the late 1950s. Since 1963, it has been available only at a clinic in Tijuana, Mexico, operated by Hoxsey's former chief nurse, Mildred Nelson. Hoxsey himself contracted prostate cancer in 1967. After treating himself unsuccessfully with his tonic, he underwent conventional surgery. He died in 1974. The treatment includes two externally used pastes and a tonic taken by mouth. Most of the herbs in the tonic have been tested for antitumor activity in cancer, with negligible results for a few and no results for the others. Some of these herbs, most notably pokeroot, have toxic side effects. The National Cancer Institute evaluated case reports submitted by Hoxsey and concluded that no assessment could be made because the records did not contain adequate information.

Young, JH: The medical messiahs.
Princeton, Princeton University Press, 1967, 1992.
Provides a comprehensive account of Hoxsey's activities.

The Hoxsey treatment.
In Gelband H et al: Unconventional cancer treatments, pp. 75–81.
Washington, DC, U.S. Government Printing Office, 1990.
Reviews the career of Harry Hoxsey and his treatment for cancer. Describes the treatment rationale and Hoxsey's views on the nature of cancer. Examines the components of the treatment and reviews results of tests on herbs used in the tonic. Mentions some toxic side effects of the treatment. Notes the lack of clinical trials of the treatment. Describes an unfavorable evaluation made during the late 1950s by a faculty group from the University of British Columbia.

Lowell JA: Hoxsey treatment still available.
Nutrition Forum 4:89–91, December 1987.
Relates an account of a visit to the Bio-Medical Center in Tijuana, Mexico, a clinic offering the Hoxsey treatment. Briefly reviews the career of Harry Hoxsey and his treatment. Describes the clinic, the course of treatment, and the costs involved. Notes hazards of using escharotic pastes, which will burn off healthy tissue as well as tumors. Describes ingredients of the tonic. Notes three patients who were treated without success by the clinic. Notes that although Mildred Nelson claimed a high cure rate, she said she did not know how many patients she treats each year.

Unproven methods of cancer management, Hoxsey method/Bio-Medical Center.
Ca-A Cancer Journal for Clinicians 40:51–55, 1990.
Examines the Hoxsey cancer treatment. Briefly reviews the career of Harry Hoxsey and the development of his treatment. Describes the ingredients of his medications and notes hazards associated with the use of some of them. Discusses investigations of the treatment that showed no evidence it was effective against cancer.

Immunoaugmentative Therapy (IAT)

Immuno-augmentative therapy was developed by Lawrence Burton, PhD, a zoologist who states that IAT can control all forms of cancer by restoring natural immune defenses. He claims to accomplish this by injecting protein extracts isolated with processes he has patented. However, experts believe that the substances he claims to use cannot be produced by these procedures and have not been demonstrated to exist in the human body. He has not published detailed clinical reports, divulged the details of his methods, published meaningful statistics, conducted a controlled trial, or provided independent investigators with specimens of his treatment materials for analysis. During the mid-1980s, several cases were reported of patients of Dr. Burton who developed serious infections following IAT. Burton now operates clinics in the Bahamas, Mexico, and Germany.

Nolen, WA. Dr. William Nolen challenges unorthodox healers.
50 Plus, pp. 43–45, 70–71, November 1983.
William A. Nolen, MD, who visited Burton's clinic in 1982, reviewed many records and had follow-up conversations with at least ten patients and some of their doctors. Dr. Nolen concluded that most of the patients had never had cancer or had tumors that typically grow slowly, while some had undergone conventional treatment that was probably responsible for any positive results.

Barnes C: Testimony before the Subcommittee on Health and Long-Term Care of the U.S. House of Representatives Select Committee on Aging.
In Pepper C et al: Quackery: a $10 billion scandal.
Washington, D.C., U.S. Government Printing Office, pp. 37–39, 1984.
Pathologist Carl Barnes, MD, describes the experience of his father-in-law who underwent treatment for lung cancer at Lawrence Burton's Bahamas facility and was told that the treatment was shrinking his tumor. The man returned home euphoric, convinced he was cured, but died two months later. Dr. Barnes noted that the x-ray film used to make this pronouncement had been overexposed, making the tumor appear smaller than it really was.

Centers for Disease Control: Cutaneous nocardiosis in cancer patients receiving immunotherapy injections – Bahamas.
Morbidity and Mortality Weekly Report 33:471–472, 477, 1984.
Reports on sixteen people who attended the immunoaugmentative therapy (IAT) clinic in the Bahamas and developed abscesses at injection sites after being treated with subcutaneous injections of human serum proteins. Describes procedure for preparation of the injections by the clinic. Notes that investigators found that none of the vials of injection material was sterile. Although they could not identify any environmental source of contamination, they noted that the protein production area where the injections were prepared was adjacent to rooms housing laboratory mice used for research.

Centers for Disease Control: Isolation of human T-lymphotropic virus type III lymphadenopathy-associated virus from serum proteins given to cancer patients – Bahamas.
Morbidity and Mortality Weekly Report 34:489–491, 1985.
Reports on the presence of the virus that causes AIDS in vials of serum proteins distributed to cancer patients at the immunoaugmentative therapy (IAT) clinic in the Bahamas. Reviews previous tests showing evidence of contamination of these vials with this virus and with hepatitis B. Notes that two of Burton's patients contracted hepatitis. Suggests that although no cases of AIDS have been discovered, Burton's

patients might be at risk of acquiring AIDS and hepatitis B infections from Burton's injectable protein materials.

Curt GA, Katterhagen G, Mahaney FX: Immunoaugmentative therapy, a primer on the perils of unproved treatments.
JAMA 255:505–507, 1986.
Describes the treatment and the theory behind it. Lists and analyzes some treatment materials used in immunoaugmentative therapy (IAT), noting evidence of contamination of some IAT products with hepatitis B. Reviews investigations of the clinic and its operations, noting conclusions that IAT is an unproven theory and that IAT products have been a source of infection with hepatitis B and possibly AIDS.

Nightingale SL: Immunoaugmentative therapy.
American Family Physician 34:159–160, 1986.
Reviews the development of immunoaugmentative therapy (IAT) and the history of the clinic Burton established to offer his treatment. Describes the treatment. Notes health hazards arising from contamination of vials of blood serum proteins with bacterial and viral infections. Notes that the clinic in the Bahamas was closed for a time after discovery of contaminated injections which were intended for use in cancer patients. Urges physicians to warn patients using IAT of health hazards arising from the use of these products.

AMA Diagnostic and Therapeutic Technology Assessment (DATTA).
Immunoaugmentative therapy.
JAMA 259:3477–3478, 1988.
Report of the American Medical Association's Department of Technology Assessment on immunoaugmentative therapy. Of 27 panelists who commented on effectiveness, none rated IAT "established," 6 (22 percent) called it "investigational," 16 (59 percent) "unacceptable," and 5 (19 percent) "indeterminate." Of 26 panelists who commented on safety, none rated IAT "established," 6 (23 percent) called it "investigational," 19 (73 percent) "unacceptable," and 1 (4 percent) "indeterminate." Report also provides a brief history of IAT.

Nightingale SL: Immunoaugmentative therapy:
Assessing an untested therapy.
JAMA 259:3457–3458, 1989.
Referring to the AMA DATTA report, an FDA official urges physicians to be aware of the hazards of IAT so they can adequately counsel patients who may be considering the treatment. Notes that although Burton once applied for FDA permission to carry out clinical studies of IAT, he did not submit an adequate protocol.

Immunoaugmentative therapy.
JAMA 260:3435–3437, 1988.
Letters to the editor from two IAT promoters and the OTA report project manager, and a response from an AMA official.

Immunoaugmentative therapy.
In Gelband H et al: Unconventional cancer treatments, pp. 127–147.
Washington, DC, U.S. Government Printing Office, 1990.
Reviews the career of Lawrence Burton, PhD, his development of IAT, and the opening of clinics to offer the treatment to cancer victims. Describes the treatment in its various forms and explains the theory behind it. Notes that some IAT products were found to be contaminated with hepatitis B and sometimes AIDS, though when some patients developed hepatitis B or AIDS, it was not determined how they were infected. Discusses the unsuccessful efforts of OTA officials to develop a protocol acceptable to Burton for testing IAT.

Marshall E: OTA peers into cancer therapy fog.
Science 249:1369, 1990.
Discusses the initiation of the OTA report and some of the controversy it engendered.

Zavertnik J. Immuno-augmentative therapy.
In Barrett S and Cassileth BR (eds): Dubious cancer treatment, pp. 63–71.
Tampa, FL, American Cancer Society, Florida Division 1990.
Presents evidence that Burton's theories are incorrect. Describes how MetPath Laboratories began testing Burton's treatment materials, but soon concluded that the project would be fruitless. Describes proponents' drive to gain legalization of IAT in Florida in 1982 and why the law was repealed two years later. Concludes that Bahamian health authorities acted irresponsibly in permitting Burton's clinic to remain open.

Questionable methods of cancer management:
Immuno-augmentative therapy (IAT).
Ca – A Cancer Journal for Clinicians 41:357–364, 1991.
Describes the professional career of Dr. Burton and the history of his treatment program. Notes that efforts by the congressional Office of Technology Assessment (OTA) to test IAT in clinical trials failed when Burton insisted that a pre-test be conducted at his clinic in the Bahamas. Debunks Burton's claims regarding the effectiveness of IAT and how it works. Notes that 35 case reports in a clinic brochure did not contain sufficient information to determine IAT's effectiveness and that most of them had received conventional treatment before undergoing IAT. Concludes that there is no scientific evidence that IAT is a safe or effective cancer therapy.

Laetrile

Laetrile, which achieved great notoriety during the 1970s and early 1980s, is the trade name for a synthetic relative of amygdalin, a cyanide-containing chemical in the kernels of apricot pits, apple seeds, bitter almonds, and some other stone fruits and nuts. Many laetrile promoters have called it "vitamin B_{17}," and claimed that cancer is a vitamin deficiency disease that laetrile can cure.

Laetrile was developed by Ernst T. Krebs, Sr., MD, and his son Ernst T. Krebs, Jr., and was first used to treat cancer patients in California in the 1950s. According to proponents, laetrile kills tumor cells selectively, while leaving normal cells alone. Although laetrile has been promoted as safe and effective, clinical evidence indicates that it is neither.

Some cancer patients who have been treated with laetrile have suffered nausea, vomiting, headache and dizziness, and a few have died from cyanide poisoning. Laetrile has been tested in at least twenty animal tumor models and found to have no benefit either alone or together with other substances. Several reviews of cases have found no benefit for the treatment of cancer in humans. And a clinical trial conducted at the Mayo Clinic and three other prominent cancer centers found no anticancer effect but found significant blood levels of cyanide in some of the patients.

Laetrile's popularity faded in the early 1980s following the Mayo Clinic study and the U.S. Supreme Court's rejection of the argument that drugs offered for terminal cancer patients should be exempt from regulation by the FDA. Laetrile is still offered as a component of "metabolic therapy" at Mexican cancer clinics.

Laetrile: The Commissioner's decision. HEW Publication No. 77-3056. Washington, DC, Department of Health, Education, and Welfare, 1977.
Following thorough review and a two-day public hearing, the FDA Commissioner concluded that (1) laetrile is not generally recognized by qualified experts as a safe and effective cancer drug, and (2) laetrile is not exempt from premarket review and thus may not be legally marketed in interstate commerce. The Commissioner's report, published on August 5, 1977, in the *Federal Register* and later as a booklet, covered the chemistry of laetrile, claims by its proponents, theories about its actions, similarities in the promotion of "unproven" cancer remedies, reasons for laetrile's use, and the freedom-of-choice issue.

Laetrile background information.
New York, 1977, American Cancer Society.
Provides a comprehensive analysis of claims made for laetrile and facts that rebut

them. Describes shifting theories about laetrile's alleged mechanism of action, propaganda techniques used by proponents, dangers of laetrile, and studies in laboratory animals.

Laetrile: The political success of a scientific failure.
Consumer Reports 42:444-447, 1977.
Debunks various ploys used to promote laetrile. Notes why testimonials are not evidence of cure and states why consumers need government protection from quackery.

Top officials cite laetrile dangers.
FDA Consumer 11:3-4, September 1977.
Cites testimony at a Congressional hearing that documented 37 cases of poisoning and 17 deaths related to laetrile. Notes that potency varies considerably from sample to sample and that some samples have been found to contain impurities and bacterial contamination.

Young JH: Laetrile in historical perspective.
In Merkle GE, Petersen JC (eds): Politics, science,
and cancer: The laetrile phenomenon.
Boulder, CO, 1980, Westview Press.
Provides a detailed history of the origins and promotion of laetrile. Lists the typical patterns of cancer unorthodoxies, including (1) exploitation of fear, (2) promise of painless and effective treatment, (3) claims of a miraculous breakthrough, (4) one cause/one therapeutic system, (5) conspiracy theory, (6) shifting claims, (7) reliance on testimonials, (8) distortion of the idea of "freedom," and (10) involvement of large sums of money.

Lerner IJ: Laetrile: A lesson in cancer quackery.
Ca – A Cancer Journal for Clinicians 31:91–95, 1981.
Describes the promotional techniques and commercial success of laetrile. Concludes that it had "achieved unprecedented triumph by capitalizing on a unique sociopolitical climate characterized by a growing hostility towards 'the establishment,' a demand for simple solutions, and frustration with the inability to solve the cancer riddle. It is also directed by sophisticated, radical political machinery, and funded by enormous profits."

Vissing MV, Petersen JC: Taking laetrile: conversion to medical deviance.
Ca – A Cancer Journal for Clinicians 31:365–369, 1981.
Reports on a study of participants in a local chapter of the Cancer Control Society, an organization that promotes questionable cancer treatments. Concludes that

friendships and sharing of experiences between users and potential users play a large role in the development of interest in laetrile and other questionable methods. Distrust of doctors also plays a role.

Herbert V: Laetrile: the cult of cyanide. In Nutrition cultism: facts and fictions. Philadelphia, 1981, The George F. Stickley Co.
Describes laetrile's chemistry and adverse effects. Provides case reports of people harmed and details the legal difficulties of laetrile's promoters.

Moertel CG, Fleming TR, Rubin J, et al: A clinical trial of amygdalin (laetrile) in the treatment of human cancer. New England Journal of Medicine 306:201-206, 1982.
Reports on a laetrile clinical trial of 178 patients. States that only one had a partial response, but died of cancer 37 weeks after beginning the therapy. Notes that many of the patients suffered side effects symptomatic of cyanide poisoning.

Relman AS: Closing the books on laetrile. New England Journal of Medicine 306:236, 1982.
Noting the above study, the journal's editor comments that, "Laetrile . . . has had its day in court. The evidence, beyond reasonable doubt, is that it doesn't benefit patients with advanced cancer, and there is no reason to believe that it would be any more effective in the earlier stages of the disease. Some undoubtedly will remain unconvinced, but no sensible person will want to advocate its further use and no state legislature should sanction it any longer. The time has come to close the books on laetrile and get on with our efforts to understand the riddle of cancer and improve its prevention and treatment."

Lerner IJ: The whys of cancer quackery. Cancer 53:815-819, 1984.
Explores reasons for the popularity of cancer quackery in general and laetrile in particular. Suggests that many people turn to unorthodox therapies either out of fear or an antiestablishment feeling. Observes that "people are not wont to defend themselves from panic with calmly reasoned scientific approaches. . . . Even when they understand it is not sensible, they are enormously tempted to indulge in magic thinking, to seize a simplistic, safe, apparently certain, perhaps mysterious answer. And this is the essence of successful quackery." Reviews tactics of promoters, ranging from the John Birch Society and similar groups to the practitioners themselves and companies that produce laetrile or otherwise profit from it. Questions the relative passivity of the medical establishment in the face of this challenge, and urges physicians to be more ready to deal with future promotion of quackery.

*Chandler RF, Phillipson JD, Anderson, LA: Cancer
chemotherapy, controversial laetrile.
Pharmaceutical Journal 232:330-332, 1984.*
Identifies laetrile and describes its chemical composition. Reviews claims of anticancer activity and discusses clinical trials showing laetrile to be ineffective in cancer treatment. Discusses laetrile's toxicity and side effects in patients, some of which are fatal.

*Nightingale SL: Laetrile: the regulatory challenge of an unproven remedy.
Public Health Reports 99:333-338, 1984.*
Reviews the attempts by promoters of laetrile, cancer patients, and others to legalize the distribution of laetrile in the United States. Discusses efforts by the FDA to ban laetrile as an unproven drug. Describes activities of the National Cancer Institute in testing laetrile for antitumor activity and safety. Discusses policy issues regarding the regulation of laetrile and other unproven drugs. Notes that any regulatory system carried out by government in a free society functions only so long and so far as the public will allow.

*Wilson B: The rise and fall of laetrile.
Nutrition Forum 5:33-40, May/June, 1988.*
Discusses the origin, rationale, promotion, and scientific evaluation of laetrile, as well as the legal and political struggle to market it. Reviews the roles of leaders of the laetrile movement. Describes the cases of children who died after their parents chose to have them treated with laetrile instead of conventional treatment. Notes that the U.S. Supreme Court rejected the argument that drugs offered to "terminal" patients should be exempted from FDA jurisdiction. Concludes that when unfavorable publicity made laetrile fade from the limelight, its prime movers added many other "miracle cures" to their arsenal and added AIDS, arthritis, cardiovascular disease and multiple sclerosis to the diseases they claim to treat.

*Laetrile.
In Gelband H et al: Unconventional cancer treatments, pp. 102-107.
Washington, D.C., U.S. Government Printing Office, 1990.*
Provides a historical perspective of laetrile, including animal and human studies and case reviews.

*Unproven methods of cancer management: Laetrile.
Ca-A Cancer Journal for Clinicians 41:187–192, 1991.*
Describes the development of laetrile and the rationale behind it. Reviews animal studies, case reviews by the National Cancer Institute, and clinical trials of the

effectiveness and safety of laetrile. Discusses laetrile's toxicity, noting some deaths. Concludes that laetrile is a toxic drug that is not effective as a cancer treatment.

Livingston-Wheeler Therapy

Virginia Livingston-Wheeler, MD, who had an interest in microbiology, postulated that cancer is caused by a bacterium she called *Progenitor cryptocides,* which multiplies and invades the body when resistance is lowered. To combat this, she claimed to strengthen the body's immune system with various vaccines (including one made from the patient's urine); a vegetarian diet that avoids chicken, eggs, and sugar; vitamin and mineral supplements; visualization; and stress reduction. She claimed to have a very high recovery rate but published no clinical data to support this. Attempts by scientists to isolate the organism she postulated were not successful. She died in 1990.

Acevedo HF, Campbell-Acevedo E, Kloos WE: Expression of human choriogonadotropin-like material in coagulase-negative staphylococcus species. Infection and Immunity 50:860–868, 1985.
Discusses a study of bacteria samples from Dr. Livingston's patients and from normal individuals to determine if any could be identified as *Progenitor cryptocides.* All five samples alleged to be *Progenitor cryptocides* were proven to be strains of other bacteria.

State acts to restrict cancer clinic.
San Diego Union, pp. B-1, B-12, February 22, 1990.
Describes how California health authorities ordered the Livingston-Wheeler Clinic to stop administering a vaccine derived from the urine of patients attending the clinic.

Unproven methods of cancer management: Livingston-Wheeler therapy.
Ca-A Cancer Journal for Clinicians 40:103–108, 1990.
Gives a history of the Livingston-Wheeler Clinic and the development of Dr. Livingston's theories and treatment. Mentions several investigations of claims of cures at the clinic and experiments testing whether the bacterium that Dr. Livingston-Wheeler allegedly discovered actually exists. Describes some legal and regulatory actions involving the clinic, including exclusion from Medicare and Medicaid (Medi-Cal) in 1986.

The Livingston-Wheeler regimen.
In Gelband H et al: Unconventional cancer treatments, pp. 107–111.

Washington, DC, U.S. Government Printing Office, 1990.
Briefly describes the career of Dr. Livingston-Wheeler's professional career, research, theories, and treatment methods. Notes her claims regarding the value of her treatment in curing cancer and some studies done to investigate these claims.

Cassileth BR, Lusk EJ, Guerry D, et al: Survival and quality of life among patients receiving unproven as compared with conventional cancer therapy. New England Journal of Medicine 324:1180–1185, 1991.
Describes how researchers at the University of Pennsylvania Cancer Center compared 78 patients with advanced cancer treated at the center with 78 similar patients given various vaccines, a vegetarian diet and coffee enemas at the Livingston-Wheeler Clinic. The study found no difference between average survival time of the two groups. However, patients in the Livingston-Wheeler program reported more problems with appetite difficulties and pain.

The effect of unproved cancer therapy in advanced cancer. New England Journal of Medicine 325:1103–1105, 1991.
Seven letters to the editor discuss the study by Dr. Cassileth and her colleagues.

Macrobiotic Diet (See pages 255-260)

Metabolic Cancer Therapy

"Metabolic therapy" is based on the idea that cancer and other chronic illnesses result from a disturbance of the body's ability to protect itself. Its most visible proponent was Harold Manner, PhD, who left his position as a biology professor to market his treatment ideas. Manner defined metabolic therapy as "the use of natural food products and vitamins to prevent and treat disease by building a strong immune system." He theorized that chemicals in food, water, and air cause large numbers of primitive cells to become cancerous. He said that when the immune system is functioning normally, the cancer cells are destroyed. But if it is weakened by poor nutrition, environmental pollutants or debilitating stress, cancer cells are uninhibited and multiply rapidly. Therefore, the way to treat cancer is by revitalizing the body's immune system with diet, supplementary nutrients, and "detoxification."

In 1982 Manner affiliated with a clinic in Tijuana, Mexico, which was later renamed the Manner Clinic. His treatment program included vegetable juices, "natural foods," intravenous laetrile, DMSO, coffee enemas, and large amounts of vitamins, minerals, enzymes, glandular extracts, and other products, and inspirational messages. Although he claimed high success rates in treating cancers, there is no evidence that he kept track of how patients did once they left his clinic. Manner died in 1988, but the clinic still operates in Tijuana.

The components of metabolic therapy vary from practitioner to practitioner. No controlled study has shown that any of its components has any value against cancer or any other chronic disease. However, many people find its concepts appealing because they do not seem far removed from scientific medicine's concerns with diet, life-style, and the relationship between emotions and bodily responses.

Barrett, S: Vitamin victims sue Harold Manner.
Nutrition Forum 1:9–10, November, 1984.
Briefly reviews the background of Harold Manner, PhD. Discusses his theories of cancer and how to cure it. Describes the experience of a boy who almost died as a result of being treated with excessive doses of Vitamin A to cure his leukemia. Notes that the youth eventually recovered and that his parents were suing Manner and his associates. [The suit was settled out of court several years later for an undisclosed sum.]

Unproven methods of cancer management: The metabolic
cancer therapy of Harold Manner, PhD.
Ca-A Cancer Journal for the Clinician 36:185–189, 1986.
Reviews the career and claims of Harold Manner, PhD. Describes Dr. Manner's publications and studies involving a few of the components of metabolic therapy. Concludes that Dr. Manner's therapy had not been shown to be effective and that some of its components posed serious health risks.

South J: The Manner seminar.
Nutrition Forum 5:61–67, December 1988.
Details the experience of a reporter attending a Manner seminar attended mostly by chiropractors and naturopaths and directed toward enlisting additional practitioners in referring patients to the Manner clinic. Gives a brief background of founder Harold W. Manner, PhD, and discusses the operations of his clinic and other enterprises. Explores the clinic's relations with referring practitioners. Describes Manner's theories and discusses details of the clinic's treatments for cancer, arthritis, and multiple sclerosis. Notes the clinic's use of live cell therapy. Notes that a representative of an insurance processing agency revealed that his agency would submit insurance claims with diagnostic codes for accepted procedures instead of indicating what treatment the patient actually received.

Lowell JA: Mexican cancer clinics
In Barrett S, Cassileth BR: Dubious cancer treatment: a report on "alternative"

*methods and the patients and practitioners who use them, pp. 53–62.
Tampa, FL, American Cancer Society, Florida Division, 1991.*
Describes various dubious tests and questionable "metabolic" treatments offered at eight Mexican clinics, most of which the author has visited. Includes information about treatment costs.

"Psychic Surgery"

*Unproven methods of cancer management: 'Psychic surgery.'
Ca – A Cancer Journal for Clinicians 40:184–188, 1990.*
Describes tricks used by "psychic surgeons" who pretend to withdraw diseased organs from the body, but who actually are handling animal entrails. Mentions several practitioners, some operating in the Philippines and others in the United States until their arrest and exposure. Concludes that "psychic surgery" is a waste of money and that using it may delay effective conventional treatment.

Unproven Psychological Approaches

Many people claim that mood is a major factor in the outcome of cancer and that improving a patient's mood can cause a cancer to regress. The techniques proposed for this purpose include imagery, visualization, meditation, and various forms of psychotherapy. A positive attitude may increase a patient's chance of surviving cancer by increasing compliance with proven treatment. But there does not appear to be any evidence that emotions directly influence the course of the disease.

The use of imagery for treating cancer patients was given impetus by publication of *Getting Well Again* [Bantam, 1978], by Stephanie Matthews-Simonton, O. Carl Simonton, MD, and James L. Creighton. The process they outline, to be repeated several times a day, begins with a period of relaxation. The patient is then instructed to visualize the tumor as a weak, disorganized mass of cells. Conventional treatment is then visualized as powerful and effective, capable of shrinking the tumor and helping the patient overcome the disease. Patients are also encouraged to visualize their immune system attacking the cancer and then imagine being healthy, energetic, and fulfilled. The Simontons have claimed that this approach can lessen fears and tension, strengthen the patient's will to live, increase optimism, and alter the course of a malignancy by strengthening the immune system. However, they have not published the results of any well-designed study to test their ideas.

Bernie Siegel, MD, author of *Love, Medicine & Miracles* [Harper & Row, 1986] and *Peace, Love & Healing* [Harper & Row, 1989], is a surgeon who espouses meditation, support-group meetings, and other psychological approaches for the treatment of cancer patients. He claims that "happy people generally don't get sick" and that "one's attitude toward oneself is the single most important factor in healing or staying well." He also states that "a vigorous immune system can overcome cancer if it is not interfered with, and emotional growth toward greater self-acceptance and fulfillment helps keep the immune system strong."

American Cancer Society: Unproven methods of cancer management: O. Carl Simonton, MD.
Ca – A Cancer Journal for Clinicians 32:58–61, 1982.
Describes the background and methods of Dr. Simonton. Notes that in 1981, consultants at two major medical centers who had reviewed his methodology concluded that his patients may experience a temporary sense of well-being and a feeling that they are "doing something" about their cancer. But the consultants also concluded that there was no scientific basis for Simonton's claims of efficacy and no logical basis for his theories.

Behavioral and psychological approaches.
In Gelband H et al: Unconventional cancer treatments, pp. 29–37.
Washington, DC, U.S. Government Printing Office, 1990.
Describes a variety of psychosocial interventions intended to help cancer patients reduce pain, control nausea and vomiting associated with chemotherapy, and cope with the stresses that cancer and its treatment may bring about. Notes that some are associated with conventional treatment, while others are not. Describes the Exceptional Cancer Patients program of Bernie Siegel, MD, the Commonweal Cancer Help Program, the psychotherapy of Lawrence LeShan, PhD, meditation, psychoneuroimmunology, mental imagery, and visualization. States that some are claimed to influence the healing process as well as making patients feel better, but no well-designed study has demonstrated any such effect. Notes that there is evidence of lengthened survival with conventional group therapy, probably because people who feel better emotionally are more likely to comply with effective treatment.

Friedlander ER: Mental imagery.
In Barrett S, Cassileth BR (eds): Dubious cancer treatment, pp. 73–78.
Tampa, American Cancer Society, Florida Division, 1990.
Describes how Dr. O. Carl Simonton evolved his imagery techniques and the claims he has made for them. Notes that if white blood cells could prevent the development of cancer, people with AIDS would get common forms of cancer rather than rare ones. Explains why the case histories presented in *Getting Well Again* provide no actual evidence that Dr. Simonton's methods are effective against cancer. Describes the approach of Dr. Bernie Siegel and notes that he too has done no research to test his notions.

Schwartz T: Doctor Love.
New York Magazine, pp. 40–49, June 12, 1989.
Describes the activities of Bernie Siegel, MD. Quotes critics who state that (1) he draws his inferences from anecdotes and testimonials, (2) uses scientific studies selectively to support his views, and (3) poses a danger that patients will abandon effective therapy because they put too much reliance in their own ability to change the course of disease.

Revici Method

Revici Cancer Control (also called lipid therapy) is based on the notion that cancer is caused by an imbalance between constructive (anabolic) and destructive (catabolic) body processes. Its proponent has been Dr. Emmanuel Revici, a physician born in Rumania in 1896. To treat the patient, Revici prescribes lipid alcohols, zinc, iron and caffeine, which he says are "anabolic," and fatty acids, sulfur, selenium and magnesium, which he classifies as "catabolic." His formulations are based on his interpretation of the specific gravity, pH (acidity), and surface tension of single samples of the patient's urine. Revici also claims success against AIDS.

Scientists who have offered to evaluate Revici's methods have never been able to reach an agreement with him on procedures to ensure a valid test. However, his method of urinary interpretation is obviously not valid. The specific gravity of urine reflects the concentration of dissolved substances and depends largely on the amount of fluid a person consumes. The acidity depends mainly on diet, but varies considerably throughout the day. Thus, even when these values are useful for a metabolic determination, information from a single urine sample would be meaningless. The surface tension of urine has no medically recognized diagnostic value.

In 1988, state licensing authorities placed Revici on 5 years' probation. The terms of his probation bar him from treating patients for cancer unless they have been: (1) diagnosed by another physician; (2) informed that Revici's treatment is unorthodox; and (3) urged to consult a cancer specialist and a psychiatrist or psychologist before signing a consent form.

Unproven methods of cancer management: Revici method.
Ca – A Cancer Journal for the Clinician 39:119–122, 1989.
Reports on the activities of Dr. Emmanuel Revici, operator of a New York-based clinic. Gives a brief biography and describes his "biologically guided chemotherapy"

for cancer and other diseases. Reviews efforts by various institutions and groups of physicians to determine if Revici's method is effective in treating cancer. Describes disciplinary actions by New York regulatory authorities and legal actions brought by former patients.

Cancer "cure" challenged.
Consumer Reports Health Letter 2:21–22, March 1990.
Describes a $1.3 million award to the estate of a woman who died from colon cancer under Revici's care. When she first consulted Revici, her tumor was the size of a walnut and probably curable by surgery. Testimony at the trial revealed that Revici told her the tumor had almost disappeared despite the fact that it was enlarging. Other evidence suggested that after the suit was filed, Revici doctored his records to suggest that the woman's cancer was far advanced when she first consulted him.

High-Dosage Vitamin C

The claim that high doses of vitamin C can prolong the life of cancer patients is based mainly on studies reported by Linus Pauling and Ewan Cameron, a Scottish surgeon. In the mid-1970s Dr. Cameron treated advanced cancer patients with 10 grams of vitamin C per day. The clinical course of 100 of these patients was then compared with that of 1,000 patients whose records were obtained from the same hospital, but who had received no vitamin C. In response to criticisms, Cameron and Pauling replaced some of the patients and controls and published another analysis. Critics still maintain that the study was invalid because the vitamin C group and the control group were labeled "untreatable" in different ways. To explore the issue further, researchers at the Mayo Clinic conducted three double-blind prospective clinical trials. These studies, involving a total of 367 patients, found no consistent benefit from vitamin C.

Cameron E, Pauling L: Supplemental ascorbate in the supportive treatment of cancer: Prolongation of survival times in terminal human cancer.
Proceedings of the National Academy of Sciences 73:3685–3689, 1976.
Claims that 100 "terminal" cancer patients given high doses of vitamin C survived an average of 4.2 times longer than 1,000 similar patients who did not receive vitamin C. The survival times of the control group was done by examining their medical records.

Cameron E, Pauling L: Supplemental ascorbate in the supportive treatment of cancer: Reevaluation of prolongation of survival times in terminal human cancer.

Proceedings of the National Academy of Sciences 75:4538–4542, 1978.
Reports the results of a comparison of the 100 vitamin C patients with 1,000 patients selected with more stringent criteria.

Creagan ET, Moertel CG, O'Fallon JR et al: Failure of high-dose vitamin C (ascorbic acid) therapy to benefit patients with advanced cancer: A controlled trial. New England Journal of Medicine 301:687–690, 1979.
Reports on a study of 123 patients given high doses of vitamin C or a placebo. Notes that there was no difference in survival between the two groups.

DeWys WD: How to evaluate a new treatment for cancer. Your Patient & Cancer 2:31, 35–36, May 1982.
Responds to the above reports in which Pauling and Cameron claimed that "untreatable" cancer patients lived longer than matched controls when given high doses of vitamin C. States that this conclusion was invalid because Dr. Cameron's patients had been labeled untreatable earlier in the course of their disease and thus would be expected to live longer.

Vitamin C goes down for the count in advanced-cancer controlled trial. Medical World News, p. 69, August 22, 1983.
Reports on double-blind study of 144 cancer patients given high doses of vitamin C or a placebo. States that average survival of the control group was a week longer than that of the vitamin C group.

Moertel CG, Fleming TR, Creagan ET, et al: High-dose vitamin C versus placebo in the treatment of patients with advanced cancer who have had no prior chemotherapy: a controlled trial: a randomized double-blind comparison. New England Journal of Medicine 312:137–141, 1985.
Reports on a study of 100 patients with advanced colorectal cancer who received either high-dose vitamin C or a placebo. States that no difference between the groups was found in the progress of the disease or survival rates of the patients.

Miscellaneous Methods

Waalen J: False screening claims undermine breast cancer detection efforts. Journal of the National Cancer Institute 82:1739–1740, 1990.
Describes a scam touted by claims "tantamount to those of a rainmaker" for lightscanning as a substitute for mammography in testing for breast cancer. The technique, also called transillumination or diaphanography, involves shining visible

and infrared light through the patient's breast to visualize internal tissues. The article notes that while "the technique may be useful in diagnosing some already-detected tumors, experts agree it does not reliably spot asymptomatic tumors, disqualifying it as a screening device." Details efforts by regulatory agencies to stop the promotion of lightscanning as a test for breast cancer.

Unreliable breast cancer screening halted.
FDA Consumer 25:42–43, November 1991.
Describes how the FDA shut down operation of Mobile Clinics of Tomorrow, Inc., a Wisconsin-based company that offered transillumination as a form of mammography for breast cancer screening. Notes that transillumination, which involves shining a light in the red and near-infrared spectrum through the breast to illuminate its interior structure, is not accurate enough to serve as a breast screening method.

Questionable methods of cancer management: Hydrogen peroxide and other "hyperoxygenation" therapies.
Ca – A Cancer Journal for Clinicians (in press).
Notes that "hyperoxygenation therapy" is based on the erroneous concept that cancer is caused by oxygen deficiency and can be cured by exposing the cancer to more oxygen than it can tolerate. The most commonly used modalities are hydrogen peroxide, germanium sesquioxide, and ozone. Although these compounds have been the subject of legitimate research, there is little or no evidence that they are effective for the treatment of any serious disease, and each has demonstrated potential for harm.

Proponent Organizations

Unproven Methods of Cancer Management: National Health Federation.
Ca – A Cancer Journal for Clinicians 41:61–64, 1991.
Reports on the activities of the National Health Federation (NHF), an organization that promotes unscientific methods and lobbies for them in the name of "health freedom." Describes how the group promotes many questionable treatments for cancer and other diseases. Mentions NHF's publications, conventions, and political and legal activities.

International Association of Cancer Victors and Friends, Inc.
Ca – A Cancer Journal for Clinicians. 39:58–59, 1989.
Reports on the activities of the International Association of Cancer Victors and Friends, Inc. (IACVF), an organization that promotes a variety of unorthodox cancer treatments. Mentions some of the therapies promoted by the group.

Zimmerman D: A case report: How Pat McGrady's 'CANHELP' helps patients with cancer.
Probe 1(2):4–7, 1991.
Analyzes a report from an information service claimed to provide information on "the latest cancer cures and where they can be found." The report, which had cost $400, had said that no effective conventional treatment was available and had recommended a restricted diet plus 100 to 150 supplement pills each day and coffee enemas. McGrady apparently was unaware of a new treatment that appeared to have extremely good results. The results had not yet been published in a scientific journal but were readily available to physicians and the public from the National Cancer Institute's information services (see below). Concluded that McGrady's advice, if followed, would have led to an unnecessary death.

Questionable Methods of Cancer Management: The Committee for Freedom of Choice in Medicine.
Ca – A Cancer Journal for Clinicians (in press).
Describes how this group is the political arm of several interlocking corporations promoting and/or marketing questionable remedies for cancer and other serious diseases. Notes that during the 1970s, when it was called the Committee for Freedom of Choice in Cancer Therapy, the organization fought for legalization of laetrile and claimed to have many members. Today the Committee appears to be a small group whose principal activities are speeches and press conferences by its leaders, protests to government agencies, and publication of a newsletter called *The Choice*.

Proponent Literature

Fink JM: Third opinion.
Garden City Park, NY, Avery Publishing Group, Inc., 1988.
An international directory "for people who want to make informed decisions about alternative cancer care programs, support groups, and informational services." Describes how the author became converted to "alternative therapy." Provides information on the background, treatment approaches, and cost of treatment at a large number of "alternative therapy centers." Also lists sources of additional information.

Moss RW: The cancer industry: Unraveling the politics.
New York, Paragon House, 1989.
Presents the author's claim that medical associations, government agencies, foundations and large corporations suppress innovation in order to maximize profits. Attacks medically accepted forms of cancer treatment and promotes the gamut of dubious ones.

Green S: Book review of The Cancer Industry.
Nutrition Forum 8:24, May/June 1991.
Saul Green, PhD, a former Sloan-Kettering researcher states that, "Readers unacquainted with the facts may find Moss's arguments disquieting, if not persuasive. . . . Having personal knowledge of many of the events he described, I found reading his versions very painful. Although the book is loaded with carefully selected facts, it is also loaded with distortions and misrepresentations."

Unproven AIDS Remedies

Acquired immune deficiency syndrome (AIDS) is a fatal disease caused by the human immunodeficiency virus. The virus is able to disrupt the functioning of the body's immune system, rendering the infected individual progressively unable to resist organisms that normally would be harmless. Although no cure has been found, a few drugs have been proven effective for helping individuals infected with the AIDS virus to live longer and have fewer complications of the disease, and many other drugs are at various stages of development in the laboratory or in human clinical trials.

Quackery and fraud related to AIDS have been rampant, with hundreds of purported remedies marketed to AIDS victims. In addition, an "underground" has developed through which drugs are imported by "buyer's clubs" for distribution to people with AIDS. These drugs are legally marketed in other countries, but not approved for general use in the United States. Some of these drugs are approved for clinical trials in this country and may eventually be approved. Although the FDA has expressed concern that some of these substances are inherently dangerous (particularly when insufficiently supervised), the agency has generally permitted them to be imported for personal use.

Fear of AIDS has also spawned a number of inappropriate promotions related to the detection or prevention of AIDS. Several companies have offered unreliable or fraudulent AIDS tests by mail. Covers for public toilets and telephone receivers have been marketed with claims that they will prevent transmission of the AIDS virus even though the virus is not transmitted in this manner.

Some AIDS activists, most notably the AIDS Coalition to Unleash Power (ACT-UP), have campaigned very aggressively to increase government and public attention to the problem of AIDS. ACT-UP has also been extremely critical of antiquackery groups, apparently because its leaders want unrestricted access to whatever "alternatives" they happen to believe in. Other AIDS groups support consumer-protection efforts because they recognize that some "alternatives" can cause adverse effects or shorten survival time.

Descriptive and Critical Literature

AIDS patients seeking alternative treatments.
Medical World News, pp. 8–9, August 22, 1983.
Describes many types of unproven treatments claimed to help AIDS patients.

Kreiger L: Phony AIDS treatments multiplying.
American Medical News 26:2, 19, October 21, 1983.
Describes how some laboratories are offering tests of immune function that are sophisticated and expensive, but actually provide little or no practical information to people concerned about AIDS.

AIDS patients initiate own trials.
Medical World News, pp. 22–25, October 28, 1985.
Describes how a few physicians are "monitoring" what happens to AIDS patients who are taking unapproved drugs.

Ticer S: 'Fast buck' artists are making a killing on AIDS.
Business Week, pp. 85–86, December 2, 1985.
Discusses the rapid proliferation and high cost of unproven and outright fraudulent remedies for AIDS and the efforts of victims to obtain the treatments.

Colburn Don: AIDS and desperation; the epidemic has spawned a range of unproven treatments.
Washington Post Health, p. 10, January 6, 1987.
Describes several quack products investigated by the FDA. Also describes how the Linus Pauling Institute stated in a fundraising appeal that vitamin C had showed promise against AIDS. Quotes a critic who said that using AIDS as a fundraising tool is "exploiting the public."

Staver S: Industry of disinformation spreads AIDS fear, MD says.
American Medical News 30:65–67, May 8, 1987.
Notes remarks by John Renner, MD, regarding the spread of fraudulent cures for AIDS, especially by practitioners of questionable background. Mentions blue-green algae, blood crystallization services, colonics, and suggestions that AIDS victims thump their thymuses to build up their immune systems or expose their genitals to sunlight. Notes the publication of misinformation about AIDS to spread fear.

Bishop K: Authorities act against AIDS cures.
The New York Times 136:20, August 30, 1987.
Describes FDA enforcement action against several bogus AIDS remedies. Notes the formation of an AIDS Fraud Task Force in California. Describes how some people view enforcement activity as a blow against quackery, while others see it as unfairly depriving AIDS patients of hope.

Segal M: Defrauding the desperate; quackery and AIDS.
FDA Consumer 19:17–19, October 1987.

Notes the wide variety of bogus products offered for the treatment of AIDS. Indicates that the FDA intends to give AIDS quackery high priority. Sidebar urges consumers to be wary of "the call of the quack" in advertising claims.

Dwyer JT, Bye RL, Holt PL, et al: Unproven nutrition therapies for AIDS: What is the evidence?
Nutrition Today 23:25–33, March/April 1988.
Compares conventional, investigational, and unproven therapies for AIDS. Discusses factors influencing choice of therapies. Lists some of the claims and possible dangers of more than thirty unproven modalities that do not deserve to be called "alternatives" because they are not as good as standard, medically accepted treatments.

Abraham L: Slick marketing tactics used to push new class of phony treatments for AIDS.
American Medical News 31:3, 36–37, April 1, 1988.
Describes a wide variety of phony AIDS products described by speakers at the 1988 National Health Fraud Conference in Kansas City, Missouri. Notes that one speaker mentioned that "many of the expert quacks in arthritis, cancer, and heart disease have now shifted into AIDS."

Plan for crackdown on fraudulent AIDS therapies.
Skin & Allergy News 19:15, May 1988.
Reports plans by the FDA to investigate fraudulent therapies for AIDS's treatment. Mentions blue-green algae, injections of hydrogen peroxide, pills derived from mice infected with AIDS, herbal capsules containing poisonous metals, a food preservative, and "sanitary" devices allegedly to prevent the transmission of AIDS. Quotes AIDS activists who want greater access to unapproved drugs and who object to the slow pace of drug trials.

Thomas P: Woman sued over soup 'cure.'
Medical World News, p. 67, June 13, 1988.
Discusses efforts by state officials in Massachusetts to stop Ann Wigmore, who reportedly called herself a "living food lifestyle specialist" and "natural healer," from claiming that her "energy enzyme soup" will restore AIDS patients to health and that she is a doctor of philosophy or a medical doctor.

Anderson A, Swinbanks D: US Protests about possible drugs for AIDS treatment.
Nature 334:3, July 7, 1988.
Reports efforts by AIDS activists to allow the importation of the unproven drug dextran sulphate into the United States for use by AIDS victims. Notes that many AIDS

victims already administer this drug to themselves, acquiring it through an underground network. Discusses research on the drug, some of it promising.

Epstein D: Underground AIDS drugs meet with FDA leniency.
Drug Topics 23:46, 48, August 15, 1988.
Notes that many people with AIDS are using drugs that are legally marketed in other countries, but not approved for sale in the United States. Discusses how AIDS patients obtain these drugs and which ones seem headed for eventual FDA approval. Confirms willingness of the FDA to permit AIDS patients to import experimental drugs for their own use as long as the product is not a useless product that is being commercialized or is directly dangerous.

Hammer J: Inside the illegal AIDS drug trade.
Newsweek 112:41–42. August 15, 1988.
Booth W: An underground drug for AIDS.
Science. 241:1279–1281, 1988.
Both articles describe how an underground market mushroomed rapidly for dextran sulfate after it had received favorable publicity. Notes the difficult problems this posed for the FDA and for a manufacturer interested in testing the drug.

Gavzer B: Why do some people survive AIDS?
Parade Magazine, pp. 4–6, September 18, 1988.
Examines people with AIDS, people who are surviving much longer than expected and who, despite suffering from AIDS, appear to be in good health. Describes changes in lifestyle and diet made by AIDS victims in the hope of living a longer and fuller life. Notes the use of unapproved drugs and unorthodox diets. Identifies groups of people at risk for developing AIDS.

MacGowan JJ: Recent occurrences in the discovery and
development of drugs to treat HIV infections.
Annals of the New York Academy of Sciences. 569:231–239, 1989.
Explores efforts to discover new drugs for AIDS treatment. Reviews activities of the National Cancer Institute and other agencies under the National Institutes of Health's aegis. Maps out the course of funding research to the trial stage for new drugs. Discusses research efforts to utilize plant extracts used by traditional medicine for treating symptoms. Describes the chemical activity of several proposed drugs.

Smith R: Doctors, unethical treatments, and turning a blind eye.
British Medical Journal. 298:1125–1126, 1989.
Reviews the case of two physicians who developed a questionable immunotherapy treatment for AIDS and then promoted it with fraudulent claims. Describes the

treatment's development by the physicians in a London hospital and their claims of its success against AIDS. Refers to an investigative journalist's article in the same issue that questions the ethics of the two practitioners and their colleagues who failed to take action against them.

Thompson R: Drugs from the underground.
Time 134:49, July 10, 1989.
Mentions the FDA decision to allow wider access to some experimental drugs. Also notes efforts by AIDS activists to obtain and test other drugs, notably Compound Q. Notes that some experts are concerned that so many AIDS patients are taking unproven drugs that it is difficult to conduct controlled studies of new drugs.

Wyss D: The underground test of compound Q.
Time 134:18, 21, October 9, 1989.
Discusses how AIDS activists conducted an underground test of Compound Q, a substance extracted from a Chinese plant, and distributed the substance to AIDS victims. Notes mixed results, which showed some patients improving while others died, apparently due to the drug itself.

Many AIDS patients using unapproved drugs—study.
American Medical News 32:21, December 22/29, 1989.
Reports the results of a recent study by researchers at the University of California showing that over one-fourth of all AIDS patients interviewed use an unapproved drug to combat AIDS. Notes the risk of dangerous side effects from the use of such drugs, some of which interact unfavorably with conventional AIDS treatments.

"Compound Q."
FDA Consumer 24:7, March 1990.
Discusses an FDA investigation of an unauthorized study of trichosanthin ("Compound Q"), an anti-AIDS drug that the agency considers too dangerous for unsupervised use. The FDA ordered Project Inform to discontinue the study (which it said had already ended), but expressed willingness to permit a study that was appropriately designed.

Kolata G: Trial of experimental AIDS drug to be continued, with revisions.
New York Times, pp. A1, A15, March 9, 1990.
Reports that the FDA permitted the above study to resume after Project Inform submitted a new protocol and Sandoz Corporation agreed to furnish the drug. Also reports that several prominent AIDS researchers lamented the FDA's decision and accused the agency of capitulating to pressure. But FDA officials replied that the new protocol was valid and had not been seen by the critics.

Martin N: AIDS fraud rampant in Houston.
Nutrition Forum 7:16, March/April 1990.
Describes how volunteers of the Consumer Health Education Council telephoned 41 Houston-area health food stores seeking an effective alternative against AIDS for their "brother" and a product that would prevent infection of the brother's wife during sex. All 41 retailers said they had products to benefit the brothers immune system, improve the wife's immunity, and protect her against harm from the AIDS virus. The recommended products included vitamins (41 stores), vitamin C (38 stores), immune boosters (38 stores), coenzyme Q_{10} (26 stores), germanium (26 stores), lecithin (19 stores), ornithine and/or arginine (9 stores), gamma-linolenic acid (7 stores), raw glandulars (7 stores), hydrogen peroxide (5 stores), homeopathic salts (5 stores), Bach flower remedies (4 stores), blue-green algae (4 stores), cysteine (3 stores), and herbal baths (2 stores). Thirty retailers said they carried products that would cure AIDS. None recommended abstinence or use of a condom.

Palca J: International doubts about a Kenyan cure.
Science 250:200, October 12, 1990.
Discusses the evidence for and against Kemron, an alpha-interferon product alleged to cure AIDS. Accompanied by another article, "African Aids: Whose Research Rules," which discusses ethical issues surrounding AIDS research in Africa.

Kolata G: Unorthodox vaccination technique may become weapon in fighting AIDS.
New York Times, p. A11, June 13, 1991.
Examines a new unorthodox technique of vaccinating AIDS victims with a protein normally manufactured by the AIDS virus in the hope that the body's immune system will respond to the attack and repel the intruder and the virus itself. Notes some positive results with tests on AIDS victims. Suggests that the discovery could open new avenues for fighting AIDS.

Brown DL: Fairfax man withdraws bid for medical license.
Washington Post, pp. C1, C3, June 22, 1991.
Reports the conviction of a Fairfax County, Virginia, physician of practicing medicine without a license after he allegedly treated AIDS patients with unconventional methods. Reports that the physician, who had applied to practice medicine in Virginia, withdrew his application after his conviction. Describes the physician's use of heavy doses of vitamins instead of antibiotics to prevent infections. Notes that he also had patients sit under green lights to cool fevers.

DeStefano G: Making a killing on AIDS: home health care and pentamidine.
New York, New York City Department of Consumer Affairs, 1991.

Reports that private high-tech home-care suppliers have been engaging in "bedside robbery" by overcharging insurance companies and government agencies for the delivery of total parenteral nutrition (TPN) to AIDS patients. [TPN is a liquid protein and fat supplement fed intravenously through a surgically implanted catheter to patients whose digestive system no longer functions normally.]

Rowlands C, Powderly WG: The use of alternative therapies by HIV-positive patients attending the St. Louis AIDS Clinical Trials Unit.
Missouri Medicine 88:807–810, 1991.
Reports that 44 of 79 (56 percent) patients said that they had tried an "alternative" remedy. The most commonly used were vitamins (46 percent of patients), herbal therapy (16 percent), imagery/meditation (14 percent), and nonapproved drugs (14 percent). The majority using these methods thought they had improved their general well-being, but readily admitted that the benefit was largely psychological. The average yearly cost was $356, but 14 of the patients spent between $500 and $2,700 and 2 patients spent more than $9,000 each.

Kassler WJ et al: The use of medicinal herbs by human immunodeficiency virus-infected patients.
Archives of Internal Medicine 151: 2281–2288, 1991.
Reports that 25 of 114 patients (22 percent) attending the AIDS Clinic of the University of California San Francisco Medical Center said they had taken one or more herbal products during the three months prior to the survey. Expressed concern that herbal extracts can produce diarrhea, liver toxicity, and other symptoms common in AIDS itself.

Barrett S: Sparks fly at health fraud conference.
Priorities, pp. 33–35, Winter 1991.
Describes how about 50 members of the AIDS Coalition to Unleash Power (ACT-UP) staged protests and attempted to disrupt the 1990 National Health Fraud Conference in Kansas City, Missouri. The protesters claimed (incorrectly) that the meeting was part of a conspiracy involving the FDA, drug companies, and the National Council Against Health Fraud to suppress alternative treatments. More than 20 protesters were arrested for trespassing.

Kolata G: Patients turning to illegal pharmacies.
New York Times, pp. A1, A10, November 4, 1991.
Notes the growth of buyers' clubs that import experimental drugs that are not authorized for sale in the United States. Most clubs cater to AIDS patients, but some supply drugs to victims of cancer, Alzheimer's disease, chronic fatigue syndrome, and other diseases.

Chelation Therapy

Chelation therapy is performed by intravenous administration of a synthetic amino acid called ethylenediamine tetraacetic acid (EDTA), along with several vitamins and other substances. A course of treatment, consisting of 20 to 50 intravenous infusions, can cost thousands of dollars.

Chelation therapy is heavily promoted as an alternative to coronary bypass surgery. Many proponents have claimed that EDTA works as a "chemical roto-rooter," pulling calcium out of atherosclerotic plaques. However, most proponents now claim that the procedure works by pulling toxic metals out of the body, thereby reducing the formation of free radicals and enabling areas of atherosclerosis to heal. There is no scientific evidence that either of these mechanisms exists or that chelation therapy is effective against atherosclerosis.

Chelation therapy is also claimed to be effective against kidney and heart disease, arthritis, Parkinson's disease, emphysema, multiple sclerosis, gangrene, psoriasis, and many other serious conditions. However, no controlled trial has shown that chelation therapy can help any of these conditions, and manufacturers of EDTA do not list them as appropriate for EDTA treatment.

In 1984 the American Medical Association's House of Delegates declared that there was no evidence to support the use of chelation therapy to treat cardiovascular disease, arthritis, atherosclerosis, cancer, and several other conditions. In 1985, the American Heart Association's Task Force on New and Unestablished Therapies concluded there is no scientific evidence to demonstrate any benefit against cardiovascular diseases.

In 1987, the FDA approved a protocol for a randomized, double-blind controlled study of chelation therapy for the treatment of intermittent claudication, a condition in which circulation to the legs is impaired. In 1989, Elmer M. Cranton, MD, a leading proponent of chelation therapy, stated that "studies are being conducted in U.S. Army hospitals by clinical investigators who are completely unbiased, with no previous connection to EDTA chelation therapy." Dr. Cranton predicted that the study would be completed in 1990. As of August 1992, however, no public report has been made, but a Danish study of chelation therapy for intermittent claudication has found no benefit.

Many vitamin concoctions have been marketed with claims that they can do the same thing as chelation therapy when taken by mouth. The FDA has ordered manufacturers to stop marketing these so-called "oral chelation" products, but a few are still doing so.

Critical Articles

Chelation therapy: A second look.
Harvard Medical School Health Letter 9:1–2, 5, July 1984.
States that chelation therapy is offered by an estimated 1,000 practitioners or clinics nationwide, typically with extravagant claims. Briefly describes the treatment and how it allegedly works. Reviews the history of the theory that EDTA binds calcium and removes it from blood vessels. Notes that even if EDTA could remove calcium from the walls of narrowed blood vessels, cholesterol and fibrous tissue would remain to obstruct blood flow. Notes that chelation therapy is expensive and highly profitable to practitioners. Concludes that chelation therapy has no proven value and, at best, is an expensive placebo.

American Medical Association. Chelation therapy.
Proceedings of the House of Delegates, pp. 272–274, 382, 430–431, December 2–5, 1984.
Reports that a computer search of the scientific and popular literature failed to find any scientific evidence that chelation therapy with EDTA is effective against cardiovascular disease, atherosclerosis, rheumatoid arthritis, cancer, and various other health problems. States that it is not accepted for diseases and conditions other than acute hypercalcemia, lead poisoning, and intoxications caused by some other heavy metals. Asserts that it is the responsibility of proponents to conduct properly controlled scientific studies, adhere to FDA guidelines for investigation of drugs, and disseminate results of scientific studies in the usually accepted channels.

American Heart Association: Questions and answers about chelation therapy.
Dallas, American Heart Association, 1985.
Describes the nature of atherosclerosis and chelation (EDTA) therapy and concludes: (1) there was no published scientific evidence demonstrating that chelation therapy is beneficial, (2) no clinical trials using modern scientific methodology support the use of chelation therapy, and (3) use of chelation therapy may deprive patients of the benefits of well-established methods of treating atherosclerotic heart disease.

Cardelli MB, Russell M, Bagne CA., Pomara N: Chelation therapy, unproved modality in the treatment of Alzheimer-type dementia.

Journal of the American Geriatrics Society 33: 548–551, 1985.
Describes case histories of two patients who underwent chelation therapy for treatment of Alzheimer's disease. Notes that the families turned to chelation therapy out of desperation when more conventional medicine was not able to treat the disease. They found that chelation therapy is not successful. Discusses shortcomings of chelation clinics in diagnosis and treatment of the disease. Mentions some uncontrolled studies on treating Alzheimer's disease with chelation therapy. Notes some hazards of chelation therapy.

Avoid 'chelation therapy' pills.
FDA Consumer 19:34, September 1985.
Warns people to be wary of "chelation therapy" pills sold through the mails, health food stores, and person-to-person with claims that they will reduce arterial plaque, improve circulation, and prevent or cure other ailments. Reports that the pills are mixtures of vitamins and minerals with no proven value. Notes that the FDA has ordered manufacturers of "oral chelation" products to stop selling them.

A Roto-Rooter it's not, avoid chelation for clogged arteries; it might harm your health.
Mayo Clinic Health Letter 4:8, April 1986.
Briefly explains how chelation therapy works. Reviews appropriate and ineffective uses. Discusses theory behind its use in removing plaque in clogged arteries, but notes the lack of evidence to support the theory. Reports cost and notes hazards of chelation therapy.

Montgomery MR: Advances in medical fraud: chelation therapy replaces laetrile.
Journal of the Florida Medical Association 73:681–685, 1986.
Reviews the characteristics of quackery and describes the rise and fall of laetrile and the rise of chelation therapy. Compares the behavior of science and quackery. Discusses the effective use of chelation therapy for treating documented heavy metal intoxication. Describes and refutes the quack rationale for chelation therapy. Notes the dangers of illegitimate chelation therapy, including those of DMSO, a recently added component.

Scott J: Chelation therapy—Evolution or devolution of a nostrum?
New Zealand Medical Journal 101:109–111, March 9, 1988.
Reviews what has happened on the "chelation front" during the previous five years. Discusses the promotion of chelation therapy in the United States, Australia, and New Zealand by traditional advocates of unorthodox medicine. Notes that "less emphasis is being placed on the alleged removal of calcium from artery walls and more on neo-magical interpretations of current biochemistry and intermediary metabolism."

*McGillem BS, Mancini GBJ: Inefficacy of EDTA chelation
therapy for coronary atherosclerosis.
New England Journal of Medicine 318:1618–1619, 1989.*
Letter to the editor describing a quantitative assessment in a patient before and after a 30-week course of chelation therapy that had cost $4,000. During this time the percentage of blockage at several points within the patient's coronary arteries increased and a segment that had been 100% occluded remained unchanged. Shortly after completing the treatments the patient had a myocardial infarction.

*Patterson R: Chelation therapy and Uncle John.
Canadian Medical Association Journal 140: 829–831, 1989.*
An intern's account of what happened when his uncle decided to seek chelation therapy instead of bypass surgery that had been recommended. While watching an educational videotape in the waiting room of a chelation therapist, the uncle suffered a sudden coronary artery occlusion. He was rushed to a hospital, where his occluded artery was cleared by angioplasty. The article also discusses the extravagant claims of proponents and why the intern had warned his uncle not to pursue chelation therapy.

*Wirebaugh SR, Geraets DR: Apparent failure of edetic acid chelation
therapy for the treatment of coronary atherosclerosis.
Annals of Pharmacotherapy 24:22–25, 1990.*
Describes the case of a patient with angina who felt much better after undergoing forty to fifty chelation treatments. One month later, however, he developed increasingly severe chest pains and was hospitalized. After angiography revealed that one of his coronary arteries was completely occluded, the patient underwent angioplasty, which restored blood flow through the artery. The author concludes that even if chelation therapy was responsible for the patient's initial relief from symptoms it did nothing to correct the underlying disease state or blockage of the patient's coronary artery. The author also reviews several reports of hazards related to chelation therapy.

*Sloth-Nielsen J, Guldager B, Mouritzen C et al: Arteriographic findings
in EDTA chelation therapy on peripheral arteriosclerosis.
American Journal of Surgery 162:122–125, August 1991.
Guldager B, Jelnes R, Jorgensen SJ, et al: EDTA Treatment of intermittent
claudication—a double-blind, placebo-controlled study.
Journal of Internal Medicine 231:261–267, 1992.*
No benefit was found in a study of chelation treatment in intermittent claudication, a condition in which impaired circulation to the legs causes pain when the person walks. A total of 153 patients received 20 intravenous infusions of either EDTA or a

placebo during a period of 5 to 9 weeks and were followed for 6 months afterward. Vitamin and mineral supplements were administered orally. The first report notes that angiograms and other tests done on 30 of the patients showed no beneficial results for chelation therapy. The second report, covering all 153 patients, notes that changes observed in pain-free walking distance and maximal walking distance on a treadmill were similar in the two groups. The study was conducted by researchers in Denmark.

Chelation therapy: Risks without benefits.
Harvard Heart Letter 3:3–5, October 1992.
Describes chelation therapy, noting proponents' claims that it is safer than surgical procedures to improve blood flow to the heart. Notes that the leading proponent group (the American College of Advancement in Medicine) lists 350 doctors as qualified to do the procedure. Analyzes research during the 1960s, which found that ten patients improved initially but appeared to have lost much of the supposed benefit four years later. Notes that most recent studies have lacked a control group, so any reported benefit could be due to a placebo effect. Concludes that those who try chelation "will be exposing themselves to a small but real risk of side effects, while the chances that this therapy will be helpful are almost surely close to nonexistent."

Proponent Literature

Walker M, Gordon GF: The chelation answer: how to prevent
hardening of the arteries and rejuvenate your cardiovascular system.
New York, M. Evans and Company, Inc., 1982.
Claims that chelation therapy enables people to "avoid degenerative diseases such as heart attack, diabetes, cancer, stroke, cirrhosis, arteriosclerosis, kidney disease, senility, gangrene, or other outgrowths of hardening of the arteries." States that chelation therapy rejuvenates the cardiovascular system "by pulling calcium out of cells in the artery walls where the calcium doesn't belong. The amino acid EDTA acts like a magnet for positively charged calcium and other metal ions." Claims that physicians doing chelation are "keeping careful clinical records and reporting an overall average 82 percent success rate in restoring blood flow in their patients' malfunctioning arteries."

Cranton EM: Bypassing bypass . . . The non-surgical treatment for
improving circulation and slowing the aging process.
Herndon, VA, Medex Publishing, 1984 [with brief update added in 1987].
Gives the author's version of the history and uses of chelation therapy. States that

chelation therapy does not strip calcium out of plaque or calcified hardened arteries, that the "roto-rooter" notion was an oversimplification used by chelation pioneers who were eager to explain the treatment in terms patients could grasp. Recommends using a low-fat diet and dietary supplements to "reverse free radical pathology, thus slowing the aging process."

Cranton EM: Protocol of the American College of Advancement in Medicine for the safe and effective administration of EDTA chelation therapy.
In Cranton EM (ed.): A textbook on EDTA chelation therapy.
Journal of Advancement in Medicine 2:269–305, Spring/Summer, 1989.
Describes the procedures for evaluating patients and administering chelation therapy. Also describes recommendations for diet, exercise, and nutritional supplementation.

Unproven Approaches to Arthritis

Arthritis, sometimes referred to as "rheumatism," is a general term applied to more than a hundred different conditions characterized by aches and pains of joints, muscles, and/or fibrous tissues. Close to forty million Americans suffer from one form of arthritis or another. Although scientific medical care cannot cure the common forms of arthritis, pain and disability can be controlled or minimized with appropriate and timely care.

Arthritis is a fertile field for quackery. As with many chronic diseases, the major forms of arthritis are subject to considerable variation in severity. If a spontaneous remission takes place following use of an unconventional measure, the individual may incorrectly conclude that the measure was effective. Many people try unconventional remedies because friends have recommended them.

Critical Literature

Schultz T, Lindeman B: The pain exploiters—a firsthand report.
on the profiteers who prey on arthritis sufferers.
Today's Health 51:30–35, 65–67, October 1973.
Details the deception taking place at two Mexican clinics and what happened to a woman who received steroids even though she had warned the doctor she couldn't tolerate them and he had told her they were something else.

Benzaia D: The misery merchants.
In Barrett S (ed.): The health robbers, 2nd edition, pp. 196–207.
Philadelphia, 1980, George F Stickley Co., 1980.
Debunks the gamut of quack treatments for arthritis and the sales pitches made for them. Notes that far more money is spent for arthritis quackery than for arthritis research.

International Medical News Service: Most arthritics try
at least one unorthodox remedy.
Family Practice News, p. 7, September 1, 1980.
Cites two surveys on the use of unproven arthritis remedies. One found that 92 of 98 arthritis patients (94 percent) interviewed in detail had tried an average of 3.7

unconventional remedies. The other reported that 123 of 384 patients (32 percent) surveyed by questionnaire had tried such remedies.

Hecht A: Hocus-pocus as applied to arthritis.
FDA Consumer 14:24–27, September 1980.
Decribes a wide range of quack treatments, some of which were very dangerous. Notes that snake venom had been promoted by a "60 Minutes" broadcast. Observes that "arthritis-strength" aspirin is little more than ordinary aspirin at a higher price. Traces the history and regulatory status of DMSO, which also had been promoted by "60 Minutes." Outlines the proven treatments for rheumatoid arthritis, osteoarthritis, and gout.

Dlesk A, Ettinger MP, Longley S, et al: Unconventional arthritis therapies.
Arthritis and Rheumatism 25:1145–1147, 1982.
Describes experiences of six arthritis patients who visited clinics in Mexico to obtain alternative remedies for arthritis. In all instances, the clinics misrepresented the treatments and dispensed steroids or other potentially life-threatening drugs without appropriate precautions. Although all of the patients felt better after the Mexican treatment, relief was short-lived and could not be sustained with domestic medication.

Price JH., Hillman KS, Toral ME, et al: The public's perceptions and misperceptions of arthritis.
Arthritis and Rheumatism 26:1023–1028, 1983.
Reports on telephone survey of a random sample of 300 respondents, which demonstrated widespread ignorance concerning the causes and treatment of arthritis. States that about half the respondents believed that arthritis could be caused by "poor diet" and "cold, wet climates." Also reports on a survey of the use of unproven treatments by 134 arthritis patients. Concludes: (1) most people relied on the mass media for information about arthritis, (2) high percentages of the general population believed that bee venom, vitamins, copper bracelets, special diets and DMSO were effective against arthritis, and (3) about half the people with arthritis had used an unproven method.

Panush RS: Controversial arthritis remedies.
Bulletin on the Rheumatic Diseases 34:1–10, 1984.
Discusses antimicrobial drugs, lasers, DMSO, vitamins and minerals, topical creams, hyperbaric oxygen, biofeedback, acupuncture, vaccines, hormones, cocaine, prayer, and venoms from snakes, ants or bees. Also describes unproven theories about diet, nutrition, and food allergy. Notes the high usage of unproven remedies by arthritis victims. Cites a large number of scientific reports.

Halpern AA: The Kalamazoo arthritis book.
Kalamazoo, MI, Alan A. Halpern, MD, 1984.
Covers all aspects of arthritis. Contains extensive discussions of nutrition fads and misconceptions, fad diets and diet books, quack gadgets, "alternative" practitioners, dietary supplements, "health foods," and many other dubious approaches to arthritis care. Provides ten tip-offs to questionable claims.

Hawley DJ: Nontraditional treatments of arthritis.
Nursing Clinics of North America 19:663–672, 1984.
Proposes five categories of nontraditional treatments ranging from those that have become part of standard care to those that are clearly fraudulent. Discusses problems with acupuncture, diets, dietary supplements, DMSO, herbs, mussel extract, and venoms.

Gray D: The treatment strategies of arthritis sufferers.
Social Science & Medicine 21:507–515, 1985.
Reports on a study of a group of arthritis victims in Australia, their knowledge and beliefs about arthritis, and the various treatments they utilize to gain relief. Mentions the wide use of self-treatment, usually liniments, lamps, and warm baths as well as prescription and nonprescription medications, patent medicines, special diets, and folk remedies. Alternative practitioners consulted included a faith healer, acupuncturists, naturopaths, iridologists, and healers promoting alternative diets and vitamins. Researchers concluded that the longer the period since onset, the wider the range of treatments used.

Louis Harris and Associates: Health, information and the use of questionable treatments: a study of the American public.
Rockville, MD, U.S. Food and Drug Administration, 1987.
Reports on a survey which found that 24 percent of 87 people with arthritis considered their condition serious or very serious and 40 percent said they had frequent pain. About one out of three said they would be willing to try anything for their condition even if it sounded silly or had a small probability of success. A similar percentage said they had tried at least one questionable method. The most frequently tried methods were vitamins (17 percent), vibrators (14 percent), special diets (12 percent), chiropractic (12 percent), alfalfa tablets (9 percent), copper bracelets (9 percent), honey/vinegar (8 percent) and cod liver or fish oil (8 percent).

Panush RS: Nutritional therapy for rheumatic diseases.
Annals of Internal Medicine 106:619–621, 1987.
Reviews published evidence and concludes that a small number (fewer than 5

percent) of individuals with rheumatoid arthritis may improve after elimination from their diet of a specific food that appears to aggravate their condition.

Unproven arthritis remedies.
Atlanta, Arthritis Foundation, 1987.
Booklet defines unproven remedies as "treatments that have not shown in repeated tests that they work and are safe." Lists common unproven remedies, noting that some are harmless but others are harmful or have unknown health effects. Discusses why people try unproven remedies and provides tips on how to spot them. Also summarizes where to turn for help.

Wolman PG: Management of patients using unproven regimens for arthritis.
Journal of the American Dietetic Association 87:1211–1214, 1987.
Discusses the popularity of unproven diet fads among arthritis sufferers who desperately seek pain relief. Lists 43 approaches involving diet or dietary supplements and comments on the effectiveness of each. Notes deficiencies in some of the diets and toxicity of vitamin megadoses. Offers suggestions for counseling arthritis patients.

Wasner CK: Unproven arthritis remedies: how to approach the problem.
Postgraduate Medicine 82:305–314, 1987.
Notes the widespread use of unproven arthritis remedies and urges better communication between physicians and their patients regarding arthritis and its treatment, whether conventional or unproven. Advises physicians to (1) assume that patients may use unproven remedies, (2) educate patients about arthritis and its symptoms, (3) emphasize the benefits of standard therapies, (4) take questions about remedies seriously, and (5) recognize patients' anger and frustration.

Fernandez-Madrid F: Treating arthritis—medicine, myth, and magic.
New York, Plenum Press, 1989.
Takes the reader on an imaginary journey through time by an arthritic patient who is treated by the ancient Mesopotamians, East Indians (Ayurvedic medicine), Chinese, Egyptians, primitive shamans, and many other types of healers. Exposes the faulty rationales for "glandulars," adrenal extracts, Liefcort, DMSO, bee stings, snake venom, and other dubious remedies. Also provides information on the nature and modern treatment of a wide range of arthritic disorders.

Cronan TA, Kaplan RM, Posner L, et al: Prevalence of the use of unconventional remedies for arthritis in a metropolitan community.
Arthritis and Rheumatism 32:1604–1607, 1989.

Reports that 382 out of 1,811 residents of San Diego County, California, contacted by telephone said that they had a musculoskeletal complaint and that 84 percent of these people had used a remedy within the previous six months that had not been prescribed by a doctor. The most commonly used such modalities were prayer (44 percent), bed rest (33 percent), nonprescribed exercise (33 percent), relaxation therapy (33 percent), liniments or salves (30 percent), whirlpool or hot tub baths (29 percent), and vitamins (27 percent). Much smaller percentages used diet (9 percent), herbs (5 percent), and other exotic approaches. The authors note that their study failed to confirm the widely held belief that individuals with arthritis devote large amounts of their personal resources to unconventional remedy use.

Jarvis WT: Arthritis: folk remedies and quackery.
Nutrition Forum 7:1–3, January/February 1990.
States that self-treatment, home-care, and friendly advice given without anticipation of financial gain can be considered folk medicine rather than quackery, even if they are erroneous—but folk medicine has often served as the basis for the commercial promotions of quackery. Cites several studies indicating widespread use of unproven arthritis remedies. Notes that a placebo effect can occur even among nonbelievers. Mentions several studies that found modest benefits with certain dietary regimens. Indicates how doctors can help people judge whether a nutritional remedy is effective.

Southwood TR, Malleson PN, Roberts-Thomson PJ, et al: Unconventional remedies used for patients with juvenile arthritis.
Pediatrics 85:150–154, 1990.
Reports on a survey which found that 37 out of 53 (70 percent) children with juvenile arthritis admitted to using an average of 2.6 unconventional remedies. Also reports three cases of children given "alternative" treatment. One developed premature puberty at age 3 following administration of Liefcort (a steroid preparation). One almost starved to death under the supervision of a naturopath. Recommends that professionals caring for juvenile arthritis patients assume that most of them will try unconventional remedies at some time.

Darlington G, Jump A, Ramsay N: Dietary treatment of rheumatoid arthritis.
The Practitioner, 234:456–460, 1990.
Analyzes the advice of twenty-one books offering dietary advice for arthritic patients. Notes that the advice varied considerably from book to book. Lists "forbidden foods." Suggests that at least a small percentage of cases of arthritis are related to food intolerance or other nutrition-related mechanism. Suggests directions for future research.

*McCaleb R, Blumenthal M: Black pearls lose luster. Prescription
drugs masquerade as Chinese herbal arthritis formula.
HerbalGram No. 22, pp. 4–5, 38–39.
Austin, Texas, American Botanical Association, 1990.*
Describes how, since the late 1970s, Oriental arthritis remedies said to be "all-natural" herbal products have been illegally marketed in the United States under the names Chuifong Toukuwan, Black Pearls, and Miracle Herb. In addition to herbs, these products have contained antianxiety agents, steroid drugs, analgesics (including one that can cause agranulocytosis), methyltestosterone, and other potent drugs not listed on their label. Some batches have contained enough diazepam to cause addiction. In 1975, four users of Chuifong Toukuwan were hospitalized with agranulocytosis and one died. The FDA has banned importation of the product. [Recently, criminal convictions were obtained against several marketers in Texas.]

*Barrett S et al: The mistreatment of arthritis.
In Health schemes, scams, and frauds, pp. 112–130
New York 1990, Consumer Reports Books.*
Discusses the major types of arthritis and a wide range of unproven treatments. Examines advertising hype for nonprescription drugs, noting that "arthritis-strength" products are overpriced. Describes effective treatments and notes that delay in getting proper care can lead to irreversible harm.

*Ringertz B: Dietary treatment of rheumatoid arthritis.
Annals of Medicine 23:1–2, February 1991.*
Notes that although little evidence has been found so far, a dietary manipulation that affects rheumatoid arthritis patients may yet be found. Discusses published reports and suggests new avenues for research.

*Kantrowitz FG: Checking out 'alternative' arthritis treatments.
Prevention 43:60–64, 116, May 1991.*
Uses a question-and-answer format to discuss the likelihood of benefit from fish oils, chiropractic and osteopathy, acupuncture, yoga, DMSO, radiation, copper bracelets, bee venom, health spas, and sex.

*Unproven remedies resource manual.
Atlanta, Arthritis Foundation, 1991.*
Provides comprehensive discussion of unproven remedies. Notes that some are physically harmless but of doubtful benefit, some may be helpful but are unproven, but some are known to be harmful. Covers "alternative" healing philosophies, diets, nutritional supplements, herbal remedies, unproven procedures, worthless diagnostic tests, and miscellaneous products. Cites many references.

Proponent Literature

Alexander D: Arthritis and common sense #2.
West Hartford, CT, Witkower Press, 1984.
Claims that the basic cause of arthritis is "poorly lubricated joints." Claims that dietary measures, especially the use of cod liver oil (which reaches the joints and lubricates them), are effective in preventing and curing arthritis.

Halpern AA: Book review: Arthritis and common sense #2.
Nutrition Forum 2:72, September 1985.
Notes that the above book has "factual errors on almost every page and an alarming tendency to endorse the work of other questionable promoters." Notes that serious scientific studies of diet and arthritis are inconclusive and certainly don't support Alexander's global conclusions. Suggests that the book's commercial success (over 1 million copies of the first edition) is due to its simplistic offer of hope combined with the fact that individuals faced with a chronic and painful illness often grasp at unproven treatments.

Kjeldsen-Kragh J et al: Controlled trial of fasting and
a one-year vegetarian diet in rheumatoid arthritis.
Lancet 338:899–902, 1991.
Describes how rheumatoid arthritis patients treated with dietary methods for thirteen months had fewer symptoms than a control group who ate normally. During the first 7–10 days, the treatment group consumed a low-calorie liquid diet with new foods added individually in an attempt to identify foods that might cause arthritis symptoms to worsen. Then these patients followed a vegetarian diet that eliminated dairy products, eggs, refined sugar, citrus fruits, and gluten-containing foods (found in wheat, oats, rye and barley) for one year. The control group ate in their usual way. Patients who appeared helped by the diet relapsed when they resumed their normal eating habits.

A ray of dietary hope for arthritis sufferers.
Tufts University Diet & Nutrition Letter 9:1–2, February 1992.
Cautions that the diet described in the above experiment can lead to nutritional shortfalls that require professional monitoring. Also notes that the results were based on the experience of only seventeen individuals and that a much larger sample would be required for confirmation.

Part IV:
Diet and Nutrition

Vitamins and "Health" Foods

Promoters of nutrition quackery are skilled at spreading fears and arousing false hopes. They promote at least five basic myths that encourage the use of health foods and food supplements: (1) it is difficult if not impossible to get the nourishment you need from ordinary foods; (2) vitamin and mineral deficiencies are common; (3) virtually all diseases are caused by faulty diet and can be prevented or remedied by nutritional means; (4) Americans are in danger of being poisoned by food additives and pesticides; and (5) personal experience is more reliable than scientific studies for telling whether something is effective.

General Information

Herbert V, Barrett S: Vitamins and "health" foods: the great American hustle. Philadelphia, George F Stickley Co., 1981.
Provides a comprehensive analysis of the activities of the "health food industry," which it defines as "promoters who greatly exaggerate the value of nutrients or use blatant scare tactics associated with a basic rejection of scientific facts." Describes how the industry is organized, how its salespeople learn their trade, how many people are involved, and how they get away with repeated lawbreaking.

*Herbert V: Megavitamins, food fads, and quack nutrition in health promotion: Myths and risks.
In Chernoff R, Lipschitz DA (eds.): Health promotion and disease prevention, pp. 45–66.
New York, Raven Press, 1988.*
Stresses that the key elements of good nutrition are moderation, variety, and balance. Discusses ways of maintaining a balanced diet. Points out deceptive claims about megavitamins. Examines allegations regarding fiber and colon cancer, cholesterol and heart disease, and calcium supplements. Discusses myths and facts about frauds, Gerovital, vitamin E megadoses, selenium supplements, life-extension formulas, zinc, hair analysis, bee pollen, RNA pills, and iron supplements.

*American Dietetic Association: Position of the American Dietetic Association: Identifying food and nutrition misinformation.
Journal of the American Dietetic Association 88:1589–1591, 1988.*
Discusses techniques used by nonscientific practitioners to persuade consumers to accept nutritional misinformation. Explains how the scientific community works to

establish scientific truths. Lists points for consumers to consider in evaluating nutrition news. Suggests ways to evaluate sources of nutritional information and locate accurate nutrition information.

Barrett S: Nutrition quackery: Recent trends and tidbits.
Nutrition Forum 7:25–29, July/August 1990.
Discusses misleading vitamin advertising, mail frauds, dubious practitioners, cancer quackery, multilevel marketing, the flow of health information through the media, the role pharmacists play in facilitating vitamin sales, how the health food industry is organized to distribute deceptive claims, and antiquackery activities.

Milner I: Devious claims: Anatomy of a marketing scheme.
Nutrition Forum 7:41–44, November/December 1990.
Describes the marketing activities of Enzymatic Therapy, Inc., of Green Bay, Wisconsin, which markets nutritional supplements, herbal extracts and "sports nutrition formulas" through health food stores. Describes how the company made no claims on product labels, but published abundant literature for distribution to consumers. Reports how the author attended a seminar for retailers, where he was given a looseleaf manual describing the company's products and how to use them to treat more than eighty diseases, including AIDS. Reports that he also received a videotape containing testimonials for a product that can "help the body nutritionally cleanse itself of the life-threatening plaque in the arteries." Notes that in 1986 the FDA ordered Enzymatic Therapy to stop using "Research Bulletins" that contained illegal claims, but that the company continued to make such claims through seminars and other publications. [In 1991 the FDA initiated action that probably will result in an injunction against further illegal claims.]

Mogadam M: Nutritional fads.
American Journal of Gastroenterology 85: 510–515, 1990.
Examines nutritional faddism promoted by manufacturers and distributors of food supplements. Offers tips on how to recognize food fads. Lists questionable weight control gadgets. Describes the promotion of fad diets, vitamin and mineral supplements, and "alternative treatments." Mentions some fad diets and commercial nutrition organizations. Lists common food additives.

Barrett S: Be wary of bogus vitamin questionnaires.
Priorities, pp. 36–39, Summer 1990.
Describes and debunks three types of questionnaires used by various segments of the health food industry: the National Vitamin Gap Test (used to frighten people into buying "nutrition insurance"); the Yeast Test (used to persuade people to buy supplements to treat nonexistent yeast infections); and the Nutritional Fitness Profile

(used as the basis for prescribing therapeutic supplement programs). Notes that nutritional professionals may use a legitimate questionnaire as part of an evaluation for dietary counseling. Warns, however, that no questionnaire is a legitimate basis for prescribing supplements.

Burros M: Are dietary supplements safe? Don't ask the F.D.A., or anyone else.
New York Times, pp. B1, B9, October 16, 1991.
Discusses the lack of enforcement action by the FDA against questionable dietary supplements. Notes that the FDA has seized some types of products, such as germanium, but even some of these remain available in health food stores. Mentions some supplements that are potentially dangerous if overused.

Food Faddism

Schafer R, Yetley EA: Social psychology of food faddism.
Journal of the American Dietetic Association 66:129–133, 1975.
Defines food faddism as an unusual pattern of food behavior enthusiastically adopted by its adherents and expressed in one of three ways: (1) acceptance of special virtues of a particular food to cure specific diseases, (2) elimination of certain foods from the diet in the belief that harmful elements are present, or (3) emphasis on "natural" foods. Discusses various ways that faddism may meet psychological needs. Describes how selective perception enables faddists to maintain their beliefs in the face of contrary evidence. Suggests how nutrition educators can use these insights in dealing with individual faddists.

Roth JA: Health purifiers and their enemies.
New York, Neal Watson Academic Publications (Prodist), 1977.
Dispassionately describes the struggle between "natural health purifiers" and the "health establishment," noting many similarities in their institutions and services. Notes how each group views the other and acts accordingly.

Deutsch R: The new nuts among the berries.
Palo Alto, Bull Publishing Co., 1977.
Provides a detailed and amusing history of the rise of food faddism in America.

Jarvis WT: Food faddism, cultism and quackery.
Annual Review of Nutrition, 3:35–52, 1983.
Defines food faddism, food cultism, and food quackery. Discusses magical thinking about food, why food faddism persists, and how nutrition education unwittingly aids food faddism. Points out that the harm done by food faddism includes not only injury

and death, but economic and psychological harm. Describes current abuses by diploma mills that sell phony credentials, pyramid sales schemes that market useless and dangerous products, dubious supplement promotions by pharmaceutical companies, mistreatment by questionable practitioners, and abuse of the First Amendment by publishers and promoters who advance nutrition misinformation as free speech. Discusses how to cope with food faddism through education, health-care delivery, and the law. Concludes that food faddism, cultism, and quackery may never be completely eliminated, but that responsible people within society must work to reduce their negative impact upon society.

Leach HM: Popular diets and anthropological myths.
New Zealand Medical Journal 102:474–477, 1989.
Observes that physicians have been encountering increasing numbers of patients who have modified their diet on the basis of a popular or fad diet book that justifies its rationale by pointing to alleged characteristics of traditional or primitive societies. Notes that the typical argument is that since the selected society shows no evidence of obesity, cardiovascular disease, etc., Western societies can eliminate these so-called "diseases of civilization" by adopting a primitive diet. Notes that a second common argument is that "diet-related diseases" occur where human societies have modified their diet so recently that they have not adapted to the new components or nutrient proportions. Discusses why arguments of this type can be challenged on anthropological grounds. Advises skepticism toward claims that the broad range of diet-related diseases stem from maladaption to particular foods.

"Nutrition Insurance"

Virtually all nutrition authorities agree that healthy individuals can get all the nutrients they need by eating a balanced variety of foods. The fear of "not getting enough" is promoted vigorously, not only by food faddists and health-food industry publicists, but also by major pharmaceutical manufacturers and trade associations. Faddists tend to stress unscientific ideas that one cannot get sufficient nourishment from ordinary foods, while the drug companies use more subtle suggestions that various people (such as people under "stress") may not be getting enough. Both groups fail to suggest how to obtain one's nutrients from foods or how to tell whether one is getting enough.

Hatfield D: Truth in advertising: Does it apply to vitamin supplements?
ACSH News & Views 5:1, 13–14, January/February 1984.
Quotes and rebuts nine scary messages in vitamin ads by major pharmaceutical manufacturers. Notes that there is no such thing as "vitamin burnout," that ordinary

exercise does not create a need for vitamin supplements, that it is not difficult to obtain vitamins from foods, and that water-soluble vitamins do not need to be replaced daily.

The vitamin pushers.
Consumer Reports 51:170–175, March 1986.
Describes how vitamin manufacturers hype their supplements for "insurance" against dietary shortfalls, protection against "stress," and better athletic performance. Notes that Lederle Laboratories' promotion of Stresstabs "for people who burn the candle at both ends" is based on misinterpretation of a 1952 National Academy of Sciences report. Notes that vitamin shortages are uncommon but that some people—especially women—need to pay attention to fluoride, calcium, and iron. Debunks myths involving vitamins C, E, and B_6. Describes how reporters visited thirty pharmacies, complaining of nervousness or fatigue. Notes that seventeen recommended a vitamin and only nine suggested seeing a doctor. Recommends that the FTC should attempt to stop misleading advertising claims for "nutrition insurance," "stress tablets," "sports vitamins," and the like.

Harper AE: "Nutrition insurance": A skeptical view.
Nutrition Forum 4:33–37, May 1987.
Notes that a large number of apparently healthy people take vitamin supplements even though deficiency diseases are rare. Describes how supplements are often promoted by misinterpreting surveys showing that some segments of the population have intakes below the Recommended Dietary Allowances (RDAs). Explains that the RDAs are not minimums and that vitamin storage in the body enables most people to achieve adequate average intakes. Describes and debunks a Council for Responsible Nutrition flyer designating eighteen "groups with proven nutrient needs." Mentions a few situations where vitamin supplementation may be appropriate and notes that supplementary fluoride is vital to help strengthen the teeth of children growing up in nonfluoridated communities. Concludes: "I see no evidence in the scientific literature that Americans generally require vitamin supplements. Rather, they need accurate nutrition information about food and health to counter the nutrition misinformation to which we are constantly exposed."

Findlay S: Squaring off over vitamins.
U.S. News & World Report 106:62–64, April 10, 1989.
States that a panel convened by the National Academy of Sciences had rejected the idea of using vitamin and mineral supplements to make up for deficits in the diet, prevent disease, or enhance health, and that the panel had come down hardest on supplements exceeding the RDAs. States that the Council for Responsible Nutrition (CRN), which represents supplement manufacturers, objected to the panel's report

and had claimed in recent ads that supplements were important because most Americans fail to eat a balanced diet. Observes that the basis of this claim was a 1978 government-funded survey which, according to CRN, had found that over a three-day period, not a single person consumed 100 percent of the RDA for each of ten nutrients. Notes, however, that the researcher who headed the project said that CRN had deliberately misinterpreted its findings, that the RDAs are set higher than most people need, and that no one in the survey had come up seriously short on all or even most of the vitamins and minerals.

"Organic Foods"

"Organically grown" foods are said to be foods grown without the use of "artificial" fertilizers or pesticides. They are promoted with false claims that "ordinary" foods are unsafe and/or less nutritious.

USDA Study Team on Organic Farming: Report and recommendations on organic farming.
Washington, DC, U.S. Department of Agriculture, July 1980.
Notes that the organic movement encompasses a spectrum of practices and philosophies. Notes that some organic practitioners won't use chemical fertilizers or pesticides under any circumstances, while others use fertilizers and also herbicides as a second line of defense. Recommends that certification programs be established "to assure that organically produced foods are properly labeled."

The "natural-organic" ripoff.
In Herbert V, Barrett S: Vitamins and "health" foods: the great American hustle, pp. 73–86.
Philadelphia, George F. Stickley Co., 1981.
Analyses and refutes the implications of a leading proponent's definition of "organically grown food." Notes that foods said to be "organic," "organically grown" or "natural" usually cost more than conventionally grown foods even though there are no significant differences in pesticide content, nutrient content, or taste. Warns that proponents of "organic" foods are working hard to obtain government endorsement and protection of their slogans.

Traiger WW, Cohen DS: New York City Department of Consumer Affairs' health food stores investigation.
New York City Department of Consumer Affairs, 1983.
Describes a three-month investigation that compares the quality and prices at 23 health food stores in New York City. Reports that the prices of 30 foods in health

food stores averaged almost double those in conventional outlets. Notes that laboratory tests found no significant pesticide levels in samples of foods from either source.

Kroger M: Food safety: what are the real issues?
Nutrition Forum 2:17–18, March 1985.
States that Americans have the most wholesome food supply in human history, but still worry that it is unsafe. Describes how a government committee polled experts to develop a list of food hazards in the order of their importance. Notes that this ranking, which places microbial toxins and food-borne infections at the top, is quite different from that generated by the media and held by the public.

Pesek J et al: Alternative agriculture.
Washington, DC, National Academy Press, 1989.
Notes that "alternative agriculture" is not a single system of farming practices, but ranges from "organic systems that attempt to use no purchased synthetic chemical inputs to those involving the prudent use of pesticides or antibiotics to control specific pests or diseases." Labels crop rotation and green manuring as "alternative" practices, even though they have been part of scientific agriculture for decades. Does not advocate "organic" farming, but seeks to reduce the use of high-cost agricultural chemicals that have undesirable features. Recommends that more research be done.

Jordon LS et al: Alternative agriculture: Scientists' review.
Ames, IA, Council for Agricultural Science and Technology, 1990.
Contains more than forty responses to the above report, most of which criticize it. Notes that neither alternative agriculture nor conventional agriculture is well-defined, that some practices are used by both, and that the major difference between the two may be more philosophical than technical.

Newsome R: Organically grown foods: A scientific status summary by the Institute of Food Technologists' expert panel on food safety and nutrition.
Food Technology 44:123–130, December 1990.
Describes the "organic" food marketplace and its relationship to consumer concerns about food safety. Describes research comparing the nutritive value, pesticide content, taste, and cost of "organically grown" and conventional foods. Concludes that the only significant difference is the higher cost of "organic" foods. States that it remains to be seen whether organic agriculture offers a viable alternative to environmentally detrimental aspects of conventional farming.

Larkin M: Organic foods get government "blessing"
despite claims that aren't kosher.

Nutrition Forum 8:25–29, July/August 1991.
Describes how proponents of "organic farming" teamed up with proponents of "alternative" and "sustainable" agriculture to gain passage of a bill to require the U.S. Secretary of Agriculture to establish organic certification standards. Discusses the difficulty in establishing meaningful standards. Concludes: "'Organic' certification. . . . will merely create more confusion and distrust in the marketplace. Foods certified as 'organic' will neither be safer nor more nutritious than 'regular' foods. They will just cost more. Instead of spending money to legitimize nutrition nonsense, our government should do more to attack its spread."

Food and Drug Administration Pesticide Program: residue monitoring 1991. Washington, DC, Food and Drug Administration, 1992.
Reports on the FDA's pesticide monitoring program, which is based on testing a wide variety of foods collected for analysis during the 1991 fiscal year [October 1990 through September 1991]. Notes that the Environmental Protection Agency sets tolerance levels, while the FDA has the authority to enforce them (except for meats, poultry and certain egg products, which are under the Agriculture Department's jurisdiction). States that of 18,214 fruits, vegetables, and other domestic or imported foods, 66.8 percent had no detectable pesticide residues, 31.6 percent had residues below the maximum federal limits, and only 1.5 percent contained violative levels. Notes that the FDA's annual Total Diet Study found that dietary intakes of pesticides for all population groups were well within international and EPA standards.

Whelan E, Stare F: Panic in the pantry.
Buffalo, Prometheus Books, 1992.
Relates the development of widely held food fears to scare tactics used by prominent faddists, "consumer advocates," and media outlets. Identifies and debunks four cornerstones of "Healthfoodland." Explains in detail why "health foods," "natural foods," and "organic foods" are not necessarily different or better than regular foods. Focuses on the nature and benefits of food additives. States that our food safety laws are outdated and unnecessarily rigid.

"Orthomolecular Medicine"

Orthomolecular medicine is defined by its proponents as "the treatment of disease by varying the concentrations of substances normally present in the human body." It is said to have begun during the early 1950s when a few psychiatrists began adding massive doses of nutrients to their treatment of severe mental problems. The original substance used was vitamin B_3 (nicotinic acid or nicotinamide), and the therapy was termed "megavitamin therapy." Later the treatment regimen was expanded to include other vitamins, minerals, hormones, and diets, any of which may be combined with conventional drug therapy and electroshock treatments. In 1968, Linus Pauling, PhD, coined the term "orthomolecular," based on the Greek word *orthos*, which means straight (or correct). This approach has been adopted by a few hundred physicians and is being used to treat a wide variety of conditions, both mental and physical.

The human body has limited capacity to use vitamins in its metabolic activities. When vitamins are consumed in excess of the body's physiological needs, they function as drugs rather than vitamins. A few situations exist in which high doses of vitamins are known to be beneficial, but they must still be used with caution because of potential toxicity. For example, large doses of niacin can be very useful as part of a comprehensive, medically supervised program for controlling abnormal blood cholesterol levels. Proponents of "orthomolecular medicine" go far beyond this, however, by prescribing vitamins to all or most of the patients they treat.

Lipton MA, Ban TA, Kane FJ, et al: Task force report on megavitamin and orthomolecular therapy in psychiatry. Washington, DC, American Psychiatric Association, 1973.
States that the concept of megavitamin therapy is loosely defined and has always been added onto existing conventional treatments for schizophrenia. States that the theoretical basis for megavitamin treatment is insufficient and that the chemical and psychological tests used by proponents to determine diagnosis and treatment response lack both reliability and specificity. Concludes: "This review and critique has carefully examined the literature produced by megavitamin proponents and by those who have attempted to replicate their basic and clinical work. . . . The credibility of the megavitamin proponents is low. Their credibility is further diminished by a consistent refusal over the past decade to perform controlled experiments and to report their new results in a scientifically acceptable fashion. Under these circumstances this Task Force considers the massive publicity which they promulgate via radio, the lay press and popular books, using catch phrases which are really misnomers like 'megavitamin therapy' and 'orthomolecular treatment,' to be deplorable."

Committee on Nutrition, American Academy of Pediatrics: Megavitamin therapy for childhood psychoses and learning disabilities. Pediatrics 58:910–912, 1976.
States that there are only a few clinical situations in which it is appropriate to administer above-RDA amounts of vitamins to children. Notes, however, that a "cult" developed with the use of large doses of water-soluble vitamins to treat mental retardation, psychoses, autism, hyperactivity, dyslexia, and other learning disorders.

Concludes that megavitamin therapy for such conditions had not been justified by documented clinical results.

Barness LA et al: Megavitamins and mental retardation.
Evanston, IL, American Academy of Pediatrics, 1981.
Position paper on the uses and abuses of megavitamins. Describes a study by Dr. Ruth Harrell that was purported to show that nutritional supplements can raise the I.Q. of mentally retarded children [*Proceedings of the National Academy of Sciences* 78:574–578, 1981]. Explains that the study's design was flawed with too many variables to yield meaningful results. Expresses doubt that a well designed study would find that megavitamins would boost I.Q. States that it is unfortunate when public funds are diverted to test poorly founded hypotheses.

Hodges RE: Megavitamin therapy.
Primary Care 9:605–619, 1982.
Notes that "with the discovery of each vitamin there has been a flurry of enthusiasm leading to a search for therapeutic benefits. If a newly discovered vitamin affected a certain physiologic function, then that vitamin would be given to patients who had any medical disorder that involved the system." Notes that there are few proven uses for megavitamins.

Bennett FC, McClelland S, Kriegsman EA, et al: Vitamin and mineral supplementation in Down's syndrome.
Pediatrics 72:707–713, 1983.
Reports that, despite its flaws, the above-mentioned study by Dr. Harrell had received considerable publicity through the mass media and in a nine-part series in *Medical Tribune*. Notes that despite skeptical statements by the American Academy of Pediatrics and the Down Syndrome Congress, many parents were giving large doses of vitamins and minerals to their retarded children. Describes how a properly designed study by the authors had found no difference in behavior or I.Q. between the vitamin/mineral group and the control group. Notes that the 15,000 IU dosage recommended in the Harrell study could be toxic to younger children if maintained for a prolonged period.

Fried JJ: Vitamin politics.
Buffalo, Prometheus Books, 1984.
Reports on a lengthy investigation in which the author traveled throughout the United States and Canada to interview proponents and critics of megavitamin therapy. Traces the origins of many of the claims for megavitamins. Notes that their promoters appear to have little interest in scientific testing of their claims.

Concludes: "Because vitamin enthusiasts believe more in publicity than they believe in accurate scientific investigation, they use the media to perpetuate their faulty ideas without ever having to face up to the fallacies of their nonsensical theories. They announce to the world that horse manure, which has latent traces of vitamin B_{12}, liberally rubbed into the scalp, will cure, oh, brain tumors. Researchers from the establishment side, under pressure to verify the claims, will run experiments and find that the claim is wrong. The enthusiasts will not retire to their laboratories to rethink their position. Not at all. They will announce to the world that the establishment wasn't using enough horse manure, or that it didn't use the horse manure long enough, or that it used horse manure from the wrong kind of horses. The process is never-ending . . . The public is the ultimate loser in this charade."

Marshall C: Vitamins and minerals: Help or harm?
Mt. Vernon, NY, Consumer Reports Books, 1985.
Comprehensive discussion of vitamins and minerals, including the history of their discovery, amounts needed, food sources, symptoms of deficiency, megavitamin claims and toxicity, and groups at risk for deficiency. Describes some of the misleading ways vitamins are promoted. Contains many case reports of individuals who were harmed by megavitamins. Discusses vitamin C and the common cold, noting that at least fifteen well-designed studies found no evidence that taking vitamin C supplements can prevent colds. Also debunks claims that megadoses of vitamins are effective against cancer, mental illness, and various other conditions.

AMA Council on Scientific Affairs:
Vitamin preparations as dietary supplements and as therapeutic agents.
JAMA 257:1929–1936, 1987.
States that healthy adult men and healthy adult nonpregnant, nonlactating women consuming a usual, varied diet do not need vitamin supplements. Notes that vitamins in therapeutic amounts may be indicated for the treatment of deficiency states, for pathological conditions in which absorption and utilization of vitamins are reduced or requirements increased, and for certain nonnutritional disease processes. Notes ways that vitamins are misused and the toxic effects that can result. Urges all health practitioners to emphasize that properly selected diets are the primary basis for good nutrition.

Bassler KH: Megavitamin therapy with pyridoxine.
International Journal for Vitamin and Nutrition Research 58:105–118, 1988.
Examines the use of megavitamin therapy. Describes several rare disorders for which treatment with vitamin B_6 is accepted in conventional medicine. Notes that the use of B_6 for rheumatic disease, carpal tunnel syndrome, Chinese restaurant

syndrome, and premenstrual syndrome is disputed and that its use for mental disorders is unconfirmed. Reviews toxicity of pyridoxine and warns that it is not appropriate for self-medication.

Barrett S: Megavitamin therapy: Claims and cautions.
Priorities, pp. 27–29, Spring 1989.
Covers vitamin C and the common cold, vitamin C and cancer, megavitamins for mental illness, vitamin E and lumpy breasts, niacin and cholesterol control, vitamin B_6 for premenstrual syndrome (PMS), and dangers of excess vitamins.

Nutrition Committee, Canadian Paediatric Society: Megavitamin and megamineral therapy in childhood.
Canadian Medical Association Journal 143:1009–1013, 1990.
Notes the widespread popularity of vitamin supplements and the advocacy of such products by different lay healers. Discusses various claims for megavitamins and research that failed to support them. Reviews toxic effects of excessive doses of vitamins and minerals. Warns that the administration of megavitamins and megaminerals involves special risks for children because the early signs of toxicity are nonspecific and may lead parents to increase dosage.

Health Food Stores

The health food industry markets thousands of products intended for therapeutic use. Although it is illegal for health food store personnel to diagnose illnesses or prescribe products to treat them, it is clear that many do so.

Stoffer SS, Szpunar WE, Coleman B, et al: Advice from some health food stores.
JAMA 244:2045–2046, 1980.
Describes how the authors surveyed ten health food stores in Michigan to see how they would advise someone taking thyroid hormone prescribed by a physician. Notes that at all ten stores the supervisor or "nutritionist" offered products, and that two advised stopping the hormone. Notes that the survey was stimulated by a patient's report that a health food store "nutritionist" had advised stopping digitoxin, a diuretic, and thyroid hormone and taking kelp and vitamin supplements instead.

Sheridan M: Singing the health food blues.
ACSH News & Views 1:10–11, February 1980.
Presents an interview with Beth Cavanaugh, former owner of a "very profitable" health food store in New Haven, Connecticut. Ms. Cavanaugh states: (1) to many people, health food plays the role of a religion; (2) some health food stores grew out

of the "hippie" movement of the sixties and its interest in love, peace, and fresh food, while others are selling things just for the money while they are perfectly aware that they don't work; (3) many such stores are operated by absentee owners who employ "dewy-eyed salespeople" who probably do believe in what they are doing; (4) radio programs in New York City are promoting sales by telling desperate people that vitamins and health foods will help them; (5) she finally quit the business because she felt it was inherently dishonest.

Meister KM: Do health food stores give sound nutrition advice?
ACSH News and Views 4:1, 8–9, 13–14, May/June 1983.
Describes how investigators from the American Council on Science and Health made 105 inquiries at stores in New York, New Jersey, and Connecticut. Asked about eye symptoms characteristic of glaucoma, 17 out of 24 suggested a wide variety of products for a person not seen; none recognized that urgent medical care was needed. Asked over the telephone about sudden, unexplained 15-pound weight loss in one month's time, 9 out of 17 recommended products sold in their store; only 7 suggested medical evaluation. Seven out of 10 stores carried "starch blockers" despite an FDA ban. Nine out of 10 recommended bone meal and dolomite, products considered hazardous because of contamination with lead. Nine stores contacted made false claims of effectiveness for bee pollen, and 10 stores did so for RNA. The investigators concluded that most health food store clerks give advice that is irrational, unsafe, and illegal.

Motil B: Advice from the health food stores: How healthy is it?
Columbus Monthly 10:79–88, January 1984.
Described what happened when nine health food stores in Central Ohio were contacted by phone or in person by researchers posing as women suffering from an undiagnosed eye condition, a mother-to-be seeking nutrition information for her pregnancy, a recent heart attack victim, and a would-be weight lifter seeking to build muscles. Concludes that although the health food store clerks appeared to be sincere, their advice was "like flipping a coin," not reliable. Urges buyers to beware.

Foods, drugs, or frauds?
Consumer Reports 50:275–283, May 1985.
A three-part article describing the dimensions of the problem of nutritional products being marketed with fraudulent claims. Explains that under federal law any product "intended for use in the diagnosis, cure, mitigation, treatment, or prevention of disease" is a drug and must be proven safe and effective in order to be legally marketed. Reports on a temporary health food "store" established by Consumers Union to gather product literature from health food manufacturers. Critiques numerous products and lists more than forty companies making illegal therapeutic

claims for their products. Notes what happened when a reporter obtained distributorships for various multilevel companies. States that the FDA's enforcement program against health frauds has been ineffective, partly due to lack of resources and partly due to lack of interest.

Anderson DH: Health food stores are harming our patients.
Medical Economics 62:27, 30, 33, December 8, 1985.
Describes how the author began asking patients about their use of vitamins, supplements, and other nonprescription medications after he learned that one of his patients had been given dangerous advice at a health food store. Describes how he then visited three local "nutrition centers" to see for himself what advice was being offered. Urges physicians to do the same and to educate patients about the risks of indiscriminate self-treatment.

Fanning O: "Training" for health food retailers.
Nutrition Forum 3:33–38, May 1986.
Describes the author's observations at a seminar for retailers given at a major health food industry trade show held in 1985. Notes that much of the seminar concerned how product information might be communicated without "prescribing" (which would be practicing medicine without a license). Describes role-playing in which a speaker gave dubious advice to a woman complaining of a breast lump. Notes that the seminar was led by Jeffrey Bland, PhD, who also supplied information through audiotapes and a magazine. States that many of Dr. Bland's ideas about individual nutrient needs run counter to those of the scientific nutrition community. Suggests that the information he distributes encourages retailers to give advice for which they are not qualified.

Aigner C: Advice in health food stores.
Nutrition Forum 5:1–3, January 1988.
The author, a registered dietitian, asked the proprietors of ten health food store in eastern Pennsylvania for advice on blurred vision, rapid weight loss to qualify for a wrestling meet, unexplained 15-pound weight loss, dolomite supplements, and bee pollen. Fewer than half the answers were correct.

Franchisor of food supplements prohibited from making false claims, under consent agreement with FTC.
FTC News, January 4, 1988.
Describes how the FTC had charged Great Earth International, the second-largest health food store chain (150 stores), with making false claims for several products. Notes that the case was settled with a consent agreement prohibiting the company from making unsubstantiated therapeutic claims in the future.

Kenney JJ: Have you seen your vitamitician lately?
Nutrition Forum 7:13, March/April, 1990.
Describes how Great Earth Vitamin Stores used a "Nutritional Fitness Profile" questionnaire containing 29 multiple-choice questions pertaining to diet, symptoms, illnesses, and lifestyle. Notes that the company had advertised that "highly trained Vitamiticians" would use the results to "tailor a nutritional support program that's a perfect fit." States that the questions, separately or together, did not provide a rational basis for any type of supplement recommendation. Describes how the author completed the test at two stores and received advice that was senseless and/or dangerous. Reports that one Vitamitician said that there was no training—"All you really have to know is how to sell supplements."

Haidet JM: Health food store probe yields poor advice plus doubletalk.
Nutrition Forum 9:6–7, January/February 1992.
The author, a student at Kent State University, made thirty phone calls to ten stores in Central Ohio for advice about headaches, kidney stones, or abnormal thirst, dizziness and fatigue. She received no appropriate advice.

Dubious Nutrition Consultants

Aronson V: You can't tell a nutritionist by the diploma.
FDA Consumer 17:28–29, July/August 1983.
Describes how the author obtained a "Nutritionist" certificate after taking a two-lesson course from Bernadean University, an unaccredited correspondence school that was not legally authorized to grant degrees. Notes that much of the information provided was invalid and that the examinations were conducted "open-book." Notes that even though she gave answers contradictory to the information in the course material, she received a high grade on the first exam and "100%" on the second. Also notes that her "nutritionist" certificate states that she graduated "Cum Laude."

Stebbins J: Pup and circumstance: Dog gets degree in mail.
Graduate places in top 2 percent without studying.
Kansas City Star, pp. 1A, 11A, January 15, 1984.
Describes the operation of the Nutritionists Institute of America, an unaccredited correspondence school in Kansas City, Missouri. Describes how a reporter obtained an "assistant nutritionist" credential for Elmar von Wetzler, a pet dog. Notes that although the school's director stated that background checks are made of all applicants, the dog was accepted even though all questions relating to educational background were not answered on the application submitted. Notes that "Elmar's" final grade average was said to be in the "upper 2 percentile range," even though the

reporter had deliberately submitted many wrong answers in preliminary tests and did not return one of the eight pages of the final exam.

Yoswick CP: How to practice nutritional counseling legally without being guilty of practicing medicine without a license.
Youngstown, OH, Cheswick Publications, 1985
States that the author is a "certified Bio-Nutritional Analyst and a Doctor of Naturopathy and Preventive Medicine," conducts a private "holistic nutritional counseling practice" in Youngstown, Ohio, and is founder and president of the Nutritional Science Association. States that "too many nutritional consultants examine, diagnose, prescribe, advise, recommend, administer, and dispense." States that "a true health counselor, operating legally . . . does not diagnose or prescribe, but offers health information to help the client to cooperate with his/her physician." Recommends offering lectures, forming a support group that can oppose restrictive legislation, having a brochure disclaiming any intent to diagnose or treat disease, using business cards stating you are a nutrition counselor, using a questionnaire to accumulate data on clients and help screen out law enforcement officials posing as patients, using a consent form, keeping complete records, joining a professional association, and carrying malpractice insurance.

Jarvis, WT: Recognizing today's nutrition quacks.
Nutrition & the M.D. 11:1–2, December 1985.
Describes the identifying characteristics of unqualified quack nutritionists. Notes that they use spurious credentials to establish their authority; use invalid diagnostic tests to convince their victims that they have special nutritional needs; make questionable prescriptions of megavitamins, herbal products, "glandular" supplements, and/or enzyme supplements; and either sell expensive supplements directly to their clients or refer them to inappropriate sites (such as a health food store) to have prescriptions filled.

Barrett S: Should 'nutritionists' be licensed? The time is right.
Postgraduate Medicine 79:11–13, February 15, 1986.
States that dietitians throughout the United States are spearheading legislation to achieve licensure for themselves and to restrict use of the word "nutritionist" to persons with recognized credentials. States that within the past five years, several individuals and organizations have developed "credentials" resembling those of established medical and nutritional organizations. Notes that unqualified individuals with such credentials are luring unsuspecting individuals into their offices where they engage in unscientific diagnosis and treatment. States that it is unrealistic to expect the public to investigate the credentials of every health practitioner they

encounter and that government should prevent individuals who do not meet professional standards from representing that they do.

*Barrett S: The American Association of Nutritional
Consultants: Who and what does it represent?
Nutrition Forum 3:49–54, July 1986.*
Describes the history and activities of the American Association of Nutritional Consultants (AANC), the American Nutritional Consultants Association, the American Nutritional Medical Association, and the American Holistic Health Sciences Association. Notes that these groups issue "professional" certificates to virtually anyone who fills out an application and pays the required fee, and that someone known to the author had obtained one from AANC by merely submitting the name and address of her pet hamster and a check for $50.

*Should nutritionists be licensed?
Prevention 38:72–75, September 1986.*
Describes how two individuals became dangerously ill as a result of advice from unqualified persons. Discusses the efforts of the American Dietetic Association and others to gain passage of laws to define nutrition practice and make it illegal without appropriate training. Notes opposition by "alternative" practitioners. Offers tips on whom to consult for good nutritional advice.

*Barrett S: Where to get nutrition advice.
Healthline 6:1–3, October 1987.*
Describes the training that enables medical and nutritional professionals to give scientifically-based advice. Lists conditions for which detailed nutrition advice is needed and notes that most of them require medical diagnosis first. Recommends avoiding practitioners who recommend vitamins for everyone or sell them in their office.

*Jarvis WT: Dubious health assessments.
Nutrition & the M.D. 15:1–3, February 1989.*
Identifies several invalid methods of health assessment used by nutrition quacks to convince their victims that they have special nutritional needs: cytotoxic testing, yeast test, Amalgameter test (related to mercury-amalgam fillings), live cell analysis, iridology, and herbal crystallization analysis. Notes that these bogus tests are enhanced by the confident style of the practitioner and other psychological factors.

*Quack plays doctor, doctor plays quack.
Consumer Reports Health Letter 2:51–2, July 1990.*

Describes the activities of Raymond J. Salani, Jr., who for several years represented himself as a nutritionist and health consultant with a PhD degree. Describes how the New Jersey Attorney General took action against Salani, based on affidavits from six former clients and four undercover investigators who had consulted Salani for various health problems. Notes that Salani's degree was obtained from Donsbach University, an unaccredited correspondence school. States that in December 1989, a Superior Court Judge characterized the PhD as "a Mickey Mouse degree" and ordered Salani to stop representing to the public that he had a doctorate. Adds that the case was concluded with a consent agreement under which Salani was prohibited from representing himself as a doctor or recommending supplements to prevent or treat any specific medical complaint (except upon physician referral).

Herbert V: Separating food facts and myths.
In Herbert V, Subak-Sharpe GJ, Hammock DA (eds.): The Mount Sinai School of Medicine complete book of nutrition, pp. 21–30.
New York, St. Martin's Press, 1990.
Discusses twenty common characteristics of quacks. Advises people who are considering going to a nutritionist to consider the following questions: (1) Do I really need a nutritionist? (2) If so, what should I expect from this person? (3) Does this counselor have an economic interest in selling tests and products? (4) Where do I find a qualified nutrition counselor?

Life-Extension Claims

Leaf A: Long-lived populations: Extreme old age.
Journal of the American Geriatrics Society 30:485–487, 1982.
Describes investigations by the author in three regions of the world whose inhabitants are claimed to live well past 100 years. Concludes that no documents support such claims and that inhabitants of these areas exaggerate their age in order to enhance their social status or to promote tourism.

Barrett S: Book review of Life Extension: A Practical Scientific Approach.
ACSH News & Views 4:14–15, November/December 1983.
Notes that the book's central premise is that animal experiments are now adaptable to humans who want to live to the age of 150. States that the book's presentation of experimental data is "biased and uncritical." Describes how the authors recommend extensive self-experimentation with drugs and dietary supplements, combined with frequent laboratory testing and consultation with a sympathetic physician. States that such a program would be costly and that no sane physician would supervise such a program.

Salholz E, Smith J: How to live forever.
Newsweek 103:81, March 26, 1984.
Slightly tongue-in-cheek report on the activities of Durk Pearson, Sandy Shaw, and their book, *Life Extension* [Warner Books, 1982], which had sold more than a million copies in less than two years. States that the pair had made more than 300 television appearances between them and had turned down offers to endorse about 100 "life extension" products. Quotes critics who state that the central premise of the book—that human life span can be increased with megadoses of nutrients—has no scientific data to support it.

Schneider EL, Reed JD Jr: Life extension.
New England Journal of Medicine 312:1159–1168, 1985
Notes that the subject of life extension had become increasingly prominent in the media. Examines the scientific evidence pertinent to claims for caloric restriction, exercise, dietary antioxidants, superoxide dismutase, centrophenoxine, levodopa, hypophysectomy, Gerovital H-3, dehydroepiandrosterone, and various immunologic interventions. Suggests that it is unlikely that a single intervention will reverse or arrest all aging processes. States that much more research is needed to elucidate the mechanisms of aging.

Can you live longer? What works and what doesn't.
Consumer Reports 57:7–15, January 1992.
Notes how the book *Life Extension* had triggered a boom in sales of nutrient products. Describes a reporter's visit to a "longevity doctor" who prescribes a diet and supplement program. Describes the activities of the Life Extension Foundation, of Hollywood, Florida, noting that its president has been indicted and charged with violating federal drug laws. Describes the nature of free radicals and the theory behind taking antioxidants to counter their effect on the body. Notes that "No one has yet proven the theory that antioxidants slow aging and fight disease by protecting the body from free radicals, although evidence is accumulating. Very few studies so far have examined the effect of supplements directly, and prospective clinical trials are still essential." Concludes that one's shot at longevity can be maximized by following the familiar risk-reduction strategies of eating a well-balanced, low-fat, high-carbohydrate diet, exercising regularly, refraining from smoking and alcohol abuse, and avoiding obesity.

Gerovital

Gerovital H3 (GH3) was developed by the late Dr. Anna Aslan, a Rumanian physician. It has been promoted by the Rumanian National Tourist Office and a few

American physicians as an antiaging substance—"the secret of eternal vigor and youth." Claims have been made that GH3 can prevent or relieve arthritis, arteriosclerosis, angina pectoris and other heart conditions, neuritis, deafness, Parkinson's disease, depression, senile psychosis, and impotence. It is also claimed to stimulate hair growth, restore pigments to gray hair, and tighten and smooth skin. The main ingredient in GH3 is procaine, a substance used for local anesthesia. Although many uncontrolled studies describe great benefits from the use of GH3, controlled trials using procaine have failed to demonstrate any benefit. Noting that para-aminobenzoic acid (PABA) appears in the urine of people receiving procaine injections, a few American manufacturers have marketed "procaine" tablets containing PABA with false claims similar to those made for GH3. The FDA has stopped the sale of several "GH3" products, but others are still marketed.

Ostfeld A, Smith CM, Stotsky BA: The systemic use of procaine in the treatment of the elderly: A review.
Journal of the American Geriatrics Society 25:1–19, January 1977.
This review, commissioned by the National Institute on Aging, discusses the pharmacological characteristics of procaine, claims for Gerovital H-3, and studies of the effects of procaine on depression, senile dementia, atherosclerosis, arthritis, skin and hair, high blood pressure, sexual and endocrine dysfunction, and various other diseases. Concludes that, except for a possible antidepressant effect, there is no convincing evidence that procaine or Gerovital has any value in the treatment of diseases in older patients. Notes that the quality of research on procaine in treating the elderly is generally very poor.

Hecht A: Time marches on despite Gerovital.
FDA Consumer. 14:16–19, March 1980.
Reviews the promotion of Gerovital or procaine hydrochloride as a rejuvenation cure by Dr. Anna Aslan in Romania and her imitators in the United States. Notes the lack of controlled studies proving its effectiveness in retarding aging and treating various diseases. Discusses the activities of Club SeneX, which set up an elaborate scheme to obtain GH3 for "club members" whose "dues" entitled them to a six-month supply prescribed by their own physician or one recommended by the club. Notes that the FDA obtained a preliminary injunction ordering an end to the scheme.

Drug with a double message.
FDA Consumer 20:32, June 1986.
Describes how the FDA stopped the sale of "Arthritis Formula Cream with Copper and Gold, "Procaine H-3 Cream," and "H-3 Formula Tablets" manufactured in a garage of a private residence. Brochures accompanying the products said they could retard aging, promote rejuvenation, and treat arthritis, rheumatism and

atherosclerosis. Despite a front-page disclaimer that the manufacturer did not endorse these claims, the FDA said they were unapproved new drugs. The products were seized by a U.S. marshal and subsequently destroyed.

Ironclad case against Gerovital.
FDA Consumer 20:34–35, April, 1986.
Relates an attempt by a paint supplier to sell drug products allegedly containing procaine hydrochloride, an unapproved drug. Describes how the FDA located the seller and, together with Colorado officials, put an end to the sales.

Rissanen V, Rissanen P, Tuomisto J: Procaine (Gerovital): No effect on the rehabilitation result in patients with back or hip disease.
Annals of Medicine 22:151–156, 1990.
Notes that Gerovital is widely used in some countries to aid in rehabilitation, but that studies of its effects have been conflicting. Describes a study of 88 patients who received Gerovital, procaine, or a placebo. No physiological or psychological benefit was found.

Some scams are hard to unplug.
Consumer Reports 51:626, 1986.
Describes how a company, ordered by the FDA to stop selling GH3, set up another company but continued to use the same toll-free number to take orders.

Raw (Unpasteurized) Milk

Raw milk, which is milk in its natural state, can be a source of bacteria that can cause undulant fever, dysentery, and tuberculosis. "Certified" raw milk should have a bacteria count below a specified standard, but it still can contain significant numbers of disease-producing organisms. In 1987, in response to a court order, the FDA ordered that milk and milk products in interstate commerce that are packaged for human consumption be pasteurized. The sale of raw milk has been banned in 27 states, but is still legal within the rest, including California, which contains the largest source.

Potter ME, Kaufmann AF, Blake PA, et al: Unpasteurized milk: the hazards of a health fetish.
JAMA 252:2048–2052, 1984.
States that meaningful differences between pasteurized and unpasteurized milk have not been demonstrated and that other purported benefits of raw milk consumption have not been substantiated. Notes that the role of unpasteurized dairy products in the transmission of infectious diseases had been established repeatedly.

Fanning O: The science and politics of raw milk.
Nutrition Forum 2:1–4, January 1985.
Describes the testimony of proponents and critics at an FDA hearing on raw milk.

Raw milk creamed by judge.
Consumer Reports Health Letter 2:14, February 1990.
Describes the judge's ruling in a lawsuit brought by the Alameda County District Attorney and Consumers Union against the Alta-Dena Certified Dairy, the nation's largest raw-milk producer. Notes that the state authorities in California had ordered recalls or issued warnings on more than forty occasions after Salmonella bacteria were found in Alta-Dena's raw milk. Reports that in 1989, after a lengthy trial, a Superior Court Judge ordered the dairy to stop advertising its product as safe as or healthier than pasteurized milk. The judge also ruled that the company's raw milk cartons must carry a conspicuous warning that the milk may contain dangerous bacteria. Notes, however, that the milk (now under the name Steuve's Natural) can still be sold without the warning until the appeal process is over.

Bolton J: Raw milk and raw nerves.
California Pediatrician 8:42–44, Fall 1992.
Reviews how the California Department of Health, Public Citizen Health Research Group, Consumers Union, American Academy of Pediatrics, and pediatrician John Bolton, MD, struggled to curb sales of raw milk. Notes that the California Director of Health ordered warning labels on all unpasteurized dairy products and that some communities in California have banned these products. Reports that in 1992 the California Supreme turned down the Steuve appeal, which means that the dairy also had to pay more than $2 million in fines, restitution, Consumers Union's legal fees, and other costs.

"Ergogenic Aids"

About a hundred companies are marketing "supplements" of vitamins, minerals, amino acids, and various other ingredients with false claims that they can help build muscles and improve athletic performance.

An ergogenic runaround for athletes.
Consumer Reports Health Letter 1:5, September 1989.
Notes that pictures of muscular athletes and endorsements from bodybuilding champions appear in ads for "ergogenic aids." Notes that some products are touted as steroid substitutes and growth-hormone releasers. Describes a scheme in which a company advertised that its products had been endorsed by a prominent panel of sports medicine professionals, who actually had not given permission for use of their

names. Quotes one of the five, a member of the President's Council on Physical Fitness, who stated: "I think the products are of no real value. A well-balanced diet can supply all the nutrients and energy that an athlete needs. The only way to reach your maximum potential as an athlete is through hard work and practice. There are no safe shortcuts or miracles in capsules or tablets." Urges the FDA and FTC to stop the marketing of "growth-hormone releasers."

Magic muscle pills!!: Health and fitness quackery in nutritional supplements. New York, New York City Department of Consumer Affairs, 1992.
Calls the bodybuilding supplement industry "an economic hoax with unhealthy consequences," and warns consumers to beware of terms like "fat burner," "fat fighter," "fat metabolizer," "energy enhancer," " performance booster," "strength booster," " ergogenic aid," "anabolic optimizer," and "genetic optimizer." Reports that investigators from the New York City Department of Consumer Affairs found that manufacturers contacted for product information were unable to provide a single published report from a scientific journal to back claims that their products did any of these things. Announces that the Department has issued "Notices of Violation" to six such companies and challenged the FDA to clean up the marketplace nationwide. Calculates that a supplement program recommended in the leading bodybuilding magazine (*Muscle & Fitness*) would cost more than $11 per day.

Philen RM, Ortiz DI, Auerbach S, et al: Survey of advertising for nutritional supplements in health and bodybuilding magazines.
JAMA 268:1008–1011, 1992.
Reports that the authors' survey of twelve popular bodybuilding magazines found advertisements for 89 brands and 311 products containing a total of 235 unique ingredients, the most frequent of which were amino acids and herbs. Among the 221 products for which an effect was claimed, 59 were said to produce muscle growth, 27 were said to increase testosterone levels, 17 were said to enhance energy, 15 were said to reduce fat, and 12 were said to increase strength. The authors advise doctors to routinely ask patients whether they are taking supplements and to report possible adverse or side effects to public health authorities.

Miscellaneous Products

The health food industry markets thousands of "supplement" products and many "health foods" through its retail outlets and by mail. Although the term "health food" cannot actually be defined, it is used to suggest that certain foods have special health-giving properties not found in "ordinary" foods. Some "health" foods are rich in various nutrients and can be a valuable part of a balanced diet. But no food has any special health-promoting property beyond those of the nutrients it contains. The first eight reports pertain to large numbers of supplement and/or health food products. The rest cover individual items that have been subjected to scientific study.

Keller CW: Report of the presiding officer on proposed trade regulation rule regarding advertising and labeling of protein supplements.
Washington, DC, Federal Trade Commission, June 15, 1978.
Reports the findings of an FTC official who investigated claims related to the marketing and use of protein supplements. Reports the official's impression that "the level of general nutrition knowledge among laymen in the United States is unfortunately low." Concludes that: (1) the use of concentrated protein supplements poses health risks to certain people; (2) relatively few Americans fail to consume enough protein; (3) there is no nutritional advantage to getting protein from supplements rather than from foods; (4) protein is not depleted in any greater degree by strenuous activity than by ordinary physical activity; (5) the small extra amounts required during rigorous athletic training are likely to exceeded by the additional protein in food consumed to provide extra calories; (6) consuming extra protein does not improve athletic performance; and (7) protein consumption, as such, offers no benefit in weight reduction.

Donegan TJ Jr, Orland MH, et al: Proposed trade regulation rule on food advertising, staff report and recommendations.
Washington, DC, Federal Trade Commission, September, 25, 1978.
Reports the FTC staff's analysis for a proposed trade regulation rule that would cover advertising claims for many types of food products. States that the terms "natural food," "organic food," and "health food" are used in misleading ways and are often misunderstood by consumers. Concludes that: (1) advertisers should be prohibited from suggesting that a food is superior in nutrient content or safety merely because it is "natural" or "organic"; (2) the term "health food" should be banned because it falsely attributes special or superior health-giving properties to certain foods and cannot be defined or qualified in any meaningful way; and (3) health-related claims that would not be legal on product labels (under FDA regulations) should be prohibited in advertising. Additional views on these matters are expressed in Dixon WD: *Proposed Trade Regulation Rule: Food Advertising, Report of the Presiding Officer,* February 21, 1978, which summarizes the views presented to the FTC by parties concerned these issues. Although no final rule was adopted, these reports are valuable because they include a thorough evaluation of the slogans used to promote many nutritional products.

Dubick MA, Rucker RB: Dietary supplements and health aids—a critical evaluation.
Journal of Nutrition Education 15:47–53, 88–93, 123–129, 1983.

A 3-part analysis of claims made for a large number of nutritional products. The first part covers niacin, vitamin B_{12}, vitamin C, vitamin A, vitamin D, vitamin E, megavitamin supplementation, dolomite and bone meal, chromium (Glucose Tolerance Factor), sea salt, selenium, and zinc. The second part covers proteins, amino acids, enzymes, gelatin, glycine, starch blockers, aspartame, tryptophan, digestive aids, superoxide dismutase, fructose, honey, choline, lecithin and dietary fiber. The final part covers acidophilus tablets, acidophilus milk, aloe vera, brewer's yeast, garlic, ginseng, herbal preparations, spirulina, wheat germ, wheat germ oil, flavonoids, gerovital, hair products, inositol, laetrile, nucleic acids, pangamic acid, para-aminobenzoic acid, and the placebo effect. Each part cites more than 100 references.

Jarvis WT: Food: Facts & fallacies A–Z.
Washington, DC, Review and Herald Publishing Association, 1985.
Booklet briefly discusses about one hundred products sold in health food stores and several other quackery-related topics.

Bender A: Health or hoax: The truth about health foods and diets.
Buffalo, Prometheus Books, 1986.
Analyzes sales techniques used by the health food industry and rebuts false claims made for many of its products.

Yetiv JZ:: Popular nutritional practices: A scientific appraisal.
San Carlos, CA, Popular Medicine Press, 1986.
Provides an extensively referenced analysis of more than one hundred nutrition topics of current concern. Includes many supplement products sold through health food stores.

Stare FJ, Aronson V, Barrett S: Your guide to good nutrition.
Buffalo, 1991, Prometheus Books, 1991
Describes current dietary guidelines and how to implement them. Tells how to recognize quack claims. Lists claims and facts for more than sixty types of products sold through health food stores.

More snake oils, scams, and wild goose chases.
In Butler K: A consumer's guide to "alternative medicine," pp. 147–230.
Buffalo, Prometheus Books, 1992.
Includes discussion of about twenty-five products sold through health food stores.

Larkin T: Bee pollen as a health food.
FDA Consumer 18:20–22, April 1984.

Describes how bee pollen is gathered. Rebuts claims that pollen "is nature's most perfect food"; can't be spoiled by bacteria; can retard aging; is "the richest source of protein known to science"; can enhance athletic performance; can relieve allergies, asthma, and hay fever; and is effective against many other ailments.

Mirkin G: Bee pollen: Living up to its hype?
The Physician and Sports Medicine 13:159–160, July 1985.
Discusses the promotion of bee pollen as a health food. Notes claims of therapeutic benefits made for it by advocates and mentions shortcomings of alleged scientific research to support these claims. Discusses the debate over methods of harvesting bee pollen and notes the lack of scientific evidence to support claims of either side. Notes that some people have developed asthma and other allergic reactions after ingesting bee pollen despite claims made by promoters that bee pollen is harmless.

Goldfinger SE: Good for what ails you?
Harvard Health Letter 16:1–2, August 1991.
Notes that many studies have examined the health effects of garlic and its derivatives in human and laboratory studies. Cautions that any evidence of benefit is preliminary and that garlic can produce bad breath, heartburn, flatulence, and can inhibit blood clotting. Notes that if it does help, it probably has to be taken fresh and in amounts large enough to drive one's companions away.

Lowell JA: Organic germanium: Another health food store junk food.
Nutrition Forum 5:53–58, September/October 1988.
Notes that the health food industry has been promoting germanium compounds as "miracle drugs." Traces the development of "organic germanium" by Japanese metallurgist Kazuhiko Asai, noting his claims regarding therapeutic benefits. Notes that some germanium compounds have been tested for anticancer activity but appear to be ineffective or too toxic for practical use. Discusses several leading promoters of germanium in the United States. Notes that in 1988 the FDA issued an Import Alert stating that germanium could be imported only for use by the semiconductor industry. [Subsequently the agency seized germanium products marketed by several American companies.]

Knuiman JT, Beynen JT, Katan MB: Lecithin intake and serum cholesterol.
American Journal of Clinical Nutrition 49:266–268, 1989.
Notes that lecithin products have been promoted for lowering blood cholesterol. Reviews twenty-four studies of lecithin supplementation to determine whether this alleged effect has been substantiated experimentally. Concludes that most of the studies were poorly designed and the rest suggest no benefit.

Adverse Case Reports

The number of individuals harmed each years by high doses of vitamins or minerals or by toxic effects of other "dietary supplements" or "health foods" is unknown. Between 1986 and 1990, the American Dietetic Association collected more than five hundred case reports of people harmed by inappropriate nutrition advice from bogus "nutritionists," health food store operators, and other sources of misinformation. The cases below illustrate the types of problems that can occur.

Smith FR, Goodman DS: Vitamin A transport in human vitamin A toxicity.
New England Journal of Medicine 294:805–808, 1976.
Describes three cases of people who developed severe toxicity from massive doses of vitamin A. One was a nine-year-old boy with sinusitus whose mother had consulted an iridologist. The iridilogist "recognized airway obstruction and hidden allergies" and referred the boy to a "nutritionist" who recommended a daily regimen of 50,000 units of vitamin A and eleven other supplements.

Barrett S: The legacy of Adelle Davis.
Environmental Nutrition 5:S3, November 1982.
Describes how a two-month-old infant was killed by the administration of potassium drops for colic, as recommended in Adelle Davis's book, *Let's Have Healthy Children*. States that the parents filed suit and collected a total of $100,000 in an out-of-court settlement with the publisher and Ms. Davis's estate. Notes that the book was recalled from the marketplace and revised by a physician aligned with the health food industry. [The manufacturer of the potassium drops subsequently settled out of court for $60,000.]

Mansfield LE, Goldstein GB: Anaphylactic reaction
after ingestion of local bee pollen.
Annals of Allergy 47:154–156, September 1981.
Describes a case of a man who purchased bee pollen at a local health food store to treat his hay fever. States that within thirty minutes after taking a teaspoonful, he experienced generalized angioedema, dyspnea, and other symptoms that required emergency care. Mentions four similar cases and recommends that vendors of bee pollen be required to warn allergic patients about possible risks.

Dalton K, Dalton MJT: Characteristics of pyridoxine
overdose neuropathy syndrome.
Acta Neurologica Scandinavica 76:8–11, 1987.
Reports on a study of 172 women who developed elevated vitamin B_6 levels while

attending a clinic that specialized in premenstrual syndrome. States that more than one hundred of them who had taken vitamin B_6 for more than six months developed neurological symptoms as a result. Notes that 20 percent had taken less than 50 mg per day and that most of the rest had taken less than 200 mg per day. Notes that although all recovered completely, cases involving higher dosages have been reported in which recovery was not complete.

Matsusaka T, Fujii M, Nakano T, et al: Germanium-induced nephropathy: Report of two cases and review of the literature.
Clinical Nephrology 30:341–345, 1988.
Describes how two Japanese men had developed kidney failure after long-term use of germanium, one for seven months and the other for 13 months. Notes eight other cases in which germanium was used for 4 to 18 months. Two of the ten people had died. Eight more cases were reported in *Clinical Nephrology* 31:219–224, 1989, and the *Japanese Journal of Medicine* 30:67–72, January/February 1991.

Lin FL, Vaughan TR, Vandewalker ML: Hypereosinophilia, neurologic, and gastrointestinal symptoms after bee-pollen ingestion.
Journal of Allergy and Clinical Immunology 83:793–796, 1989.
Notes that some people have suffered ill effects from ingesting bee pollen purchased from health food stores. Describes a case of a woman who was treated at a military hospital after consuming bee pollen in order to increase her energy. The patient, who had no prior history of allergic reactions, developed general malaise, headache, nausea, abdominal pain, diarrhea, generalized itching and rash, and was found to be allergic to several pollens.

Bluhm R et al: Aplastic anemia associated with canthaxanthin ingested for 'tanning purposes.'
JAMA 264:1141–1142, 1990.
Reports that a 20-year-old woman took high doses of canthaxanthan and developed aplastic anemia, a serious condition in which the production of blood cells is impaired. Notes that previous reports have linked canthaxanthin use to hepatitis, generalized itching, hives, and eye problems.

Vitamin A cases settled for record sum.
Nutrition Forum 7:31, July/August 1990.
Reports how two children with ichthyosis (a hereditary condition in which the skin is hard and scaly) developed symptoms of vitamin A poisoning from large doses prescribed by a chiropractor. Notes that one child had damage to the growth centers of several of her bones and wound up with a short leg and scoliosis as a result. Notes that the other child sustained permanent damage to his liver and spleen. Reports that

suits filed against the chiropractor and two vitamin companies were settled out of court for a total of almost $900,000.

Dyer JE: Gamma-Hydroxybutyrate: A health-food product producing coma and seizure-like activity.
American Journal of Emergency Medicine 9:321–324, 1991.
Reports adverse effects in sixteen patients who consumed gamma hydroxybutyrate, a health–food product claimed to aid dieting or bodybuilding by releasing growth hormone. Notes that symptoms included weakness, confusion, incontinence, hallucinations, incoordination, agitation, dizziness, seizures, and respiratory problems. Notes that the product continues to be sold even though it is banned. Urges physicians to be aware of the product's symptoms.

Kamb ML, Murphy JJ, Jones JL, et al: Eosinophilia-myalgia syndrome in L-tryptophan-exposed patients.
JAMA 267:77–82, 1992.
Reports on the incidence of eosinophilia-myalgia syndrome (EMS) among patients of a psychiatrist who had prescribed the amino acid L-tryptophan to more than 450 patients during 1989. Reports that 47 definite cases and 68 possible cases occurred among 418 patients whom the researchers interviewed, and that most had received it for the treatment of depression. Notes that the illness produces muscle and joint pain, hair loss, skin changes, and/or localized numbness, tingling or weakness, accompanied by an elevated eosinophil count. States that those who became ill had used brands traceable to a Japanese company that had manufactured the L-tryptophan used to make the retail products, suggesting that the problem was caused by a contaminant in the manufacturing process. Notes though June 1990, the U.S. Centers for Disease Control, using strict criteria, had collected reports of 1,531 cases of EMS among L-tryptophan users. [L-tryptophan had been widely promoted for insomnia, depression, premenstrual syndrome (PMS), and overweight, even though it had not been proven safe and effective for these purposes. To date, 38 deaths from EMS have been reported.]

Anderson SA, Raiten DJ (eds.): Safety of amino acids used as dietary supplements.
Washington, DC, Federation of American Societies for Experimental Biology, July 1992.
Notes that the eosinophilia-myalgia syndrome epidemic has raised questions about the safety of amino acids sold as dietary supplements. Notes that these products were "used primarily for pharmacological purposes or enhancement of physiological function rather than for nutritional purposes." States that little scientific literature exists on most amino acids ingested as single or multiple-ingredient capsules,

tablets, or liquid products. Notes that no scientific rationale has been presented to justify the taking of amino acid supplements by healthy individuals. Concludes that safety levels for amino acid supplement use cannot be established at this time and that a systematic approach to safety testing is needed.

Criticism of Individual Proponents

Rynearson EH: Americans love hogwash.
Nutrition Reviews 32 (Supplement No. 1):1–14, July 1974.
Severely criticizes Adelle Davis, Carlton Fredericks, the Hypoglycemia Foundation, J.I. Rodale, the Zen macrobiotic diet, and the overpromotion of vitamin E. Hopes that physicians and nutrition scientists will become more interested in attacking nutrition misinformation and cultism.

Barrett S: Book review of Your Personal Vitamin Profile, *by Michael Colgan.*
Nutrition Forum 1:14, November 1984.
Notes that the book jacket claims that "the author's work has been recognized throughout the world," but does not say by whom. Notes that the table of contents states that vitamin supplements can inhibit aging and prevent heart disease, cancer, diabetes, and herpes. Calls attention to the warning on the copyright page that "any application of the advice herein is at the reader's sole discretion and risk." Observes that "the author cites hundreds of reputable reports, but the scientists who wrote them would certainly disagree with his advice." Describes how the author recommends how to determine one's "individual biochemical equation," starting with a basic 28-nutrient formula and adding various amounts of these and other nutrients for each positive answer to more than fifty questions. (For example, a 125-pound woman who lives in a big city, takes the Pill, and gets colds is advised to take 1500+1000+500+1000 mg of vitamin C and 300+0+100+100 IU of vitamin E daily." States that most readers who follow the prescribed schedule for each nutrient would waste hundreds of dollars per year.

Lowell JA: Some notes on Linus Pauling.
Nutrition Forum 2:33–36, May 1985.
Describes the writings and other activities of Linus Pauling, PhD. Notes how Dr. Pauling had coined the term "orthomolecular" and postulated that many people needed above-RDA amounts of vitamins and minerals to maintain good health. Describes how Pauling is aligned with the health food industry. Notes that he persists in claiming that large doses of vitamin C can prevent colds and cure cancer even though scientific studies have refuted these claims.

Lowell JA: An irreverent look at the Vitamin Bible *and its author.*
Nutrition Forum 3:46–47, June 1986.
Criticizes the writings of Earl Mindell, who helped found the Great Earth chain of health food stores. Describes how Mindell acquired a "PhD" in nutrition from an unaccredited school. Notes that information sheets written by Mindell have been used to promote product sales in health food stores.

Forester JD, Thompson SLT: The legacies of Paavo Airola.
Nutrition Forum 4:9–11, February 1987.
Describes the notions of naturopath Paavo Airola, author of many books sold through health food stores. Describes how the publisher says that the books will boost sales of vitamins, minerals, other supplements, herbs, and natural foods, as well as juicers, seed grinders, and flour mills, all of which are recommended in Airola's writings.

Lund DS: MD surrenders license; author, medicine's critic.
American Medical News 30:21, March 27, 1987.
Describes how "nutritional advocate" Lendon Smith, MD, permanently surrendered his medical license to the Oregon Board of Medical Examiners after having been charged with "obtaining any fee by fraud or misrepresentation" and "making a fraudulent claim." Indicates that the charges involved allegations that Dr. Smith had signed documents authorizing insurance payments for patients who were seen by chiropractors, homeopaths, and other nontraditional practitioners at "nutrition-oriented" clinics with which Smith was affiliated. Also describes disciplinary action he faced during the mid-1970s.

South J: Can nutripathy transform the world?
Nutrition Forum 4:57–61, September 1987.
Discusses Gary Martin and his widely advertised correspondence school, the American College of Nutripathy. States that Martin defines nutripathy as "the condensation of most all natural healing and counseling. . . . the basics boiled down from literally hundreds of different therapies and techniques." Reports that Martin is listed in the Yellow Pages under "nutritionists" and that patients who consult him are asked to submit urine and saliva samples for testing. Notes that this test procedure was developed about fifty years ago by Cary Reams, a self-proclaimed biophysicist who was prosecuted during the 1970s for practicing medicine without a license. Notes that the various "degrees" offered by Martin's school include "PhD's" in nutritional philosophy and nutripathic philosophy. States that the school is unaccredited and that state regulatory agencies were attempting to shut it down. Also states that Martin is selling products with claims that make them unapproved and misbranded drugs.

Barrett S: Book review of Design Your Own Vitamin and
Mineral Program, *by Shari Lieberman, MA, RD.*
Nutrition Forum 4:64, September 1987.
Observes that the book is claimed to provide "the most comprehensive, unified, and scientifically sound picture of what vitamins and minerals can—and cannot—do for you." Notes that the author claims incorrectly that "you cannot get all the nutrients you need from today's food" and that "the RDAs are the nutritional equivalent of today's minimal wage." Describes how the author postulates higher "Optimal Daily Allowances" and suggests that "nutrition should be our first line of defense if an illness or condition is not life-threatening." Notes that the author states that in her private practice she counsels fifty people each week who come to her with a variety of problems and needs. Notes that in 1985, the American Dietetic Association censured the author for failing to adhere to accepted standards.

Parton N: Self-claimed nutrition expert faked credentials, probe finds.
Vancouver Sun, pp. B1, B5, September 13, 1988.
Reports on an investigation of the credentials of Alexander G. Schauss, who operates the American Institute for Biosocial Research, in Tacoma, Washington, and edits the *International Journal of Biosocial Research.* Notes that Schauss is interested in relationships between diet and behavior and had written a book called *Nutrition and Criminal Behavior.* States that Schauss listed himself as "Dr." and "Ph.D." in city and telephone directories but had no such degree. States that in 1981 Schauss had registered in a doctoral program at an unaccredited school and sometimes identifies himself as "Ph.D. (c)," explaining when queried that "c" means "candidate." Notes that seven other claims Schauss made about his professional background and activities appeared to be false.

Conlin J: Bring us your tired, your sickly, your gullible and hypochondriacal rich.
Spy, pp. 58–66, 73–74, March 1989.
Traces the careers of Stuart Berger, MD, author of *Dr. Berger's Immune Power Diet* [New American Library, 1985], and Robert Giller, MD, author of *Medical Makeover* [William Morrow and Co., 1986], both of whom attribute a wide variety of common symptoms to hidden allergies. States that both use hair analysis and prescribe large doses of vitamins to many patients. Describes what happened to two reporters who visited Dr. Giller as patients. Notes that he prescribed vitamin B_{12} shots for many of his patients.

"Experts" to Be Wary of.
In Butler K: A consumer's guide to "alternative medicine," pp. 29–62.
Buffalo, Prometheus Books, 1992.
Criticizes the ideas of ten people who have written popular books promoting

unproven nutritional methods: Paavo Airola, Adelle Davis, Kurt Donsbach, Carlton Fredericks, Robert Mendelsohn, Earl Mindell, Gary Null, Kristin Olsen, Durk Pearson and Sandy Shaw.

Health Food Industry Organizations and Activities

Barrett S: CRN: responsible or irresponsible?
Nutrition Forum 4:38–39, May 1987.
Examines the formation, composition, and activities of the Council for Responsible Nutrition, a trade association for manufacturers and wholesale distributors of dietary supplements. Notes that several of the group's members are violating its code of ethics by making misleading advertising claims.

Barrett S: Dietary Supplement Coalition (DSC) is formed to fight FDA.
Priorities, pp. 24–25, Fall 1989.
Describes how supplement manufacturers have banded together to defend against certain FDA regulatory actions. Notes that five of the seven founding members have made improper claims for their products.

Tannenhaus N: A visit to Natural Foods Expo.
Nutrition Forum 7:47–48, November/December 1990.
Reports on a major trade show for the health food industry. Notes that the meeting had about 12,000 visitors and 826 exhibit booths filled by 657 manufacturers. Suggests that the most dangerous provider of advice was the Cancer Control Society, which offered information and referrals for "alternative" approaches to cancer, arthritis, and other diseases. Notes that additional misinformation was provided at seminars and in literature that was distributed by many companies.

Barrett S: Proposed labeling rules stir controversy.
Nutrition Forum 9:9–14, March/April 1992.
Notes passage of the Nutrition Labeling and Education Act (1990), which orders the FDA to issue regulations for the labels of foods and dietary supplements. Explains why the health food industry is upset about regulations the agency proposed in response to the law. Notes formation of the FDA Dietary Supplement Task Force to explore how dietary supplements should be defined and regulated. Reports testimony given by critics and supporters at a public hearing on these issues.

Barrett S: Another "vitamin war" has begun.
Priorities, pp. 28–32, Summer 1992.
Describes how the Nutritional Health Alliance was formed to stop legislation and new

rules that would enable the FDA to curb sales of many of the products sold in health food stores. Notes that the industry hopes to generate at least one million letters to Congress.

Supplement rules, RDIs delayed by Congress.
Nutrition Week 22:3, October 9, 1992.
Describes how Senator Orrin Hatch (R-UT) gained passage of an amendment establishing a 13-month moratorium on implementing new rules for dietary supplements.

Proponent Literature

The health food industry is supported by a cadre of writers who promote the ideas that everyone needs to take vitamin supplements, that many people should take above-RDA amounts, and/or that supplements are appropriate for the treatment of virtually every health problem. Many books and articles written by such writers make unproven claims for vitamins and "health foods" that would be illegal on product labels but are permitted in print under the doctrine of freedom of the press. The largest supplier of books to the industry, Nutri-Books Corp., of Denver, Colorado, carries more than 1,500 titles. Its merchandising manual for retailers states: "Books and articles created the nutritional foods industry. They are still at work, creating new customers every moment of every hour! They are the number one product promoters of our industry. . . . They tell your customers what your products will do for them. . . . Very often this is information you may not be able to give—or may not be permitted to discuss." The first book described below traces the growth of the health food industry. The next two books prescribe an abundance of supplements for virtually every health problem. The final article, from *Time* magazine, is being widely used to promote the sale of antioxidant supplements.

Murray F, Tarr J: More than one slingshot: How the
health food industry is changing America.
Marlborough House Publishing Co., Richmond, VA, 1984.
Describes the origins and many of the political battles fought by the health food industry. Emphasizes the events leading to passage of the Proxmire Amendment to the Food, Drug, and Cosmetic Act, which weakened the FDA's ability to regulate the marketing of vitamin and mineral supplements. Describes the origins of the National Nutritional Association, the leading trade association for health food retailers, manufacturers, and distributors. Notes how a 1964 court decision enables retailers to sell books which contain claims that would be illegal on product labels. Falsely suggests that several critics of the health food industry have financial motives for their criticism.

Dunn LJ: Nutrition almanac, 3rd edition.
New York, McGraw-Hill, 1990.
Presents the author's views on various nutrients and herbs. Lists vitamins, minerals, and other supplements the author recommends for more than a hundred diseases and conditions. Previous editions written or coauthored by the author's father, John D. Kirschmann, were published by McGraw-Hill in 1975, 1979, and 1984. The cover states that over 2.5 million copies of these editions were sold.

Balch JF, Balch PA: Prescription for nutritional healing: a practical A–Z reference to drug-free remedies using vitamins, minerals, herbs & food supplements.
Garden City Park, NY, Avery Publishing Group, 1990.
Provides the authors' views of the various supplements and herbs found in health food stores. Provides diagnostic guidelines and treatment suggestions for more than 250 common ailments and disorders. Lists manufacturers of the types of products recommended. Includes recommendations for chelation therapy, hair analysis, color therapy, coffee enemas, and many other unproven and unscientific methods. Promoted by the publisher as "a complete and authoritative self-help approach to dealing with health disorders using the nutritional, herbal, and supplemental therapies sold in your store."

Toufexis A: The new scoop on vitamins.
Time 139:54–59, April 6, 1992.
Provides a confusing look at research tidbits and speculations about vitamins, garnished by hedged statements by the article's author. Suggests that "almost every week brings new hints that extra doses of vitamins may help you stay healthy longer, especially if you can't stand broccoli and Brussels sprouts." States that the FDA's proposed Reference Daily Intake (RDI) standard for food labels "flies in the face of research that suggests benefits from higher doses of vitamins." [The article was published as a cover story headlined "The Real Power of Vitamins – New research shows that they may help fight cancer, heart disease, and the ravages of aging." The National Nutritional Foods Association (NNFA) labeled publication of the article "a watershed event for the industry. . . . the most positive public relations tool that the industry has been able to use in years." NNFA sent a copy to every member of Congress as part of its campaign to prevent implementation of proposed FDA food labeling regulations. Multiple copies were distributed to health food stores to give to their customers, and the article's author spoke at the annual NNFA convention.]

Dubious Diagnostic Tests

This section discusses six kinds of tests used by unscientific practitioners as the basis for prescribing dietary supplements, herbs, and/or homeopathic remedies. Hair analysis has limited usefulness for screening populations for heavy metal poisoning and is a legitimate subject for further research, but it is not valid for determining the body's nutritional status. The other five tests play no role in scientific health care.

Applied Kinesiology

Applied kinesiology is a system of diagnosis and treatment developed by chiropractor George J. Goodheart during the mid-1960s. Its proponents claim that every organ dysfunction is accompanied by a specific muscle weakness, which enables diseases to be diagnosed primarily through muscle-testing procedures. Its practitioners—most of whom are chiropractors—also claim that nutritional deficiencies, allergies, and other adverse reactions to food substances can be detected by placing substances in the mouth so that the patient salivates. "Good" substances will make specific muscles stronger, whereas "bad" substances will cause specific weaknesses. Treatment then consists of vitamin supplements or a special diet. In double-blind studies, one investigator found no difference in muscle response from one substance to another, while others have found no difference between the results with test substances and with placebos. Applied kinesiology should be distinguished from kinesiology (biomechanics), the scientific study of movement.

Friedman MH, Weisberg J: Applied kinesiology—double-blind pilot study. Journal of Prosthetic Dentistry 45:321–323, 1981.
Describes a series of double-blind tests conducted with college students whose arm muscle strength was tested before and after "muscle-strengthening" or "muscle-weakening" techniques and ingestion of sugar, vitamin E, or candy. During a final test the students were told that eating the candy would probably make them test stronger. In the first two tests, techniques that applied kinesiologists claim will increase or decrease muscle strength produced no overall change. In the second two tests, while ingestion of sugar caused a majority of students to test weaker, simple suggestion reversed this trend.

Triano JJ: Muscle strength testing as a diagnostic screen for supplemental nutritional therapy: A blind study.

Journal of Manipulative Physiology and Therapeutics 5:179–182, 1982.
Describes how several groups of twenty-five patients said to have a weak latissimus dorsi muscle were subjected to muscle-testing by chiropractors who were "certified" in applied kinesiology. Using a double-blind protocol, four types of nutritional products were placed under the patients' tongue or in an unopened packet on the patient's abdomen. No product showed a consistent relationship with reported "strengthening" of the muscle.

Goodheart GJ, Poortinga G, Triano JJ: Letters to the editor.
Journal of Manipulative Physiology and Therapeutics 6:87–90, 1983.
Responding to the above article, Dr. Goodheart and another practitioner accuse Dr. Triano of bias and poor experimental design. He replies that Dr. Goodheart had endorsed the protocol at a planning session and had even volunteered to be a tester.

Kenney JJ, Clemens R, Forsythe KD: Applied kinesiology
unreliable for assessing nutrient status.
Journal of the American Dietetic Association 88:698–704, 1988.
Describes a study in which three experienced kinesiologists performed independent testing to evaluate eleven subjects for "deficiencies" of thiamin, zinc, and vitamins A and C. The results were then compared with each other and with standard biochemical measurements of nutrient status and computerized testing of muscle strength. Notes that the three testers agreed with each other in only 12 out of 44 cases, whereas random guessing would have been predicted to produce agreement in 11 out of 44 cases. Notes that no correlation was found between the kinesiologists' assessments and the laboratory measurements. Concludes that "the use of applied kinesiology to evaluate nutrient status is no more useful than random guessing."

Commercial Hair Analysis

Hair analysis is a test in which a sample of a person's hair is sent to a laboratory for measurement of its mineral content. Commercial hair analysis involves the use of a single procedure to determine values for many minerals simultaneously. This type of analysis is used by chiropractors, "nutrition consultants," physicians who do chelation therapy, and other "alternative" practitioners who claim that hair analysis can help them diagnose a wide variety of diseases and can be used as the basis for prescribing dietary supplements. These proponents claim that hair analysis is useful for evaluating a person's general state of nutrition and health and is valuable in detecting predisposition to disease. They also claim that hair analysis enables the practitioner to determine whether mineral deficiency, mineral imbalance or heavy metal pollutants in the body may be the cause of a patient's symptoms. In 1984, there were about fifteen laboratories doing commercial hair analysis in the United States. Today there are probably about ten.

Although hair analysis has limited value as a screening device for heavy metal exposure, it is not considered reliable for evaluating the nutritional status of individuals. In 1974, the AMA Committee on Cutaneous Health and Cosmetics noted that "the state of health of the body may be entirely unrelated to the physical and chemical condition of the hair.... Although severe deficiency states of an essential element are often associated with low concentrations of the element in hair, there are no data to indicate that low concentrations of an element in the hair indicate low tissue levels or that high concentrations reflect high tissue stores. Therefore... metal levels in hair would rarely help a physician select effective treatment."

Other commentators have noted the following problems with hair analysis interpretation:

• Hair mineral content can be affected by exposure to various substances such as shampoos, bleaches and hair dyes. No analytic technique enables reliable determination of the source of specific levels of elements in hair as bodily or environmental.

• The level of certain minerals can be affected by the color, diameter and rate of growth of an individual's hair, the season of the year, the geographic location, and the age and gender of the individual.

• Most commercial hair analysis laboratories have not validated their analytical techniques by checking them against standard reference materials. Moreover, the techniques typically used to prepare samples for analysis introduce errors for many of the elements being determined.

• Normal ranges of hair minerals have not been defined.

• For most elements, no correlation has been established between hair level and other known indicators of nutrition status. It is possible for hair concentration of an element (zinc, for example) to be high even though deficiency exists in the body.

• Hair grows slowly (1 cm/month), so even hair closest to the scalp is several weeks old and thus may not reflect current body conditions for purposes of health diagnosis.

- The use of a single multielemental hair analysis test as the sole means of diagnosis violates basic tenets of medical practice that laboratory findings should be considered together with the patient's history and physical examination. In addition, laboratory errors occur.

For these reasons, multielemental analysis of human hair is not considered a valid technique for identifying an individual's current bodily excesses or deficiencies of essential or nonessential elements. Nor does it provide a valid basis for recommending vitamins, minerals, or other dietary supplements.

In December 1984, the AMA House of Delegates adopted a resolution opposing the use of hair analysis to determine the need for medical attention. In 1987, the Association's Council on Scientific Affairs issued a report noting the wide divergence of opinion on the merits of hair analysis and the lack of adequate information regarding its merits. The report called for further research and recommended that hair analysis be reserved for experimental study to assess its potential value for various purposes.

During the past few years, some interest has been expressed in the use of hair analysis to detect whether individuals are abusing drugs. The National Institute for Drug Abuse argues that there is too little information on hair analysis to support its widespread use in drug testing. In 1990 the FDA issued a Compliance Policy Guide stating that analysis of hair by radioimmunoassay (RIA) for the presence of abused drugs is "an unproven procedure unsupported by the scientific literature or well controlled studies or clinical trials."

Hambidge KM: Hair analyses: worthless for vitamins, limited for minerals. American Journal of Clinical Nutrition 36: 943–949, 1982.
Thorough discussion of the factors influencing the outcome and significance of hair analysis. Reviews uses of hair analysis by "alternative" practitioners for diagnosis of nutritional deficiencies and disease states. Concludes that hair analysis is worthless for most of these applications.

Fenner L: Hair analysis? May as well be bald. FDA Consumer 17:16–17, April 1983.
Discusses how commercial hair analysis laboratories would analyze hair specimens sent by mail and issue reports suggesting that vitamin and mineral supplements were needed. Notes that hair analysis was also used by chiropractors, "nutrition counselors," and "holistic" physicians as a diagnostic aid. Notes that some labs also

diagnose nonexistent medical problems. Discusses factors that make hair analysis unreliable for diagnosing nutritional deficiencies.

Freifeld K, Engelmayer S: Hair analysis: Are you being scalped?
Health 15:33–34, 36, 42–43, July 1983.
Describes how one of the article's authors sent identical hair samples to three commercial hair analysis laboratories, which reported widely differing results and recommendations for dietary supplements. Discusses the theory behind hair analysis, costs involved, and types of practitioners who use it for diagnosis. Notes flaws in the procedure, such as the lack of standards to measure trace elements in hair and the possibility of contamination by pollutants and hair-care products. Mentions government attempts to regulate hair analysis firms. Reports response by laboratories to criticism. Notes legitimate uses of hair analysis.

Rivlin RS: Misuse of hair analysis for nutritional assessment.
American Journal of Medicine 75:489–493, 1983.
Explores the potential use of hair analysis, noting its potential advantages compared to urine and blood tests. Discusses some pitfalls of hair analysis, including contamination by sweat, environmental conditions, and hair-care products. Concludes that hair analysis may be useful in toxicology (for measuring heavy metal concentrations) but not for evaluation of nutritional status.

Brody JE: Scrutiny of hair-analysis scam reveals that the public is getting scalped.
Chicago Tribune, Section 5, p. 9, November 3, 1983.
Examines commercial hair analysis by nutrition consultants, health food retailers, and other "alternative practitioners." Describes the procedure and discusses examples of people who were given inappropriate advice based on hair analyses. Reports on two patients who were advised that they had lead poisoning and should undergo chelation therapy. Argues that hair analysis is unreliable, noting that hair-care products can leave residues of substances that would be toxic within the body but are harmless on the hair.

Hair analysis halted by FTC.
Nutrition Forum 1:12, November 1984.
Describes how the Federal Trade Commission obtained a temporary restraining order against a commercial laboratory that was the largest advertiser of hair analysis to the public. Describes how six identical hair samples sent to the laboratory under different names generated reports with widely inconsistent findings. The laboratory also made supplement recommendations that varied greatly from one report to another. [Several months later the court issued a permanent injunction forbidding

direct marketing to the public but permitting the procedure to be done if ordered by a health professional. However, the laboratory went out of business.]

Hair analysis—a potential for medical abuse.
Proceedings of the AMA House of Delegates, p. 382, December 2–5, 1984.
Resolution adopted by the American Medical Association's House of Delegates opposing the use of hair analysis to determine the need for medical attention and urging the Association to inform the public and government agencies of the potential for health fraud.

Sherertz, EC. Misuse of hair analysis as a diagnostic tool.
Archives of Dermatology 121:1504–1505, 1985.
States that hair analysis may have some potential usefulness but should be regarded primarily as a research tool.

Barrett S: Commercial hair analysis: Science or scam?
JAMA 254:1041–1045, 1985.
Explains why hair analysis has a poor reputation among scientific practitioners. Describes an experiment in which the author sent hair samples from two healthy teenagers to thirteen commercial laboratories that perform multimineral hair analysis. Reports how the study showed discrepancies in the laboratories' reports of mineral levels in the hair samples and their interpretations of these mineral levels. Notes that the laboratories made unfounded and conflicting claims that the subjects were afflicted with various diseases and should take various dietary supplements. Concludes that commercial hair analysis is unscientific, economically wasteful, and probably illegal.

Walsh, WJ, Hickok G, Waters S: Commercial hair analysis: Science or scam?
JAMA 255: 2603–2604, 1986.
Letters to the editor from three individuals with commercial involvement in hair analysis attack the above article. The first acknowledges that serious abuses of hair analysis are widespread, but claims that Dr. Barrett used improper sampling to prepare his specimens. The second claims that "hair analysis has provided the clue that led to proper diagnosis in many thousands of patients." The third admits that "many laboratories measuring hair elements are giving spurious results," but he berates Dr. Barrett for publishing the laboratory ratings (high, normal, low) instead of the raw data. Dr. Barrett replies that the technique used for specimen preparation had been proven valid by an FDA laboratory experiment and that the data in the published article were sufficient to draw his conclusions. He also wonders why the proponents had neither published their alleged data in scientific journals nor reported the abuses to appropriate law enforcement officials.

AMA Council on Scientific Affairs: Informational report of the Council on Scientific Affairs. Commercial hair analysis.
Reports of the Council On Scientific Affairs, pp. 261–265, February, 1987.
Reviews previous AMA actions regarding hair analysis. Discusses historical background, noting the widespread use and abuse of hair analysis. Notes various factors influencing hair characteristics and the absence of standards for normal values. Notes that misinterpreting test results can harm patients by suggesting nonexistent problems. Urges physicians and dietitians to caution patients about the misuse of hair analysis as a basis for recommending dietary supplements. Notes that an AMA official has urged congressional oversight of federal enforcement agency activities.

Klevay LM, Bistrian BR, Fleming CR, et al: Hair analysis in clinical and experimental medicine.
American Journal of Clinical Nutrition 46:233–236, 1987.
Notes that each year about 9000 papers on trace elements are published, with about 75 of them dealing with trace elements and hair, yet few studies have shown a correlation between the minerals in hair and those in body organs. Concludes that "hair analysis seems potentially useful in experimental medicine but its use in clinical medicine for diagnosis, prognosis and therapy will remain limited until validation by the standard methods of clinical investigation is achieved." An accompanying statement by the Committee on Clinical Issues in Health and Disease of the American Society for Clinical Nutrition notes that (1) beneficial effects of therapy based on hair analysis have not been found; (2) measurement of some elements, such as iron, is superfluous because hair analysis has not been found superior to traditional methods of assessing nutrition status; (3) measurements of single elements, such as arsenic, may be useful if an abnormal exposure is suspected; and (4) simultaneous measurement of several elements is likely to produce falsely positive results.

Gest T: Does he or doesn't he? New drug tests target hair.
U.S. News and World Report 108:58, May 28, 1990.
States that some law enforcement agencies and employers had been using hair analysis to detect drug abuse. Notes that this use raises privacy issues and that "scientists have yet to give hair analysis their stamp of approval."

Holden C: Hairy problems for new drug testing method.
Science 249:1099–1100, 1990.
Examines the use of hair analysis to test for drug use by individuals. Notes that a company called Psychemedics was performing such tests. Discusses questions raised

regarding the test's accuracy. Notes opposition by critics, including some government agencies.

Haddy TB, Czajka-Narins, DM, Sky-Peck HH, et al: Minerals in hair, serum, and urine of healthy and anemic black children.
Public Health Reports 106: 557–563, 1991.
Discusses a study comparing the levels of various minerals in the hair, serum, and urine of normal children and children with iron overload, iron-deficiency anemia, or thalassemia trait. A total of 48 children were tested. Concludes that the data do not support the use of hair analysis as a screening test for body iron levels in children.

Electroacupuncture

Electroacupuncture according to Voll (EAV), which is also called electrodiagnosis, is performed with a device claimed to measure energy flow along "acupuncture meridians." The various generations of the device include the Vega, Dermatron, Accupath 1000, and Interro. Proponents claim these devices can determine the cause of any disease by detecting the "energy imbalance" causing the problem. The first such device was developed during the 1970s by Reinhold Voll, MD, a West German physician. The device has been marketed in many versions, all of which operate in similar ways. The basic mechanism is a galvanometer, which measures changes in the electrical resistance of the patient's skin. One wire from the device goes to a brass cylinder covered by moist gauze, which the patient holds in one hand. A second wire is connected to a probe, which the operator touches to "acupuncture points" on the patient's other hand or foot. This completes a low-voltage circuit and the device registers the flow of current. The information is then relayed to a gauge that provides a numerical readout. The most recent versions make sounds and provide the readout on a computer screen. The treatment selected depends on the scope of the practitioner's practice and may include acupuncture, diet, vitamin supplements, homeopathic remedies, and/or surgery. In the United States, the devices are most popular among homeopaths, but are used by a few dentists, medical doctors, and chiropractors. Regulatory agencies have seized several types of electroacupuncture devices.

Barrett S: My visit to the Nevada Clinic.
Nutrition Forum 4:6–8, January 1987.
Describes how the author went through the Nevada Clinic's diagnostic procedure, based primarily on testing with an Interro. He reported that readings over 60 on a computer screen are interpreted as "inflammation," readings of 48 to 60 as normal,

and readings below 48 as "degeneration," which may signify cancer or atherosclerosis. The device was programmed so that charts and tables could be placed on the screen to help the doctor select the homeopathic remedies said to balance disturbed "energy flow" in the patient's body. Other devices were used to check for allergies and possible toxicity from the author's mercury fillings. During testing with the Interro, the author noted that the harder the probe was pressed against his finger or toe, the higher the reading on the computer screen. After testing, the author was informed that he had "electromagnetic blockages ... temporomandibular joint stress, probable subclinical allergies, and possible mild early preclinical arthritis." The proposed treatment included vitamin B_{12} injections and homeopathic remedies.

Medical Practitioners Disciplinary Committee: Professional misconduct findings against Dr. D W Steeper.
New Zealand Medical Journal 103:194–195, April 25, 1990.
Describes in detail allegations from three patients against a homeopathic physician who used a Vega device to diagnose allergies in three infants. In each case the device had been applied to the mother with the child on the mother's lap or roaming about the examining room. The doctor also diagnosed "miasms," which, if not removed, would prove fatal later in life. The committee noted that "alternative medicine" was not on trial, but the doctor's actions comprised professional misconduct. The committee ordered that he be censured, pay a penalty of NZ$900 plus NZ$25,000 for costs and expenses, and follow certain standards of care for three years.

Herbal Crystallization Analysis

This test is performed by adding a solution of copper chloride to a dried specimen of the patient's saliva on a slide. The resultant crystal patterns are then matched to those of dried herbs to determine supposed body problem areas and the herbs for treating them. The test has been banned in New York State and is not widely performed. In 1984, Dr. Stephen Barrett prepared specimens by licking one slide with the left side of his tongue and the other slide with the right side of his tongue and submitted them under different names to a herbal crystallization laboratory for analysis. The resultant reports indicated multiple health problems but differed about which organs had the problems.

Lingual Vitamin C Test.

This test is performed by placing a drop of 2,6-dichloro-indophenol on the tongue and noting the time required for the color to change from blue to pink. Proponents claim that this indicates whether there is enough vitamin C in the body. However, two published studies have demonstrated that the test is not valid.

Randolph P, Wilson TJ, Roth GD, et al: Evaluation of
the lingual ascorbic acid test.
Journal of Oral Medicine, 29:8–12, January–March 1974.
Reports that no correlation was found between lingual test result and serum ascorbic acid concentration in fifty male dental students.

Stults VJ, Sapiro KTS, Clemens RA, et al: Evaluation of a
lingual test for vitamin C status.
Journal of Oral Medicine 42:229-232, October–December 1987.
Describes an experiment in which seventeen volunteers were tested with the Vitamin C Self Test Kit, a lingual test, after which a sample of their blood was analyzed using high-pressure liquid chromatography. States that the test subjects also kept a 24-hour food diary for the day preceding the tests. Notes that no significant correlation was found between the lingual test result and the serum concentration or dietary intake of vitamin C.

Live-Cell Analysis

Live cell analysis is carried out by placing a drop of blood from the patient's fingertip on a microscope slide under a glass coverslip to keep it from drying out. The slide is then viewed with a dark-field microscope to which a television monitor has been attached. Both practitioner and patient can then see the blood cells, which appear as dark bodies outlined in white. The practitioner may also take Polaroid photographs of the television picture for himself and the patient. Proponents of live cell analysis claim that it is useful in diagnosing vitamin and mineral deficiencies, tendencies toward allergic reactions, liver weakness, and many other health problems. There is no scientific evidence that this is true.

Lowell JA: Live cell analysis: high-tech hokum.
Nutrition Forum 3:81–85, November 1986.
Details the claims made for live cell analysis and why they are false. Observes how one practitioner failed to clean his slides properly and another neglected to focus his microscope.

Fad Diagnoses

A small percentage of physicians and dentists are making diagnoses with which the vast majority of their colleagues disagree. These diagnoses are commonly applied to people who experience fatigue, insomnia, irritability, faintness, depression, and various other stress-related complaints. Three of these conditions—hypothyroidism, hypoglycemia, and chronic fatigue syndrome—are medically recognized diseases that "alternative" practitioners diagnose far too often. The other three diagnoses—"environmental illness, "candidiasis hypersensitivity," and "mercury amalgam toxicity" are not recognized by the scientific community. Practitioners who are "true believers" typically use invalid tests, diagnose these conditions in most or all of their patients, and charge high fees. Instead of testing their ideas with well-designed research, they have been marketing them to the public through books, magazine articles, talk show appearances, and lectures.

"Environmental Illness"

"Clinical ecology," which is not a recognized specialty, is based on the notion that multiple symptoms are triggered by hypersensitivity to common foods and chemicals. Advocates of this belief describe themselves as "ecologically oriented" and consider their patients to be suffering from "environmental illness," "cerebral allergy," "allergy to everything," "twentieth century disease," or "multiple chemical sensitivity (MCS)," which can mimic almost any other illness. The signs and symptoms are said to include depression, irritability, mood swings, inability to concentrate or think clearly, poor memory, fatigue, drowsiness, diarrhea, constipation, sneezing, running or stuffy nose, wheezing, itching eyes and nose, skin rashes, headache, muscle and joint pain, urinary frequency, pounding heart, and swelling of various parts of the body.

Clinical ecologists claim that hypersensitivity develops when the total load of physical and psychological stresses exceeds what a person can tolerate. They state that potential stressors include practically everything that modern humans encounter, such as urban air, diesel exhaust, tobacco smoke, fresh paint or tar, organic solvents and pesticides, certain plastics, newsprint, perfumes and colognes, medications, gas used for cooking and heating, building materials, permanent press and synthetic fabrics, household cleaners, rubbing alcohol, felt-tip pens, cedar closets, tap water, and electromagnetic forces.

To diagnose "ecologically related" disease, practitioners take a history that emphasizes dietary habits and exposure to environmental chemicals they consider harmful. Various nonstandard tests and elimination and rotation diets are used with the hope of identifying foods that cause problems. The primary test is "provocation" and "neutralization," in which the patient reports symptoms that occur within ten minutes after suspected substances are administered under the tongue or injected into the skin. If any symptoms occur, the test is considered positive and lower concentrations are given until a dose is found that "neutralizes" the symptoms.

Once the diagnosis is made, patients generally are instructed to modify their diet and to avoid such substances as scented shampoos, aftershave products, deodorants, cigarette smoke, automobile exhaust fumes, and clothing, furniture and carpets that contain synthetic fibers. In severe cases, patients may spend several weeks in environmental control units designed to remove them from exposure to airborne pollutants and synthetic substances that might cause adverse reactions. Extreme restrictions can include staying at home for months and avoiding physical contact with family members.

Several prominent medical groups have denounced the concept of "environmental illness" and the methods used to diagnose and treat it as speculative and unproven. Critics believe that most people diagnosed with "environmental illness" have psychosomatic disorders in which they react to stress by developing multiple symptoms. Although it is clear that some individuals are hypersensitive to environmental chemicals, there is no scientific evidence that "multiple chemical sensitivity" has an allergic or immunologic basis. In 1992, a National Research Council subcommittee indicated what research would be needed to establish or refute the validity of this diagnosis as conceived by clinical ecology practitioners.

Brodsky CM: 'Allergic to everything': a medical subculture.
Psychosomatics 24:731–742, 1983.
Discusses patients of clinical ecologists, focusing on eight patients who had been examined by conventional physicians who found nothing physically wrong. The patients then turned to clinical ecologists who attributed their ailments to allergic reactions to various substances around them. Describes the lifestyle changes made by these alleged allergy victims, all of whom stopped working and relocated so they could be outdoors. Notes that some had experienced symptoms before their alleged exposure to harmful substances at work.

Thomson GM et al: Report on the ad hoc committee
on environmental hypersensitivity disorders.

Toronto, Ontario Ministry of Health, August 1985.
Zimmerman B et al: Report on the Advisory Panel
on Environmental Hypersensitivity.
Ontario, Ministry of Health, September 1986.
The committee report describes the concepts of clinical ecology and the evidence, if any, supporting them. The advisory panel reviewed this report and concluded that "scientific support for the mechanisms that have been proposed to underlay the wide variety of dysfunctions are at best hypothetical. Moreover the majority of techniques for evaluating the patients and the treatments espoused are unproven."

Stewart DE, Raskin J: Psychiatric assessment of patients with "20th-century disease" ("total allergy syndrome").
Canadian Medical Association Journal 133:1001–1006, 1985.
Concludes that psychiatric disorders were found in 18 patients with "20th century disease" referred to the authors for psychiatric evaluation. Suggests that the condition is not a new illness but a fashionable name for a condition known to physicians for centuries and previously called hysteria, asthenia, soldier's heart, hypoglycemia, and candidiasis.

Terr AI: Environmental illness: A clinical review of 50 cases.
Archives of Internal Medicine 146:145–149, 1986.
Analyzes 50 cases of people diagnosed by clinical ecologists as victims of environmental illness. Although all had been diagnosed as "environmentally ill," Dr. Terr could find no unifying pattern of symptoms, physical findings or laboratory abnormalities. Eight of the patients had not gotten their symptoms until after they had consulted the clinical ecologist because they had been worried about exposure to a chemical. Eleven had symptoms caused by preexisting problems unrelated to environmental factors, and 31 had multiple symptoms. Their various treatments included dietary alterations (74 percent), food or chemical extracts (62 percent), an antifungal drug (24 percent), and oxygen given with a portable apparatus (14 percent). Fourteen of the patients had been advised to move their home to a rural area, and a few were given vitamin and mineral supplements, gamma globulin, interferon, female hormones and/or oral urine. Despite treatment, twenty-six patients reported no lessening of symptoms, twenty-two were clearly worse, and only two improved.

Wiederholt WC et al: Clinical ecology: A critical appraisal.
Western Journal of Medicine 144:239–245, 1986.
Task force report concludes that "clinical ecology does not constitute a valid medical discipline" and should be considered "experimental" only when its practitioners begin to use scientifically sound experimental methods. Also expresses

concern that unproven diagnostic tests can lead to misdiagnosis that results in patients becoming psychologically dependent, believing themselves to be seriously and chronically impaired.

Anderson JA et al: Position statement on clinical ecology.
Journal of Allergy and Clinical Immunology 78:269–271, 1986.
Position paper defines clinical ecology and describes the symptoms attributed to environmental illness and the treatment prescribed for these symptoms. Notes the lack of evidence to support the claims made regarding sensitivity to environmental substances, and the lack of controlled studies to support the diagnosis or treatment of environmental illness. Concludes that although the idea that the environment is responsible for a multitude of health problems is very appealing, "to present such ideas as facts, conclusions, or even likely mechanisms without adequate support is poor medical practice."

Selner JC, Staudenmayer H: The relationship of the environment and food to allergic and psychiatric illness.
In Young SH, Rubin JM, Demon H (eds.): Psychobiological aspects of allergic disorders, pp. 102–146.
New York, Praeger, 1986.
Traces the history and practice of clinical ecology and dissects flaws in the proponents' thinking. Describes the work of the authors, who are not clinical ecologists but operate an environmental unit in Denver, Colorado. Concludes that: (1) people do exist who are very sensitive to various microorganisms, noxious chemicals, and common foods; (2) the key question is whether multi-system disease can be caused by generalized allergy to environmental substances; (3) when a physician is confronted by a patient claiming to be "allergic to everything," the diagnosis can usually be traced to the influence of a proponent of clinical ecology; (4) there is no scientific evidence that an immunologic basis exists for such a symptom pattern; (5) clinical ecologists assume that if even a trace of any chemical is found in the patient's environment, that chemical can be held responsible for any symptom; (6) clinical ecologists appear to lack the motivation or intellectual capacity to test their theories scientifically; (7) clinical ecologists offer a philosophy of certainty, often reassuring patients during an initial phone contact that their diagnosis is obviously ecologic disease; (8) patients with genuine allergies to noxious chemicals do not have multi-system complaints without associated physical or laboratory findings; (8) many patients with symptoms of "environmental illness" find "healers" who tell them they are "universal reactors" to environmental substances; (10) this explanation of their experience and symptoms that makes sense to them and enables them to avoid facing their real problem—which is psychiatric in nature; (11) using well designed double-blind tests with more than a

hundred patients, the authors were able to demonstrate that most people said to be "universal reactors" develop multiple symptoms in response to the testing process without being allergic to any of the individual substances administered; and (12) once patients understand that this can happen, psychotherapy may cure them. Also notes that "ecologists claim a unique identity with victims of the environment by declaring themselves, or members of their families, similarly affected. . . . This is a powerful bonding tool which snares patients into a . . . cult interdependence in which facts are irrelevant."

Terr AI: Clinical ecology.
Journal of Allergy and Clinical Immunology 79:423–426, 1987.
Examines the concept of clinical ecology, noting changes in the theory of disease. Summarizes results of a study of 50 cases of patients diagnosed by clinical ecologists as chemically sensitive, but discovered by other physicians to be afflicted with other physical diseases or mental disorders. Argues that there is no scientific evidence of the existence of 20th-century disease or environmental illness.

Terr AI. Clinical ecology in the workplace.
Journal of Occupational Medicine 31:257–261, 1989.
Reviews the cases of 90 individuals who filed for workman's compensation based on claims of work-related environmental illness. Reports alleged causes of environmental illness diagnosed by clinical ecologists and the diagnosis of other physical or mental disorders, including legitimate occupational illness, by other physicians who were not clinical ecologists. Discusses methods used by clinical ecologists to diagnose illness, noting that in almost two thirds of the cases, symptoms treated by clinical ecologists existed before the patient's presumed occupational exposure. Notes that 32 of the 90 patients had also been diagnosed as suffering from "candidiasis hypersensitivity."

Terr AI: Clinical ecology.
Annals of Internal Medicine 111:168–178, 1989.
Position paper of the American College of Physicians defines clinical ecology and describes the theory and symptoms of environmental illness. Lists and describes methods of diagnosis and treatments. Reviews studies, mostly uncontrolled, done by clinical ecologists to evaluate their methods of diagnosis and therapy. Concludes that evidence to support the theory and practice of clinical ecology is inadequate and indicates how advocates could carry out more rigorous tests.

Kahn E, Letz G: Clinical ecology: Environmental medicine or unsubstantiated theory?
Annals of Internal Medicine 111:104–106, 1989.

Summarizes criticisms of clinical ecology and notes that it has the attributes of a cult, including tendencies to attack organized medicine and to rely on testimonials and anecdotes as evidence.

Selner JC: Workup of the chemically sensitive patient.
Masters in Allergy 1:8–16, Summer 1989.
Describes a protocol for distinguishing between real chemical intolerance inappropriately-diagnosed "environmental illness."

Jewett DL, Fein G, Greenberg MH: A double-blind study of
symptom provocation to determine food sensitivity.
New England Journal of Medicine 323:429–433, 1990.
Describes a double-blind study in which 18 patients each were given three injections of suspected food extracts and nine of normal saline over a three-hour period. In unblinded tests, these patients had consistently reported symptoms when exposed to food extracts and no symptoms when given saline injections. But during the experiment, they reported as many symptoms following saline injections as they did after food extract injections, indicating that their symptoms were nothing more than placebo reactions. The symptoms included nasal stuffiness, dry mouth, nausea, fatigue, headaches and feelings of disorientation or depression.

Whitley G: Is the 20th century making you sick?
D Magazine, pp. 46–49, 73–80, August 1990.
Traces the theories and controversial career of William Rea, MD, who is considered the leading clinical ecologist.

Black DW et al: Environmental illness: A controlled study
of 26 subjects with '20th century disease.'
JAMA 264:3166–3170, 1990.
Reports that 15 (65%) of 23 individuals diagnosed as environmentally ill met criteria for a current or past emotional disorder compared to 13 of 46 (28%) age- and sex-matched control subjects. Concludes that psychiatric diagnoses should be considered for patients with multiple ill-defined symptoms for which an explanation is not apparent.

Huber PW: No immunity: Chemicals cause everything.
In Huber PW: Galileo's revenge: Junk science in the courtroom.
New York, 1991, Basic Books.
Describes how clinical ecologists testifying as experts in cases of alleged illness due to chemical exposure have resulted in huge undeserved verdicts for plaintiffs. Suggests that clinical ecologists are "perfectly adapted to modern-day testifying"

because they are "adept at prevaricating, playing on credulity, scoring verbal points, forgetting inconvenient data, and dredging up convenient anecdotes."

AMA Council on Scientific Affairs: Multiple chemical sensitivity syndrome.
Report of the Council on Scientific Affairs, 1991.
Provides a referenced summary of claims and scientific reports related to environmental illness, candidiasis hypersensitivity, chronic fatigue syndrome, and sick-building syndrome. Based on reports in the peer-reviewed scientific literature, the Council on Scientific Affairs concluded: (1) there are no well-controlled studies establishing a clear mechanism or cause for multiple chemical sensitivity syndrome, (2) there are no well-controlled studies confirming the efficacy of the diagnostic and therapeutic modalities relied upon by those who practice clinical ecology. The council also noted that proponents of a new test, procedure, or treatment, should bear the burden of proving through appropriate peer-reviewed controlled trials that it is effective for its intended purposes.

Medical malpractice – treatment of paranoid schizophrenia by "clinical ecology" – wrongful death – punitive damages.
The New York Jury Verdict Reporter 10(23):1–2, 1991.
Describes a jury award of $489,000 in actual damages and $411,000 in punitive damages to the estate of a man who committed suicide after several years of treatment by a prominent clinical ecologist. Testimony at the trial indicated that although the man was a paranoid schizophrenic who thought "foods were out to get him," the doctor had diagnosed him as a "universal reactor" and advised that, to remain alive, he must live in a "pure" environment, follow a restrictive diet, and take supplements. During the trial the doctor admitted that since 1974, when he began practicing clinical ecology, he had diagnosed every patient who consulted him as environmentally ill. [In September 1992, after a lengthy investigation, the New York State Health Department's Board for Professional Medical Conduct recommended that the doctor's license be revoked.]

Talmage DW et al: Biologic markers in immunotoxicology.
Washington, DC, National Academy Press, 1992.
Reports the findings of a National Research Council subcommittee that investigated possible relationships between chemical exposure and depressed immunity. Distinguishes between hypersensitivity, which is an immunologically based host response to a compound or its metabolic products, and multiple chemical sensitivity (MCS) syndrome, which has not been shown to have an immunologic basis. Notes that this diagnosis is applied to individuals who develop adverse reactions at doses below presumed toxic levels, but the existence of MCS has been challenged in the scientific and medical communities and that the "paucity of solid scientific data has

severely clouded objective scientific understanding of this syndrome, including its clinical diagnosis and objective treatment." Notes that "the use of anecdotal reports without standardized case definitions and attention to alternative explanations will not resolve the current controversies surrounding this issue." States that "a crucial step in resolving the intense controversy in the area of chemical sensitivity will be the development of refined terminology. A series of well-designed studies . . . is required to address this problem." Recommends: (1) replacing the term MCS, whenever possible, with a specific diagnosis; (2) epidemiologic research focused on the prevalence of MCS, and (3) studies under controlled environmental conditions to confirm or eliminate immune-system dysfunction as a cause of MCS. [A follow-up report, described at the end of this section, was generated by a workshop in which proponents participated.]

Barrett, S: Unproven "allergies": An epidemic of nonsense.
New York, American Council on Science and Health, 1993.
Provide a thorough review of promotion and criticism of the concepts of "environmental illness" and "candidiasis hypersensitivity." Urges state licensing boards to examine the activities of the physicians involved and determine whether the overall quality of their care is sufficient for them to remain in medical practice.

"Candidiasis Hypersensitivity"

Candida albicans (sometimes referred to as monilia) is a fungus normally present in the mouth, intestinal tract and vagina. Under certain conditions, it can multiply and infect the surface of the skin or mucous membranes. Such infections are usually minor, but serious and deeper infections can occur in patients whose resistance has been weakened by other illnesses. However, promoters of "candidiasis hypersensitivity" claim that even when infection is absent, the yeast can cause or trigger multiple symptoms such as fatigue, irritability, constipation, diarrhea, abdominal bloating, mood swings, depression, anxiety, dizziness, unexpected weight gain, difficulty in concentrating, muscle and joint pain, cravings for sugar or alcoholic beverages, psoriasis, hives, respiratory and ear problems, menstrual problems, infertility, impotence, bladder infections, and prostatitis. The treatment may include dietary changes, supplements, and antifungal drugs (nystatin and/or ketoconazole).

According to its promoters, 30 percent of Americans suffer from "candidiasis hypersensitivity." Many clinical ecologists view it as an underlying cause of the "environmental illness" that they postulate. It is also being touted as an important factor in AIDS, rheumatoid arthritis, multiple sclerosis, and schizophrenia as well as "hypoglycemia," "mercury amalgam toxicity" and chronic fatigue. According to proponents, signs of actual infection (such as vaginal discharge) or the ability to prove the presence of Candida organisms by culturing them are not necessary for making the diagnosis.

The leading promoters of "candidiasis hypersensitivity" are C. Orian Truss, MD, of Birmingham, Alabama, and William G. Crook, MD, of Jackson, Tennessee. As their ideas became widely publicized, health food industry manufacturers jumped on the bandwagon and began producing "anti-Candida" products which were sold in health food stores and prescribed by chiropractors in their offices. In the process, the distinction between "candidiasis hypersensitivity" and "yeast infection" became blurred, so that today both terms are used loosely and interchangeably by various proponents.

Tabor E: Potential toxicity of ketoconazole.
Journal of Infectious Diseases 152:233, 1985.
Letter noting that symptomatic liver toxicity occurs in some patients taking ketoconazole, with an incidence between 1 in 10,000 and 1 in 15,000. The hepatitis is usually resolves when the drug is stopped, but at least four fatal cases have been reported. [This report is significant because ketoconazole is often inappropriately prescribed by proponents of "candidiasis hypersensitivity."

Quinn JP, Venezio FR: Ketoconazole and the yeast connection.
JAMA 255:3250, 1986.
Reports four cases of young women with chronic fatigue, anxiety, depression, and other nonspecific complaints who believed that they had disseminated candidiasis and were taking nystatin or ketoconazole. Notes that all had read *The Yeast Connection* and brought the book to their appointment. Expresses concern that patients with no discernible organic disease would be given antifungal drugs, particularly ketoconazole, which can cause hepatitis. Notes that one of the patients taking ketoconazole did develop hepatitis that resolved when the drug was stopped.

Haas A et al: The "Yeast Connection" meets chronic mucocutaneous candidiasis.
New England Journal of Medicine 314:854–855, 1986.
Reports the case of a 2-year-old boy who actually had a serious candidiasis infection and was ineptly treated by a proponent of "candidiasis hypersensitivity." The treatment included two days of testing, electronic acupressure of the hands and feet, skin tests to inhalant allergens, and a candida skin test that suggested the correct diagnosis. Treatment with nystatin was started, and blood transfusions from the parents, isoprinosine therapy, and sheep-cell infusions (at a Mexican clinic) were also recommended. Before going to Mexico, however, the parents consulted the

authors, who treated the child appropriately with ketoconazole, which cleared up the infection. The authors comment that the expensive treatment offered by "yeast connection" advocates is not only inappropriate for nonexistent infection; it is also inappropriate for actual yeast infection.

American Academy of Allergy and Immunology. "Candidiasis hypersensitivity syndrome."
Journal of Allergy and Clinical Immunology 78:271–273, 1986.
Describes candidiasis hypersensitivity syndrome and its theory as reported by C. Orian Truss, MD, and William G. Crook, MD. Lists various aspects of the treatment used for the syndrome. Recommends that the concept be viewed as speculative and unproven and points out elements of the treatment program that are potentially dangerous.

Blonz ER: Is There an epidemic of chronic candidiasis 'in our midst?"
JAMA 256:3138–3139, 1986.
Notes rising interest in "candidiasis sensitivity" by commercial interests marketing products to control the yeast and practitioners who treat patients with "anti-Candida" therapy. Notes weaknesses in the proponents' theories but urges that well designed studies be carried out so the public can be protected from "entrepreneurial adventurism" or the possibility that a real condition is being overlooked.

Yeast: Raising questions. Harvard Medical School
Health Letter 12:1–3, February 1987.
Discusses the theory behind clinical ecology and *Candida albicans* overgrowth infections as the cause of multiple symptoms. Reviews symptoms attributed to yeast growth and diet regimens, lifestyle changes, and drugs recommended for treating it. Discusses scientific objections to the theory and treatment. Concludes that "there is no more reason to believe that candida is responsible for an epidemic of chronic disease in otherwise normal people than there ever was to believe that the moon was made of green cheese. Meanwhile the world's basements are full of moldy books that once made health claims as broad—and unsubstantiated—as those made in *The Yeast Connection.*"

Renfro L, Feder, HM Jr., Lane TJ, et al: Yeast connection among 100 patients with chronic fatigue.
American Journal of Medicine 86:165–168, 1989.
Describes a study of 100 patients with chronic fatigue, eight of whom expressed the belief that their problem was due to the "yeast connection." No significant differences were found between the two groups except that those who thought they

had a yeast problem were more likely to be taking vitamins or seeing an "alternative" practitioner.

FDA Stops Yeastop.
FDA Consumer 24:36, March 1990.
Reports on FDA regulatory action against Yeastop, a supplement concoction promoted by its manufacturers for controlling infections of *Candida albicans*. The firm alleged that Yeastop was not a drug but a dietary supplement and promised to remove medical claims from the packaging. When they failed to do so, a quantity of the product was seized and destroyed.

Dismukes WE., Wade J, Scott L, et al: A randomized, double-blind trial of nystatin therapy for the candidiasis hypersensitivity syndrome.
New England Journal of Medicine 323:1717–1723, 1990.
Notes that the antifungal drug nystatin did no better than a placebo in relieving systemic or psychological symptoms of 42 women said to be suffering from "candidiasis hypersensitivity syndrome."

Bennett JE. Searching for the yeast connection.
New England Journal of Medicine 323:1766–1767, 1990.
Speculates that part of the reason for public acceptance of the diagnosis of "candida hypersensitivity" is that doctors pay insufficient attention to patients who have multiple symptoms but no physical or laboratory findings to explain them. Suggests that no matter what studies are done to test the claims of the proponents, they will reject any negative results by saying that the tests were improperly designed.

Chronic Fatigue Syndrome

Chronic fatigue syndrome (CFS) is an illness characterized by debilitating fatigue and several flu-like symptoms such as pharyngitis, enlarged lymph nodes, low-grade fever, muscle and joint pains, headache, difficulty concentrating, and exercise intolerance. The profound fatigue usually comes on suddenly and persists throughout the course of the illness. It is included in this section on "fad diagnoses" because a small percentage of physicians are diagnosing CFS in most or all patients who complain to them about fatigue.

Chronic fatigue syndrome: a pamphlet for physicians.
NIH Publication No. 90-484.
Bethesda, MD, National Institutes of Health, 1990.

Describes the findings that should be present to make an appropriate diagnosis of CFS. Notes that although chronic fatigue is a common complaint among patients, CFS is probably an uncommon cause of chronic fatigue. Notes that no laboratory test can establish the diagnosis of CFS, but certain tests are advisable to rule out other causes of fatigue.

Chronic fatigue: all in the mind?
Consumer Reports 55:671–675, October 1990.
Describes the dilemma of people with chronic fatigue and the difficulty in pinning down a diagnosis. Summarizes the CDC criteria for diagnosis. Calls CFS "a magnet for quacks" and describes what happened when the reporter visited three New York City physicians listed on the "Physicians Honor Roll" published by a CFS organization.

Katzenstein L: Sick & tired: Chronic fatigue syndrome
shows signs of yielding its secrets.
American Health 11:51–56, May 1992.
States that although many people with severe fatigue are told "it's all in your head," mounting evidence supports the idea that CFS is a real disorder. Cautions that expensive approaches involving herbs or dietary supplements are unlikely to be helpful. Advises where to get reliable information.

Dooley DP: Commercial laboratory testing for chronic fatigue syndrome.
JAMA 268:873–874, 1992.
Letter to the editor discusses an ad from a prominent laboratory for a test panel said to aid in the diagnosis of CFS. Comments that CFS probably has multiple causes, with fatigue being a final common manifestation. Notes that the CDC diagnostic criteria were designed for epidemiological case definition rather than definitive diagnosis. States that there is no consistent or diagnostic laboratory profile and that "commercial marketing of irrelevant laboratory tests, performed outside of approved investigator protocols, is useless to both physicians and patients, expensive, and distracting."

"Hypoglycemia"

"Hypoglycemia" (low blood sugar) is sometimes used as a diagnosis to explain various symptoms of nervousness or fatigue. Doctors who are "true believers" in hypoglycemia are apt to diagnose it in a large number of their patients. However, it is actually quite rare and should be diagnosed only after careful interpretation of blood sugar tests. The only way to reliably diagnose hypoglycemia is to prove that blood sugar is low whenever symptoms occur during the patient's usual living pattern. The most practical way to do this is probably with a home testing device.

Bennion L: Hypoglycemia: fact or fad?
New York, Crown Publishers, 1985.
Describes the true causes of hypoglycemia and when to suspect they are present. Thoroughly discusses the misdiagnosis of hypoglycemia based on the patient's history alone or misinterpretation of a glucose tolerance test. Explains that this test is useless or misleading for diagnosing most cases of hypoglycemia because intravenous injection of 50–100 grams of concentrated sugar solution is an abnormal situation that is unrelated to the circumstances of most patients' symptoms. Low blood sugar levels without symptoms occur commonly in normal individuals fed large amounts of sugar and are of no diagnostic significance.

"Mercury-Amalgam Toxicity"

A few hundred dentists claim that the mercury in silver-amalgam fillings is toxic and causes multiple sclerosis, arthritis, headaches, Parkinson's disease, emotional stress, and many other health problems. They recommend that mercury fillings be replaced with either gold or plastic ones and that vitamin supplements be taken to prevent trouble during the process. These dentists typically use an industrial mercury detector to indicate that "toxic" amounts of mercury are being released. To use the device, the dentist asks the patient to chew vigorously for ten minutes, which may cause tiny amounts of mercury to be released from the fillings. Although this exposure lasts for just a few seconds and most of the mercury will be exhaled rather than absorbed by the body, the machines give a falsely high readout, which the anti-amalgamists interpret as dangerous. The proper way to determine mercury exposure is to measure blood or urine levels, which indicate how much has been absorbed by the body. Scientific testing has shown that the amount of mercury absorbed from fillings is only a small fraction of the average daily intake from food and is insignificant. The American Dental Association Council on Ethics, Bylaws and Judicial Affairs considers the unnecessary removal of silver amalgam fillings "improper and unethical."

On December 23, 1990, CBS's "60 Minutes" aired a report called "Poison In Your Mouth," which interspersed remarks from an American Dental Association representative with statements by three amalgam critics and four patients who claimed to have made a remarkable recovery from arthritis or multiple sclerosis after their amalgam fillings were removed. The most powerful segment featured a woman who said that her symptoms of multiple sclerosis had disappeared overnight. The broadcast frightened many listers into seeking removal of their mercury fillings. Many magazines and newsletters published responses indicating why it was misleading.

The mercury scare.
Consumer Reports 51:150–152, March 1986.
Describes the visit of a Consumer Reports editor to a dentist who measured the mercury vapor level in his mouth and advised him to have his silver fillings replaced immediately. Explains why the test used by the dentist is invalid and how scientists have determined that the mercury-amalgam filings pose no threat to a person's health. Notes the background of several leading anti-amalgamists. Advises consumers that "if a dentist wants to remove your fillings because they contain mercury, hold on to your wallet." [The dentist consulted by the reporter later had his license revoked for professional misconduct after a patient complained that he had removed mercury-amalgam fillings from her teeth after telling her that the mercury was poisoning her.]

Mackert JR Jr: Dental amalgam and mercury.
Journal of the American Dental Association 122:54–61, August 1991.
Notes that extensive studies in humans with and without amalgam fillings have revealed no statistically significant differences in organ function or immune cell distribution. Also notes that the contribution of dental amalgam to the total daily dose is minor.

Mandell ID: Amalgam hazards: an assessment of research.
Journal of the American Dental Association 122:62–65, August 1991.
Notes that although mercury vapor in high concentration can have adverse effects on several organ systems, there is no evidence of risk at the levels generated by chewing with amalgam fillings.

Barrett S: Toxic television: the mercury amalgam scam.
Priorities, pp. 35–37, Fall 1991
Labels the "60 Minutes" broadcast "the most irresponsible report on a health topic ever broadcast on network television." Notes that the removal of fillings temporarily raises body mercury load, so that no "overnight cure" could possibly be caused by mercury removal.

The mercury in your mouth.
Consumer Reports 56:316–319, May 1991.
Provides a detailed rebuttal to the "60 Minutes" program. Explains why the design of a study of mercury toxicity in sheep was improper and not related to the use of

mercury-amalgam filings in humans. Notes that removing good fillings, particularly large ones, can damage tooth structure and may injure the nerve, requiring root canal therapy to save the tooth.

The mercury scare.
Consumer Reports 56:512, August 1991.
Letter to the editor from the daughter of a woman who, soon after the "60 Minutes" program, had spent $10,000 having her mercury fillings replaced because she hoped this would cure her of amyotrophic lateral sclerosis ("Lou Gehrig's disease"). Notes the "monumental disappointment" the woman and her whole family experienced as they "lived through one more false hope."

Jacob JA: N.Y. court upholds pulling of license
American Dental Association News, February 3, 1992.
Reports that a state appellate court upheld a new York Board of Regents decision to revoke the license of Joel Berger, DDS [the dentist who had been visited in 1985 by the *Consumer Reports* reporter]. The revocation took place after a woman complained that Dr. Berger had removed her amalgam fillings after telling her that mercury poisoning from the fillings was responsible for her leg and arm pain. Notes that Dr. Berger planned to appeal to a higher court.

Proponent Literature

Truss CO. The missing diagnosis.
The Missing Diagnosis, Inc., Birmingham, 1983.
Maintains that "chronic yeast infection with systemic allergic and toxic effects is a widespread problem." Recommends avoidance of carbohydrates, foods with a high yeast content, antibiotics, immunosuppressant drugs, and birth control pills. Recommends treatment with nystatin and a *Candida albicans* vaccine.

Baker S: An epidemic in disguise.
Omni 7:85, 86, 88, 120, 122, 126, March 1985.
Describes several cases which Dr. Truss reported had been suffering from serious symptoms until he diagnosed their problem as "candidiasis hypersensitivity" and treated it accordingly. Reports the views of one critic who observed that Dr. Truss has not tested his theory in a double-blind study. Reports Dr. Truss's response that it would be unethical for him as a private practitioner to conduct double-blind studies.

Crook, WG. The yeast connection—a medical breakthrough.
Professional Books, Jackson, TN, 1983, 1984, 1986.

Expounds Dr. Crook's beliefs that problems with *Candida albicans* are responsible for a myriad of symptoms and health problems. Describes his "anti-candida diet" and other treatment approaches. Contains two questionnaires purported to be screening tests for yeast problems.

Huggins HA, Huggins SA: It's all in your head.
Colorado Springs [no publisher identified], 1985.
Claims that people "sensitive" to mercury in fillings can develop emotional problems (suicidal depression, anxiety, irritability), neurological disorders (facial twitches, muscle spasms, epilepsy, multiple sclerosis), cardiovascular problems (unexplained rapid heart rate, unidentified chest pains), collagen diseases (arthritis, scleroderma, lupus erythematosus), allergies, digestive problems (ulcers, regional ileitis), and immunologic disorders (which he claims include leukemia, Hodgkin's disease, and mononucleosis). Recommends that mercury fillings be replaced with other materials and that vitamin supplements be taken to prevent trouble following amalgam removal.

Langer SE, Scheer JF: Solved: The riddle of illness.
New Canaan, CT, Keats Publishing, Inc., 1984.
The book's foreward maintains that "some sixty-four different symptoms are associated with one root cause—hypothyroidism—an ailment so widespread and sometimes so difficult to detect that a vast percentage of the population unknowingly suffers from it." The authors claim that the most accurate way to diagnose hypothyroidism is to take one's underarm temperature upon awakening in the morning—that readings below 97.8° for two consecutive days usually establish the diagnosis.

Samet J et al: Multiple chemical sensitivities: Addendum to
Biologic Markers in Immunotoxicology.
Washington, DC, National Academy Press, 1992.
Presents material from a workshop conducted by the National Research Council to develop an agenda for research on "multiple chemical sensitivity." Most of the contributors were proponents. One contributor traces the history of clinical ecology and notes that the papers collected in this book have not undergone peer review. Another contributor mentions several critical reports and notes that meaningful research on "multiple chemical sensitivity" cannot be conducted until clear criteria for such a diagnosis can be defined. The rest of the participants describe their theories and/or experiences with patients. There was general agreement that more research is needed, and various protocols were outlined.

Dubious Allergy Concepts and Practices

Many diagnostic and therapeutic approaches to real or purported allergies have been severely criticized by the scientific community. The articles abstracted in this section cover cytotoxic testing, skin titration, IgE testing for food allergies, urine autoinjection, the misdiagnosis of food allergies, and carotid body resection. The diagnosis and treatment of "environmental illness" and "candidiasis hypersensitivity" are covered elsewhere in the book under fad diagnoses.

General Discussions

American Academy of Allergy: Position statements—Controversial techniques.
Journal of Allergy and Clinical Immunology 67:333–338, 1981.
Summarizes the case against cytotoxic testing, provocation-neutralization, skin titration (Rinkel method), and autogenous urine immunization. In the skin titration method of immunotherapy, increasing concentrations of antigen extract are injected into the skin. The weakest dilution producing a positive skin reaction is then used as the basis for calculating dosages for treatment. For autogenous urine injection, urine is collected, sterilized by boiling or filtration, and injected intramuscularly into the patient.

Spector SL et al: Controversial and unproven techniques
Position statement from the ACCP Section on Allergy and Clinical Immunology.
Chest 86:132–133, 1984.
Summarizes the case against cytotoxic testing, provocation-neutralization, and autogenous urine immunization.

The potential for quackery and questionable treatment
in asthma and allergy medicine.
Washington, DC, The Asthma & Allergy Foundation of America, 1985.
Notes that the management of allergy should include careful history-taking and physical examination, allergy tests when necessary, environmental avoidance where practical, and use of medications with proven track record and insignificant side effects. Criticizes cytotoxic testing, provocation and neutralization, and urine autoinjection.

Anderson JA et al: Position statement on unproven procedures for
diagnosis and treatment of allergic and immunologic diseases.

Journal of Allergy and Clinical Immunology 78:275–277, 1986.
Position paper defines the conditions necessary for testing unproven procedures for the diagnosis and treatment of allergic and immunologic diseases. Notes that the responsibility for testing unproven procedures should rest with their proponents and that controlled trials are necessary.

Sethi TJ, Kemeny DM, Tobin S, et al: How reliable are commercial allergy tests? Lancet, pp. 92–94, January 10, 1987.
Describes an experiment in which blood and hair samples from nine people who were allergic to fish and nine people who were not were sent to five different commercial laboratories that offered "allergy diagnosis." All five labs were unable to diagnose fish allergy, reported many allergies in the nonallergic subjects, and provided inconsistent results on duplicate samples from the same subject.

Selner JC, Condemi J: Unproven diagnostic and therapeutic techniques for allergy, 3rd edition.
In Middleton E Jr (ed.): Allergy: Principles and practices, pp. 1,571–1,597. St. Louis, C.V. Mosby Company, 1988.
Discusses various aspects of adverse food reactions, the Feingold diet, clinical ecology, cytotoxic testing, the Rinkel technique, provocation-neutralization testing and "environmental illness." Describes the valid use of an environmental control unit to distinguish between true sensitivity and other types of responses to foods or environmental chemicals.

Shapiro GG, Anderson JA: Controversial techniques in allergy.
Pediatrics 82:935–937, 1988.
Describes and criticizes nine dubious practices related to the diagnosis and treatment of allergies. It notes that assessment of serum immunoglobulin E (IgE) to specific foods is not valid because the production of IgE to food antigens has not been proven pathologic by controlled trials. The article also criticizes the remote practice of allergy, in which the patient's blood is sent to a laboratory for RAST testing and the results are used as the basis for prescribing allergy shots. This process is invalid because the diagnosis of allergy cannot be made reliably without correlating allergy tests with the patient's history and other data. In most cases, avoidance of allergens and proper drug treatment preclude the need for immunotherapy.

VanArsdel PP Jr, Larson EB: Diagnostic tests for patients with suspected allergic disease: Utility and limitations.
Annals of Internal Medicine 110:304–312, 1989.
Notes the distinction between true allergies and other types of sensitivities to foreign

substances. Notes that for a skin-testing to be appropriate, there must be a reasonable probability that the patient's reaction is mediated by IgE antibodies. States that oral challenge with a suspected food may have value for diagnosing idiosyncrasy if the test is properly designed. States that RAST testing is valid but should be used primarily for research. Briefly discusses several other tests.

Cytotoxic Testing

Cytotoxic testing, also called cytotoxicity testing, leukocyte antigen sensitivity testing, Bryan's test, the Metabolic Intolerance Test, or sensitivity testing, was promoted during the early 1980s by storefront clinics, laboratories, nutrition consultants, chiropractors, and medical doctors. Advocates claimed it could determine sensitivity to food, which they blamed for asthma, arthritis, constipation, diarrhea, hypertension, obesity, stomach disorders, and many other conditions. Those administering cytotoxic testing often used it to design a personalized diet program, which included a range of vitamins and minerals that they sold.

To perform the test, about 10 cubic centimeters of a patient's blood were placed in a test tube and centrifuged to separate the white cells (leukocytes). These were mixed with plasma and sterile water and applied to a large number of microscope slides, each of which had been coated with a dried food extract like that used by allergists for skin testing. The cells were then examined under a microscope at various intervals over a two-hour period to see whether they had changed their shape or disintegrated—supposedly signs of allergy to the particular food.

Cytotoxic testing was never proven reliable by controlled studies, and some studies found it to be highly unreliable. Enforcement actions taken by state and federal agencies appear to have driven cytotoxic testing from the marketplace during the mid-1980s, but some promoters still use "food sensitivity" similar tests.

Barrett S, Monaco GP: Cytotoxic testing.
Nutrition Forum 1:17–19, December 1984.
Describes the promotion of cytotoxic testing during the early 1980s. Cites scientific studies showing that the test is unreliable. Mentions efforts by government agencies to discourage cytotoxic testing.

Hecht A: Lab warns cow: Don't drink your milk.
FDA Consumer 19:31–32, July-August 1985.
Describes what happened when investigators from the FDA and the New York health department mailed two blood samples to a firm doing cytotoxic testing. The first specimen was from a physician who had no allergies or health problems. The

second was blood from a cow. In both cases, the lab reported allergies to a large number of foods. The New York Attorney General obtained a restraining order and California authorities initiated action also.

Bartola J: Cytotoxic test for allergies banned in state.
Pennsylvania Medicine 88:30, October 1985.
Reports that the Pennsylvania Department of Health's Bureau of Laboratories banned cytotoxic testing within Pennsylvania and stated that any laboratory caught doing the test would have its permit revoked.

Power failure for the 'Immune Power' diet.
Consumer Reports 51:112-113, February 1986.
Debunks the theories expressed by Stuart Berger, MD, in *Dr. Berger's Immune Power Diet*. Notes that Dr. Berger claimed that his dietary regimen would lead to "health, weight loss and super energy." Describes his recommendations for: (1) "detoxifying" the body by identifying hidden allergies and eliminating the offending foods, (2) losing excess weight, and (3) "rebuilding" the immune system with an array of vitamins and other supplements. Notes that the *Harvard Medical School Health Letter* said that the book was "selling a collection of quack ideas about food allergies that have been around for decades." Notes that Dr. Berger relied on cytotoxic testing to identify supposed allergies.

New York Academy of Medicine Committee on Public Health:
Statement on cytotoxic testing for food allergy (Bryan's test).
Bulletin of the New York Academy of
Medicine 64:117–119, January-February 1988.
Position paper on cytotoxic testing. Concludes that there is no scientific basis for expecting that the test could detect food allergy.

Misdiagnosis of Food Allergies

Robertson DAF, Ayres RCS, Smith CL, et al: Adverse consequences arising from misdiagnosis of food allergy.
British Medical Journal 297;719–720, September 17, 1988.
States that food allergy is rare, but there is a widespread belief—supported by the popular press and "alternative" practitioners—that sensitivity to specific foods is a common cause of a variety of symptoms. Reports on four cases in which alternative practitioners diagnosed food allergy in patients whose actual problems were metastatic liver cancer, Crohn's disease, villous atrophy of the duodenum, and anorexia nervosa.

Taylor S et al: Food allergies.
New York, American Council on Science and Health, 1989.
States that many Americans mistakenly believe they suffer from some form of food allergy. Describes the various ways in which individuals can react adversely to foods. Notes that many reactions are idiosyncrasies rather than true allergies.

Allergies: real or bogus?
In Barrett S et al: Health schemes, scams, and frauds, pp. 78–96.
New York, Consumer Reports Books, 1990.
Notes that a survey found that 43 percent of adults said that they have some type of adverse reaction to foods. States, however, that fewer than 2 percent of adults have true food allergies, and that what people believe are food allergies often are individual idiosyncrasies without a detectable physical basis. States that desensitization shots may help some people, but should not be used unless: (1) neither medication nor avoidance of suspected foods is effective, (2) the symptoms disrupt the person's life and have persisted for at least two years, and (3) evidence exists that shots can work against the particular allergies. Notes that a pamphlet of the American Academy of Otolaryngic Allergy states that the list of possible disorders that can be caused by food allergies is almost endless.

Carotid Body Resection

Carotid body resection (glomectomy) is a controversial operation in which one or both carotid bodies are surgically removed for the purpose of relieving the sensation of shortness of breath (dyspnea). The procedure has been performed on patients with asthma and chronic obstructive lung disease (emphysema and bronchitis). The carotid bodies play an important role in stimulating respiration in response to low blood oxygen levels.

In the early 1960s, a surgeon reported good results in several thousand patients who had undergone unilateral glomectomy. Subsequent research found that the procedure was no more effective than a sham operation. Unilateral glomectomy fell into disrepute, but another surgeon began claiming that bilateral glomectomy was effective. However, critics state that the bilateral procedure has not been proven effective by controlled studies and that it makes the body dangerously unresponsive to lack of oxygen.

National Center for Health Services Research and Health Care
Technology Assessment: Bilateral carotid body resection.

Health Technology Assessment Report Number 12, Department of Health and Human Services, 1985.
Describes the anatomy and physiology of the carotid bodies. States that bilateral carotid body resection has not been documented in any clinical trial and has the potential for life-threatening episodes due to loss of the ventilatory response to hypoxia. Concludes that the operation may be hazardous and should not be regarded as safe and effective until data from properly controlled studies indicate otherwise.

Anderson JA et al: Carotid body resection.
Journal of Allergy and Clinical Immunology 78:273–275, 1986.
Position statement of the American Academy of Allergy and Immunology (AAAI). Notes that glomectomy had a surge in popularity during the 1960s but virtually disappeared from major medical centers in the United States following publication of a critical AAAI position statement. Notes that a few individuals still performed the procedure and that some follow-up studies cast doubt on its long-term safety and efficacy. Notes examples of patients who suffered life-threatening asthma attacks following the operation. Recommends that glomectomy be reserved for experimental use only in well designed prospective trials.

Stulberg MS, Winn WR: Bilateral carotid body resection for the relief of dyspnea in severe chronic obstructive pulmonary disease, physiologic and clinical observations in three patients.
Chest 95:1123–1128, 1989.
Traces the history of glomectomy, noting that controlled studies of unilateral carotid body removal had shown that it was no more effective than a sham operation. Notes that some proponents then recommended bilateral glomectomy but provided no controlled studies to document improvement. Reports on three patients who had the bilateral procedure performed by Benjamin Winter, MD, the leading American proponent. States that all three patients, who later died, had claimed significant relief following the operation even though their blood levels of oxygen and carbon dioxide had worsened. Urges rigorous research to study the effects of such an operation in relieving extreme dyspnea in chronic lung diseases.

Bencini C, Pulera N: The carotid bodies in bronchial asthma.
Histopathology 18:195–200, 1991.
Reports that a study of fifty carotid bodies removed from patients with asthma were compared with ten obtained during autopsies of people who did not have asthma. States that certain differences were found, but their significance is unknown.

Diet and Behavior

Many books and articles in the popular press have claimed that various dietary components play a major role in determining a person's behavior. Perhaps the best known theory of this type was articulated in the early 1970s by Benjamin Feingold, MD, who claimed that hyperactivity in children was related to their intake of salicylate-containing foods and food additives. In the ensuing years, other people have claimed that sugar, "junk foods," milk, and nutrient deficiencies can make people upset and are even a factor in juvenile delinquency and adult criminal behavior. Some proponents even claim that hair analysis can detect mineral deficiencies or toxicity related to criminal behavior. Proponents have published the results of studies purported to back their claims—mostly in journals published by promoters of "alternative" methods. However, scientific analyses of these studies have shown that they are not well-designed.

General Literature

Rix KJB, Pearson DJ, Bentley SJ: A psychiatric study of patients with supposed food allergy.
British Journal of Psychiatry 145:121–126, 1984.
Reports that British investigators were unable to find any evidence that food hypersensitivity played a role in the mood disturbances or other psychological symptoms of 23 consecutive patients seeking treatment at an allergy clinic. Nineteen of these patients, whose parents believed that their mental symptoms were related to food hypersensitivity, turned out to have no allergies at all. The outcome of treatment appeared to depend on the degree of belief that symptoms had an allergic basis. The majority of patients in whom food allergy was excluded accepted the physician's findings and improved with supportive counseling. But some patients insisted they must have hidden food allergies and engaged in dangerous dietary restriction in an attempt to identify foods they should avoid.

Diet and behavior: A multidisciplinary evaluation.
Nutrition Reviews, May 1986.
A collection of 33 papers on diet and behavior presented at an international symposium on diet and behavior cosponsored by the AMA and the International Life Sciences Institute–Nutrition Foundation. The editors conclude: "There was general agreement that diet does affect behavior, but that the effects demonstrated to date had are subtle. Diet has not been established as a significant etiologic factor or as

having therapeutic potential in the management of abnormal behavior. Clearly, on the basis of existing evidence, it is premature to utilize information about the effect of diet on behavior to influence health policy."

Meister K: Diet and behavior: A state-of-the-art report.
Nutrition Forum 2:11–13, February 1985.
Summarizes what took place at the symposium described above. Notes that most speakers were cautious about conclusions and warned that research on diet and behavior must be carefully designed. Notes, however, that a few speakers reported results based on seriously flawed experiments.

Diet and behavior.
Dairy Council Digest, July/August 1985.
Summarizes research findings, citing 75 references. Concludes: (1) diet has been demonstrated to exert short-term effects on specific behaviors, but most of these are subtle; (2) no evidence supports the view that hypoglycemia, excess dietary sugar, food additives, food allergies, and vitamin and mineral deficiencies or excesses are related to juvenile delinquency or criminal behavior; and (3) little evidence suggests that food additives, food allergy, refined sugar, or caffeine causes hyperactivity in children or that megavitamin therapy corrects this behavioral disorder.

Schiffman SS, Buckley CE, Sampson HA, et al: Aspartame and susceptibility to headache.
New England Journal of Medicine 317:1181–1185, 1987.
Describes a double-blind test on 40 people who reported experiencing headaches repeatedly after consuming products containing aspartame (NutraSweet). Notes that the incidence of headaches after aspartame administration (35 percent) was not significantly different from that after a placebo (45 percent). Concludes: "This finding emphasizes the importance of double-blind studies to assess adverse reactions to a food or food ingredients." The study illustrates how people often misjudge whether ingesting a particular food or food substance is responsible for a symptom or behavior that follows.

Meister KA: Diet and behavior.
New York, American Council on Science and Health, 1987.
Discusses misinformation associated with the subjects of diet and hyperactivity, misdiagnosed hypoglycemia, and diet and crime. Also covers eating disorders and the effects of malnutrition, meal-skipping, and caffeine intake. Concludes: "The issue of diet and behavior is fraught with uncertainty and misunderstanding, due partly to exaggerations by misguided enthusiasts and partly to the incomplete understanding scientists have of the subtle ways in which nutrients influence action."

Diet and behavior: A series of regional forums.
Washington, DC, The Sugar Association, 1992.
Reports on presentations at a series of meetings sponsored by the American Dietetic Association's National Center for Nutrition and Dietetics. Covers consumer perceptions and current scientific knowledge related to food habits, food safety, and the alleged behavioral effects of food additives, sugar, and artificial sweeteners. One speaker noted that consumer confidence in the American food supply had dipped temporarily after the Alar scare and Chilean grape incidents.

Feingold Diet

In 1973 Benjamin Feingold, MD, a pediatric allergist from California, proposed that salicylates, artificial colors, and artificial flavors were causes of hyperactivity. To treat or prevent this condition, he suggested a diet that was free of these additives. His 1975 book, *Why Your Child is Hyperactive,* spelled out his claims and dietary strategies.

The Feingold Association of the United States (FAUS), which has local chapters throughout the country, claims that fidgetiness, poor sleep habits, short attention span, self-mutilation, antisocial traits, muscle incoordination, memory deficits, asthma, bedwetting, headaches, hives, seizures, and many other problems may respond to the Feingold program. FAUS publishes a food list, a medication list, a monthly newsletter, and a handbook describing its recommended program.

Adherence to the Feingold diet requires a drastic change in family life-style and eating patterns. Homemade foods prepared "from scratch" are necessary for many meals. Feingold strongly recommended that the hyperactive child help prepare the special foods and encouraged the entire family to participate in the dietary program. Many parents who have followed Feingold's recommendations have reported an improvement in their children's behavior. However, controlled studies do not support the Feingold hypothesis.

The September 1992 issue of the Feingold Association's newsletter, *Pure Facts,* claimed that teachers and children have been noted to suffer from the effects of chemicals used in construction, furnishing, housekeeping, maintenance, renovation, pest control, food service, and classroom activities at their schools. An article entitled "The Sick Building Syndrome" stated that one child was repeatedly disciplined for reacting to his teacher's perfume, another child became abusive toward his mother because of the school's newly-painted lunchroom, and that another child required tutoring because of a very bad reaction to a leak in the school's oil furnace. Claims like these are similar to those made by clinical ecologists.

Wender EH, Lipton MA: The National Advisory Committee on Hyperkinesis and Food Additives – Report to The Nutrition Foundation, June 1, 1975. Washington, DC, The Nutrition Foundation, 1975.
Notes that the term "hyperactivity" had not been clearly defined and may be a common feature among several unrelated diagnostic subgroups. Describes the difficulties involved in conducting research intended to measure behavioral changes in children. Notes that Dr. Feingold had not performed a controlled experiment to test his hypothesis and the success rate he claimed in his book was similar to the rate found in a study of hyperactive children on long-term drug therapy who stopped taking the drug. Notes that the Feingold diet called for elimination of many commonly eaten foods, not all of which contain food additives, and that no single substance or group of substances that the diet specifically removed had been identified. Concludes that the Feingold hypothesis was vaguely stated and had no scientific foundation. Recommended guidelines for scientific testing of Feingold's hypothesis.

Wender EH, Lipton MA: The National Advisory Committee on Hyperkinesis and Food Additives – Final report to The Nutrition Foundation. Washington, DC, The Nutrition Foundation, 1980.
Notes that the vagueness of Dr. Feingold's claims made it difficult to design appropriate studies either to confirm or refute his assertions. States that Dr. Feingold has not specified which chemicals and at what concentration are to be allowed or excluded from the "additive-free" diet. Notes that Dr. Feingold's recommendations for including or excluding foods on the basis of their salicylate content were based on erroneous assumptions about the levels of salicylate found naturally in many of the foods. Notes, too, that the diet excluded some "artificial food flavorings" that were identical to chemicals found in natural foods. Reviews published data and concludes that seven carefully designed experiments had failed to support the Feingold hypothesis, and that the few changes described in some reports had no practical significance. Concludes that the failure to support Dr. Feingold's claim of dramatic improvement in 32 to 60 percent of cases "suggests that the Feingold regimen produces a therapeutic effect that has nothing to do with the removal of specific food additives. . . . a placebo response." Concludes that Feingold's hypothesis provides no reason to change public policy about the use of artificial food colorings by the food industry. Also concludes that the Feingold hypothesis had been sufficiently refuted that there was no reason to continue giving high funding priority to research in this area.

Defined diets and childhood hyperactivity.
JAMA 248:290–292, 1982.
Reports on a National Institutes of Health Consensus Conference held in January 1982. States that defined diet should not be used universally in the treatment of childhood hyperactivity. States that dietary treatment may be worth trying if thorough and appropriate evaluation of the child and family and consideration of traditional therapeutic options have taken place. Advises further research, including study of possible adverse biological and psychosocial effects of dietary intervention.

Sheridan M, Meister KM: Food additives and hyperactivity
New York, American Council on Science and Health, 1982.
Summarizes research related to the Feingold hypothesis and concludes that it lacks scientific support. Notes that if a limited relationship exists between hyperactivity and the ingestion of certain food colors, it would affect only a small number of children. Concludes: "Because the Feingold diet does no physical harm, it might appear to be helpful in some instances due to its impact on family interactions. However, any potential benefits should be weighed against the potentially harmful impact of teaching children to blame food ingredients for their difficulties when other factors are more likely to be responsible." Also notes that the spread of inaccurate health information is inherently undesirable.

Kaplan BJ, McNicol J, Conte RA, et al: Dietary replacement
in preschool-aged hyperactive boys.
Pediatrics 83:7–17, 1989.
Describes an elaborate double-blind ten-week study of 24 children, during which about half of the children exhibited behavioral improvement. Notes, however, that "not a single parent believed that participation in this study had transformed their child into an easy to manage person."

Diet and Criminal Behavior

Gray GE, Gray LK: Diet and juvenile delinquency.
Nutrition Today 19:14–22, May/June 1983.
Notes that books and articles have suggested that reactive hypoglycemia, food allergies, and dietary inadequacies and excesses may all play a role in causing antisocial behavior. Describes the serious methodological flaws in research reports making such claims. Notes that a few correctional agencies have implemented dietary programs and that their cost can be very high. Concludes that there is no credible evidence to suggest that dietary change or megavitamin therapy alters the behavior of delinquents.

Position paper of the American Dietetic Association on diet and criminal behavior.
Journal of the American Dietetic Association 85:361–362, 1985.
States that there is no valid evidence to support the claim that diet is an important determinant of violence and criminal behavior. Warns that inappropriate dietary treatment based on unfounded beliefs can: (1) result in nutritional deficiencies or excesses; (2) detract from efforts to identify and effectively prevent and correct true causes of aberrant behavior; (3) lead to the dangerous belief that diet, rather than the individual, has control over and responsibility for the individual's behavior; and (4) result in the waste of limited public funds.

Sugar and Hyperactivity

Behar D, Rapoport JL, Adams AJ, et al: Sugar challenge testing with children considered behaviorally "sugar reactive."
Nutrition and Behavior 1:277–288, 1984.
Reports on double-blind tests in which 21 boys whose parents considered them to have adverse behavioral reactions to dietary sugar were challenged with glucose, sucrose, and a placebo. Neither sugar appeared to produce behavioral excitation or other significant changes in behavior, attention span, or memory. For the group as a whole, sugar ingestion actually produced a slight but significant decrease in motor activity.

Kruesi MJP, Rapoport JL, Cummings EM, et al: Effects of sugar and aspartame on aggression and activity in children.
American Journal of Psychiatry 144:1487–1490, 1987.
Reports on a study that compared 18 children ages 2 to 6 whose parents considered them "sugar-responders" and 12 of their playmates with no such history. During the baseline period, the "sugar-responsive" children appeared to be more disturbed and hyperactive. Double-blind challenges with aspartame, saccharin, sucrose, and glucose produced no significant effect on aggression or observer's ratings of behavior. Concludes that it is unlikely that sugar and aspartame are significant causes of disruptive behavior, but disturbed children said to be sugar-responsive may represent a group for whom families are searching for help.

Roshon MS, Hagen RL: Sugar consumption, locomotion, task orientation, and learning in preschool children.
Journal of Abnormal Child Psychology 17:349–357, 1989.
Reports that in a study of 12 children, no differences were found between the activity

level, attentiveness, or attention span of six children who were given sugar and six children given a placebo (aspartame).

Aylsworth J: Sugar and hyperactivity.
Priorities, pp. 31–33, Winter 1990.
States that despite the lack of evidence linking sugar and hyperactivity, many parents of misbehavior-prone children are still restricting dietary sugar. Notes the role of the media in perpetuating misinformation on this issue.

Gan DA. Sucrose and unusual childhood behavior.
Nutrition Today 26:8-14, May/June 1991.
Examines claims that childhood behavior is related to sucrose intake. Concludes that "speculations that ingestion of sucrose (or sugar) causes either hyperactivity in children or delinquent behavior in adolescents are not based on sound scientific evidence. Rather, they are based on anecdotes and incorrect interpretation of scientific data."

Macrobiotics

Macrobiotics is a quasireligious philosophical system founded by George Ohsawa [1893–1966]. "Macrobiotic" means "way of long life." The system advocates a vegetarian diet in which foods of animal origin are used as condiments rather than as full-fledged menu items. The optimal diet is said to be achieved by balancing "yin" and "yang" foods.

Ohsawa claimed to have cured himself of serious illness by changing from the modern refined diet then sweeping Japan to a simple diet of brown rice, miso soup, sea vegetables, and other traditional foods. He wrote that refined sugar and excess animal protein are two main causes of all illness, including cancer and mental illness. He outlined a 10-stage Zen macrobiotic diet in which each stage became progressively more restricted. The diet was claimed to enable individuals to overcome all forms of illness, which Ohsawa said were due to excesses in diet. In 1971, the AMA Council on Foods and Nutrition said that followers of the diet, particularly the highest level, stood in "great danger" of malnutrition and noted that several deaths had been reported. Current proponents espouse a diet that is less restricted but still can be nutritionally inadequate. They recommend whole grains (50–60 percent of each meal), vegetables (25–30 percent of each meal), whole beans or soybean-based products (5–10 percent of daily food), nuts and seeds (small amounts as snacks), miso soup, herbal teas, and small amounts of white meat or seafood once or twice weekly.

Today's leading proponent is Michio Kushi, a former student of Ohsawa, who founded and is president of the Kushi Institute in Brookline, Massachusetts. He also established *East West Journal*, a monthly magazine now called *East West Natural Health*. According to Institute publications, the macrobiotic way of life should include chewing food at least fifty times per mouthful (or until it becomes liquid), not wearing synthetic or woolen clothing next to the skin, avoiding long hot baths or showers (unless you have been consuming too much salt or animal food), having large green plants in your house to enrich the oxygen content of the air, and singing a happy song every day. *East West Natural Health* promotes a wide variety of "alternative" methods and tends to be critical toward scientific medicine and various public health measures. Books and magazines, special food items, macrobiotic cooking classes, and other macrobiotic products and services are obtainable through local health food stores and regional macrobiotic teaching centers ("East West Centers"). General bookstores also carry books by Michio Kushi and other proponents.

Macrobiotic diets have been promoted for maintaining general health and for preventing and "relieving" cancer and other diseases. Kushi's books contain case histories of people whose cancers have supposedly disappeared after they adopted macrobiotic eating. However, there is no scientific evidence of any such benefit, and the diet itself can cause cancer patients to undergo serious weight loss.

Recent studies showed that Dutch children who were fed macrobiotic diets were smaller and weighed less than other children who eat normally. Infants on macrobiotic diets often develop rickets and have deficiencies of vitamin B_{12} and iron. A New England study found similar deficiencies of vitamin B_{12} in children and adults in a macrobiotic community. As with the Dutch studies, these children tended to be smaller, shorter, and to weigh less than children fed normal diets.

Nutrient Inadequacies

van Staveren WA, Dagnelie PC: Food consumption, growth, and development of Dutch children fed on alternative diets.
American Journal of Clinical Nutrition 48:819–821, 1988.
Reviews four studies of children following diets espoused by the ecological, anthroposophic, and macrobiotic movement. Notes that all three movements espouse breast-feeding for a longer time than the usually recommended six months. Concludes that macrobiotically-fed children are probably most at risk.

Dagnelie PC, van Staveren WA, van Klaveren JD, et al: Do children on macrobiotic diets show catch-up growth? A population-based cross-sectional study in children aged 0–8 years.
European Journal of Clinical Nutrition 42:1007–1016, 1988.
Reports on a study of 243 Dutch children. Notes that from 6–8 months onward, growth stagnation occurred in both sexes, but was most marked in girls. Notes that some improvement occurred between eighteen months and five years, but the children often failed to achieve full recovery from the previous set-back. States that additional studies would be needed to determine whether the growth stagnation has any health consequences.

Dagnelie PC, van Staveren WA, Vergote FJVRA, et al: Nutritional status of infants aged 4 to 18 months on macrobiotic diets and matched omnivorous control infants: A population-based mixed-longitudinal study.
European Journal of Clinical Nutrition 43:325–338, 1989.
Reports on a Dutch study comparing the growth in fifty-three macrobiotic children with fifty-seven omnivorous control infants. Notes that the children had lower birth

rates and slower growth and psychomotor development than children who ate normally. Major skin and muscle wasting was observed in sixteen macrobiotic children and one omnivorous child.

Dagnelie PC., van Staveren, WA., Vergote FJVRA, et al: Increased risk of vitamin B-12 and iron deficiency in infants on macrobiotic diets. American Journal of Clinical Nutrition 50:818–824, 1989.
Compares the incidence of deficiencies of vitamin B_{12} and iron in fifty macrobiotic infants with those of fifty-seven infants fed omnivorous diets. Reports that the macrobiotic children had a high incidence of deficiencies of vitamin B_{12} and iron. States that most macrobiotic teachers had accepted recommendations for regular consumption of fish with a high vitamin B_{12} concentration.

Dagnelie PC, Vergote FJVRA, van Staveren WA, et al: High prevalence of rickets in infants on macrobiotic diets. American Journal of Clinical Nutrition 51:202–208, 1990.
Compares the incidence of rickets in fifty-three macrobiotic children ages 10–20 months with that of fifty-seven matched control infants on omnivorous diets. Notes that fifteen macrobiotic infants developed signs of rickets during the first phase of the study, due mainly to the omission of dairy products. Reports that some parents made dietary modifications as a result of this and other studies.

Inadequate vegan diets at weaning. Nutrition Reviews 48:323–326, 1990.
Notes that during the 1970s there were reports of malnutrition among infants and young children of new vegetarians who followed macrobiotic diets. Briefly describes the teachings of George Ohsawa. Reviews results of studies showing a higher incidence of rickets and other nutritional deficiencies among macrobiotic children. Also notes lower birth weights and growth rates in children fed macrobiotic diets. States that "macrobiotic leaders appear to be slow in responding to the adverse nutritional implications of these diets for young infants."

Miller DR, Specker BL, Ho ML, et al: Vitamin B-12 status in a macrobiotic community. American Journal of Clinical Nutrition 53:524–529, 1991.
Reports on the status of vitamin B_{12} in 110 macrobiotic adults and 42 macrobiotic children who lived in Boston or in Middlesex, Connecticut. Notes that about half of the participants showed evidence of at least marginal vitamin B_{12} deficiency and that the children tended to be shorter and to weigh less than would be expected for their age. Notes that the B_{12} content of sea vegetables is high, but that individuals who reported consuming more of them did not have better B_{12} status than those who did not.

Unproven Therapeutic Claims

Arnold C: The macrobiotic diet: A question of nutrition.
Oncology Nursing Forum 11:50–53, May/June 1984.
Describes the nutritional value of the macrobiotic diet advocated by the East West Foundation, noting that it can produce nutritional deficiencies in healthy populations and aggravate the compromised state of cancer patients. Contrasts the macrobiotic diet and standard nutritional regimen for malnourished cancer patients and shows that the macrobiotic diet is nearly opposite to what these patients require.

Bowman BB, Kushner RF, Dawson SC, et al: Macrobiotic diets for cancer treatment and prevention.
Journal of Clinical Oncology 2:702–711, 1984.
Describes the theories of George Ohsawa and Michio Kushi. Reviews the basic components of macrobiotic diets and the rationale for using these foods. Discusses known deficiencies in vitamins, minerals, and trace elements and notes potential adverse effects. Notes cases of people who have become seriously ill or children who have failed to develop properly because of following macrobiotic diets. Discusses the role of nutrition in cancer prevention and treatment. Concludes that there are no valid data on the effectiveness of macrobiotic diets in treating cancer, but there are legitimate concerns about their safety and nutritional adequacy for cancer patients.

Londer R: Cure by diet?
Health 17:54, 56–57, 72, October 1985.
Discusses concerns of critics who note the hazards of diets lacking calcium, zinc, iron and other nutrients. This is an especially serious matter for cancer patients. Mentions claims by some patients that they were cured of cancer by macrobiotic diets, noting a lack of proof. Argues that proper diet is important but is not a substitute for proven treatment.

Lindner L: The new, improved macrobiotic diet.
American Health 7:71–72, 76, 78, 80, 83, 85–86, May 1988.
Notes changes in the macrobiotic diet in response to deficiencies in the original one proposed by George Ohsawa who, at one point, insisted on one composed only of brown rice. Describes the current diet as more healthful, but still lacking in important nutrients. Notes that many followers of the macrobiotic movement do not allow enough flexibility to make up for deficiencies. Reviews arguments of critics that the diet is too restrictive and dangerous. A sidebar describes what happened when the author went as a "patient" to a "senior consultant" at the Kushi Institute. He was told that: (1) his heart was enlarged because he ate too much fruit, (2) his kidneys were weak, (3) he was slightly hypoglycemic (4) deposits of fat and mucus

were starting to build up in his intestines, (5) cold drinks could freeze the deposits and cause kidney stones, and (6) he should avoid chicken because it is linked with pancreatic cancer and melanoma. The consultation cost $200.

Unproven methods of cancer management: Macrobiotic diets for the treatment of cancer.
Ca-A Cancer Journal for Clinicians 39:248–251, 1989.
Reviews the history of the macrobiotic diet movement and proponents' claims that it is effective against cancer. Notes that "the only reports of efficacy are testimonials by patients, many of whom received conventional therapy in addition to following a macrobiotic diet." Discusses health hazards of macrobiotic diets, especially for cancer patients.

Dwyer J: The Macrobiotic diet: No cancer cure.
Nutrition Forum 7:9–10, March/April, 1990.
Briefly describes macrobiotic diets and the rationale behind them. Lists guidelines for foods to be consumed or avoided in a macrobiotic diet. Notes that the macrobiotic diet can satisfy the desire of some patients to be involved in their own care and can also provide a social support system. Notes that macrobiotic proponents falsely suggest that medical authorities agree with their dietary treatment. Discusses the case of a woman with a vocal cord tumor who adhered to a macrobiotic diet for a year rather than pursuing conventional medical treatment.

Raso J: A Kushi seminar for professionals.
Nutrition Forum 7:17–21, May/June 1990.
Describes a visit to a five-day seminar at the Kushi Institute in Becket, Massachusetts. Gives a brief history of the macrobiotic movement. Explains the theory of macrobiotics, noting its ties to Chinese philosophy. Describes the sessions led by Michio Kushi and others, some of whom claimed to have been cured of cancer by macrobiotic diets. Reports that astrological conditions, weather conditions, and a long list of other bizarre factors were said to be relevant to diagnosing patients. Notes the hazards of macrobiotic diets, especially when compared to other diets that are nutritionally superior. Mentions the case of Anthony Sattilaro, MD, whose books *Recalled by Life* and *Living Well Naturally* had suggested that macrobiotics had cured him of prostate cancer. Notes that Dr. Sattilaro had undergone conventional therapy but credited macrobiotics for his improvement. Also notes that despite his claims that he had been pronounced cured, he died several years later from the disease.

Gelband H et al: Macrobiotic diets.
In Gelband H et al: Unconventional cancer treatments, pp. 58–66.

Washington, DC, U.S. Government Printing Office, 1990.
Explores macrobiotic diets. Reviews the history of the development of macrobiotic diets. Discusses the Zen-based macrobiotic philosophy behind macrobiotic diets and explains the rationale behind the role of macrobiotic diets in cancer treatment. Lists dietary guidelines describing foods to be eaten or avoided. Describes possible adverse effects, noting nutritional deficiencies. Reviews the few studies discussing macrobiotic diet in treatment of cancer, noting flaws. Concludes that more studies are needed.

Multilevel Marketing

Multilevel marketing (also called MLM or network marketing) is a form of direct sales in which independent distributors sell products, often in their customers' home or by telephone. Most distributors hope to profit not only from their own sales, but also from those of other distributors they recruit.

Several dozen MLM companies are involved in the sale of health or nutrition products. No knowledge of health or nutrition is required to become a distributor. Completion of a one-page application and purchase of a distributor's kit costing $25 to $50 are usually the only requirements. Distributor kits typically include a sales manual, product literature, order forms, and a subscription to a magazine or newsletter published by the company. Distributors can buy products "wholesale," sell them "retail," and recruit other distributors who can do the same. When enough distributors have been enrolled, the recruiter is eligible to collect a percentage of their sales. Companies suggest that this process provides a great money-making opportunity. However, it is unlikely that people who don't join during the first few months of operation or become one of the early distributors in their community can build enough of a sales pyramid to do well.

Most multilevel companies that market health products claim that their products can prevent or cure a wide range of diseases. A few companies merely suggest that people will feel better, look better, or have more energy if they supplement their diet with extra nutrients. When clear-cut therapeutic claims are made in product literature, the company is an easy target for government enforcement action. Some companies run this risk, hoping that the government won't take action until their customer base is well established. Other companies make no claims in their literature but rely on testimonials, encouraging people to try their products and credit them for any improvement that occurs.

Most multilevel companies tell distributors not to make claims for the products except for those found in company literature. (That way the company can deny responsibility for what distributors do.) However, many companies hold sales meetings at which people are encouraged to tell their story to the others in attendance. Some companies sponsor telephone conference calls during which leading distributors describe their financial success, give sales tips, and describe their personal experiences with the products. Testimonials may also be published in company magazines, audiotapes or videotapes. Testimonial claims can trigger enforcement action, but since it is time-consuming to collect evidence of their use, few government agencies bother to do so.

Government enforcement action against multilevel companies has seldom been vigorous. These companies are usually left alone unless their promotions become so conspicuous and their sales volume so great that an agency feels compelled to intervene. Even then, few interventions have substantial impact once a company is well established.

Critical Literature

Friendly salespeople.
In Herbert V, Barrett S: Vitamins and "health foods": the great American hustle. Philadelphia, George F. Stickley Co., 1981.
Describes the early years of multilevel marketing of health products and the history and sales approaches of Shaklee Corporation, Amway Corporation, and Neo-Life Corporation. Describes how people are misled into thinking that products are helpful and how people can be persuaded to become MLM distributors.

Fitzgerald S, Mekeel P: King of the nutrition peddlers.
Lancaster (PA) New Era, May 26-27, 1981.
Describes meetings in which "people stand up at meetings and in the best spirit of an old-fashioned revival tell how Shaklee products have rid them of arthritis, saved their marriage, enabled them to have two bowel movements a day, and kept them from breaking a leg when they fell off a ladder." When the reporters inquired about becoming distributors, they were advised to begin by purchasing a regimen of products costing $600 a year.

Dale KC: "We don't prescribe," but . . . .
ACSH News & Views 3:12-13, September/October 1982.
Describes how the author obtained a Shaklee distributorship and attended sales meetings where she encountered claims that vitamin E might make one live longer, that B-complex was good for coffee jitters, and that alfalfa has "miraculous" benefits. She observed a large variety of testimonial claims and found that Shaklee's multivitamin sold for 3 to 7 times as much as comparable products at a drugstore.

The dubious distributors: An inside look at the booming nutrition-supplement business.
Consumer Reports 50:280-282, May 1985.

Describes the experiences of a reporter who became a distributor for several MLM companies and was encouraged to make false and illegal claims for their products.

Fanning O: Herbalife criticized at Senate hearings.
Nutrition Forum 2:65–68, September 1985.
Fanning O: "Herbalife hearings," part II.
Nutrition Forum 2:73–77, October 1985.
Describes portions of hearings held by a U.S. Senate subcommittee that investigated the dangers of very-low-calorie (VLC) diets. Describes expert testimony indicating hazards of some products and testimony by Herbalife officials indicating that product users had a high incidence of side effects. Editor's sidebar describes misleading claims made when marketing of Herbalife and the Cambridge diet (another VLC product) began.

Herbalife agrees to pay $850,000 penalty.
Nutrition Forum 4:15, February 1987.
Describes how Herbalife International and its president, Mark Hughes, agreed to pay $850,000 to settle charges by the California Attorney General that the company had made false medical claims and engaged in an illegal pyramid-style marketing scheme.

Stare FJ: Marketing a nutritional "revolutionary breakthrough."
New England Journal of Medicine 315:971–973, 1986.
Attacks United Sciences of America's promotion of "optimal health and vital energy through state-of-the art nutrition." Debunks claims for the company's "four revolutionary breakthrough formulas" and describes how, when he asked for documentation of various claims, the company's medical director offered to meet with him and encouraged him to apply for a research grant from the company.

Barrett S: Health or hype? A report on United Sciences of America.
New York, American Council on Science and health, 1987.
Provides extensive details of this MLM company's rapid rise using high-tech videotapes and an alleged endorsement by a prominent scientific advisory board to market its products. Then tells how state and federal enforcement actions drove the company out of business.

Barrett S: Be wary of medical endorsements.
ACSH News & Views 8:3–4, May/June 1987.
Describes the use of endorsements by United Sciences of America. Notes the author's conclusion that "vitamin endorsements by doctors—no matter how prestigious they

are—should be viewed with extreme caution. All I have seen so far have included claims that were unproven and also illegal."

Eisenberg R: The mess called multilevel marketing.
Money, June 1987.
A detailed investigation of the multilevel industry and some of the companies selling health products. Illustrates the great enthusiasm of some distributors and the shattered dreams of others. Concludes that the FTC should do more to curb misleading sales practices by multilevel companies and that and the FDA should do more to halt fraudulent claims for nutrition products.

Paros M: Can Super Blue Green help save the world?
Nutrition Forum 5:17–19, March 1988.
Relates the author's experience in trying blue-green algae products marketed by Cell Tech, Inc. Describes the manufacturer's and distributor's exaggerated claims. Discusses government enforcement actions against another company run by the brother of Cell Tech's president. Notes side effects from the consumption of blue-green algae and its lack of significant nutrients.

Barrett S: Sunrider warnings issued.
Nutrition Forum 5:31-32, April 1988.
Describes illegal therapeutic claims made by Sunrider International and government regulatory actions involving the company.

Krajick K: The stay-young hucksters.
Longevity 1:56–60, 62, August 1989.
Describes how the parents of a 4-year-old girl with an inoperable brain tumor put her on a $900-a-month Sunrider regimen with the hope of curing the cancer. When the tumor went into remission (following radiation therapy), Sunrider distributors began telling prospective clients that their products had cured it. Although the child died of her disease several months later, the parents continued to receive phone calls from families of cancer patients inquiring about the "cure." Also describes an enforcement action taken against Rockland Corporation for making illegal claims for its product, Body Toddy.

Barrett S: The multilevel mirage.
Priorities, pp. 38-40, Summer 1991.
Describes questionable claims made by Enrich International, Omnitrition International, Inc., Matol Botanical International, Sunrider International, and Light Force. Advises consumers to avoid multilevel products altogether because "those that have nutritional value . . . are invariably overpriced and may be unnecessary as

well. Those promoted as remedies are either unproven, bogus, or intended for conditions that are unsuitable for self-medication." Urges government agencies to police the multilevel marketplace aggressively, using undercover investigators and filing criminal charges when wrongdoing is detected.

Raso J: Bottled hype: The story of Km.
Nutrition Forum 8:33-37, September/October 1991.
Provides a detailed history of Matol Botanical International and its main products, Km, which contains potassium and several herbs. Describes how distributors market Km with claims that are illegal and violate official company policy. Describes what the author observed at two large company-sponsored meetings.

Stern RL, Grover MB. Pyramid power?
Forbes, pp.139–148, November 11, 1991.
Describes various legal difficulties faced by Nu Skin International, a multilevel company that sold skin-care products and had predicted sales of $500 million for 1991.

Raso J: The shady business of Nature's Sunshine.
Nutrition Forum 9:17–23, May/June 1992.
Provides a detailed history of Nature's Sunshine Products, an MLM company that sells more than 400 herbal, homeopathic, and supplement products. Describes what happened when the author attended a training program for distributors. Describes how the company encourages distributors to use iridology and muscle-testing [described elsewhere in this book] as a basis for recommending products. Notes that despite elaborate disclaimers, the company and its distributors are breaking the law.

Barrett S: Sunrider and the law.
Priorities, Fall 1992.
Reports that a woman who suffered hair loss, tooth discoloration, and nausea was awarded $650,000 in actual and punitive damages in a trial in which she charged Sunrider with racketeering. Describes how Sunrider products were marketed with claims that they were derived from ancient Chinese manuscripts. Describes how the story was proved to be a complete fabrication.

Vegetarianism

Much of the world's population is primarily vegetarian due to circumstances beyond their control. People in underdeveloped countries have limited access to flesh foods, but usually utilize animal products that are available. Vegetarianism is gaining popularity in Western societies because vegetarians appear to suffer less from diseases that are prevalent in industrialized societies. Such differences may be more related to the greater life expectancies of industrialized countries, but there is some evidence that diseases associated with obesity (coronary artery disease, hypertension, diabetes) are less common among vegetarians, who tend to weigh less than nonvegetarians. Some people espouse vegetarianism out of concern for the environment, animal rights, attitudes toward violence, and other philosophical and ethical issues. Still others eat less flesh food for economic reasons.

Vegetarian diets can be classified into six categories: semivegetarian, which includes milk, eggs, dairy products, poultry and fish, but excludes red meat; pesco-vegetarian, which allows dairy foods, eggs, and fish, but no other flesh foods; lacto-ovo-vegetarian, which allows milk, eggs, and dairy products, but excludes all flesh foods; lacto-vegetarian, which allows milk and dairy products, but excludes eggs and flesh foods; ovo-vegetarian, which excludes dairy products and all flesh foods; and, vegan, which allows no animal products (except honey), relying exclusively on plant products for nutrition. This classification does not take into account the diverse practices within each group, such as the taking of dietary supplements, the emphasis or avoidance of certain foods, or the use of scientific health care. Food fortification makes it possible even for vegans to have nutritionally adequate diets if they are careful and rational in their planning.

Vegetarian diets are healthful and nutritionally adequate when appropriately planned. However, extreme vegetarians may consume a diet that is nutritionally inadequate and can harm the health and stunt the growth of their children. Some also fail to use medical care for serious diseases. Extremism appears to be most likely when individuals become vegetarians for strongly-held philosophical or religious reasons. Extremists may fail to see obvious signs of ill-health in themselves and their dependent children—with disastrous results. People who adopt vegetarian diets for practical reasons such as to save money, to lower body weight, to put greater variety in the diet, out of general health consciousness, or those who are occasional backsliders, may be at lower risk for the adverse effects of vegetarianism.

Caution is in order for those who are seeking the objective truth about the possible benefits or hazards of vegetarian eating. Many people who conduct research and write about vegetarian diets are themselves philosophically-committed vegetarians whose biases prevent them from reporting adverse effects as rigorously as they do beneficial findings. Until recent years, there has been a notable lack of skepticism among vegetarian researchers. Science without skepticism is pseudoscience. Whether real differences in health outcome exist when all factors are roughly equal (i.e., genetics, calories, grains, fruits, vegetables, dairy products, etc.) except the source of the entree (flesh versus non-flesh) has not been resolved, or even seriously addressed.

This section contains general information about the risks and benefits of vegetarian eating. For references to serious harm related to vegetarian eating, see the discussion of macrobiotic diets elsewhere in this book.

General Information

American Dietetic Association. Position of the American Dietetic Association: Vegetarian diets—technical support paper.
Journal of the American Dietetic Association 88:352–355, 1988.
States that vegetarian diets are healthful and nutritionally adequate when appropriately planned. Notes that since vegetarianism encompasses a wide variety of eating patterns, nutrition assessment of such diets is difficult without knowing specific food avoidances and health-related attitudes and practices. Discusses health benefits and potential nutritional deficiencies of vegetarian diets.

Dwyer JT: Health aspects of vegetarian diets.
American Journal of Clinical Nutrition 48:712–738, 1988.
Surveys studies of the health benefits and risks of vegetarian diets compared to nonvegetarian diets. Suggests that lifestyle factors such as not smoking may have as much effect as vegetarianism in reducing the risk of certain diseases. Suggests that while vegetarians may have less risk of obesity, diabetes, gallstones, and certain cancers, there is less evidence of benefits in preventing various other diseases. Concludes that a prudent nonvegetarian diet can incorporate many of the advantages of vegetarian diets while maintaining other advantages.

Jacobs C, Dwyer JT: Vegetarian children: Appropriate and inappropriate diets.
American Journal of Clinical Nutrition 48:811–818, 1988.

Notes that dietary needs for children change as children grow older. Describes dietary needs for children in early infancy, later infancy, preschool age, grade school age, and adolescence. Discusses hazards associated with certain diets, noting instances of malnutrition, rickets, and other diseases resulting from inadequate diets. Suggests ways of avoiding dietary deficiencies. Concludes that well-planned vegetarian diets can provide adequate nutrition, though this is difficult for the person following a vegan diet. Mentions possible benefits of vegetarian diets.

Freeland-Graves J: Mineral adequacy of vegetarian diets.
American Journal of Clinical Nutrition 48:859–862, 1988.
Reviews research on mineral adequacy of vegetarian diets. Discusses levels of zinc, calcium, iron, manganese, selenium, and copper in vegetarian diets and vegetarians. Compares vegetarians with nonvegetarians and with other groups of vegetarians. Notes that data is conflicting with some vegetarian diets providing adequate levels of minerals while others are inadequate. Concludes that most vegetarians probably have adequate mineral levels, but that potential problems exist. Suggests that vegetarians can make wise choices of foods to maintain adequate levels of minerals.

Acosta PB: Availability of essential amino acids and nitrogen in vegan diets.
American Journal of Clinical Nutrition 48:868–874, 1988.
Notes that vegan children often fail to grow as well as their omnivorous counterparts despite protein intakes that exceed the RDA. Discusses the effects of high-fiber diets in reducing the intake of amino acids and other nutrients. Concludes that while more research is needed, children subjected to vegan diets may need to consume more protein to achieve normal growth and health.

Johnston PK: Counseling the pregnant vegetarian.
American Journal of Clinical Nutrition 48:901–905, 1988.
Notes that children have different dietary needs from those of adults. Suggests ways that nutritionists and physicians can counsel pregnant vegetarians and vegetarian mothers of young children about nutritional needs of their children and help them make appropriate dietary changes to meet these needs. Urges a nonjudgmental attitude toward their dietary beliefs.

Smith MV: Development of a quick reference guide to accommodate vegetarianism in diet therapy for multiple disease conditions.
American Journal of Clinical Nutrition 48:906–909, 1988.
Describes the development of a guidebook to help vegetarians adapt to diet therapy for twelve disease conditions.

Kestin M, Rouse IL, Correll RA, et al: Cardiovascular disease risk factors in free-living men: comparison of two prudent diets, one based on lactoovovegetarianism and the other allowing lean meat.
American Journal of Clinical Nutrition 50:280–287, 1989.
Reports on an Australian study comparing cardiovascular risk factors in a lacto-ovovegetarian diet, a low-fat diet allowing lean meat, and a standard diet. Discusses results showing that both the lacto-ovovegetarian and the lean meat diets lower cholesterol levels and blood pressure compared to the standard diet. Notes a slight advantage for the lacto-ovovegetarian diet in lowering cholesterol, but no difference in reducing blood pressure for the lacto-ovovegetarian and the lean meat diets. Notes that the men in the study preferred the lean meat diet over both the lacto-ovovegetarian and the standard diet.

Lombard KA, Olson AL, Nelson SE: Carnitine status of lactoovovegetarians and strict vegetarian adults and children.
American Journal of Clinical Nutrition 50:301–306, 1989.
Discusses a study analyzing the status of carnitine in groups of adults and children following a lactovegetarian, strict vegetarian, or mixed diet. Describes selection of subjects for the study from members of the Seventh-day Adventists and collection of data for the study. Lists statistics on group characteristics, protein nutritional status, plasma, and urinary carnitine. Discusses results which show that people following diets with low amounts of carnitine have lower reserves of carnitine but also excrete less of it. Plasma concentrations of carnitine are within the normal range, though the study does not report whether or not vegetarian children are at risk for nutrition deficiency.

O'Connell JM, Dibley MJ, Sierra J, et al: Growth of vegetarian children: The Farm study.
Pediatrics 84:475–481, 1989.
Discusses the growth and health of 404 children living at The Farm, a collective Tennessee community that followed a vegan diet that included fortified soy milk, nutritional yeast, and other vitamin and mineral supplements. Notes that the children were within average growth limits for their age, though slightly smaller than the U.S. growth reference. Concludes that children raised on a vegan diet can achieve adequate growth if there is proper attention to weaning foods and nutrient intake.

Hodgkin G: Diet manual—including a vegetarian meal plan, 7th edition.
Loma Linda, CA, Seventh-day Adventist Dietetic Association, 1990.
Provides up-to-date nutritional guidance including scientifically-based vegetarian

meal planning. Covers normal nutrient needs, nutrition for pregnancy and lactation, pediatric diets, GI diets, renal diets, cardiac diets, diabetic and related diets, mineral modified diets, diets for acute care, nutrition and immunity, nutrition support and enteric feedings, geriatric and rehabilitation diets, test diets, nutrition and drugs, and nutrition for exercise and weight control.

Burr M: Vegetarianism and health.
The Practitioner 234:62, 64, January 15, 1990.
Examines reasons why vegetarians have fewer health problems than nonvegetarians. States that the interpretation of research results is complicated by the fact that vegetarians also tend to adopt a healthier lifestyle. Discusses several studies comparing vegetarians and nonvegetarians, noting links between eating meat and eggs and certain diseases. Notes that cholesterol reduction among vegetarians is not simply due to the exclusion of meat because an increase in vegetable fiber may also be important. Concludes that it may be possible to obtain the health benefits of a vegetarian diet without totally excluding lean meat.

Thorogood M, Roe L, McPherson K, et al: Dietary intake and plasma lipid levels: lessons from a study of the diet of health conscious groups.
British Medical Journal 300:1297–1301, 1990.
Reports on a study evaluating the diets and cholesterol levels of health-conscious people following four distinct diets: vegan, vegetarian, fish eaters, and meat eaters. Discusses results which show no significant differences in cholesterol levels among the four groups. Notes that all follow a health-conscious diet, with meat eaters consuming less meat and fish than the general population, and all groups restricting their intake of fat. Concludes that health-conscious people can select a diet that fulfills most of the current dietary recommendations regardless of whether or not they eat meat.

Sabate J, Lindsted KD, Harris RD, et al: Anthropometric parameters of schoolchildren with different life-styles.
American Journal of Diseases of Children 144:1159–1163, 1990.
Compares the height and weight of children attending Seventh-day Adventist schools and public schools. Discusses results which show that Seventh-day Adventist children are taller and leaner than children in the general population. Reports that they consume meat, dairy products, eggs, and "junk food" less frequently and fruits and vegetables more frequently than public school children. Notes also that children of nonsmoking Seventh-day Adventists are taller than children of smoking parents in the general population. Concludes that a health-oriented lifestyle in childhood and adolescence can sustain physical growth.

Pedersen, AB, Bartholomew MJ, Dolence LA, et al: Menstrual differences due to vegetarian and nonvegetarian diets.
American Journal of Clinical Nutrition 53:879–885, 1991.
Examines the relationship of diet to menstrual regularity in vegetarian and nonvegetarian women. Concludes that vegetarian women are significantly more likely to have irregular periods than nonvegetarian women. Suggests that vegetarian women may have lower reproductive capability.

Dingott S, Dwyer J: Benefits and risks of vegetarian diets.
Nutrition Forum 8:45–47, November/December 1991.
Lists types of vegetarian diets. Lists and discusses benefits and risks of vegetarian diets, citing references to key studies. Notes typical health practices associated with various types of vegetarian diets. Provides tips on foods to ensure adequate intakes of iron, calcium, zinc, and vitamin D.

Farley D: Vegetarian diets: the pluses and the pitfalls.
FDA Consumer 26: 20–24, May 1992.
Points out that vegetarian diets meet many of the recommendations of more grains, fruits and vegetables and less fats made in the U.S. Surgeon General's 1988 report on nutrition and health. Also cautions that there are certain risks associated with vegetarian diets that exclude all animal foods, including eggs and dairy products. Discusses possible associations between diet and cancer. Provides advice on switching slowly to a vegetarian diet to avoid intestinal discomfort due to increased bulk, and points out the need for vegans to supplement with vitamin B_{12} and engage in careful meal planning.

Questionable Approaches to Weight Control

Thousands of questionable diets, devices, pills, powders, and programs have been claimed to help people become slimmer. Most fad diets can produce weight loss due to calorie restriction, but the weight usually returns when the dieter resumes previous eating patterns. Some diets are dangerous because they lack vital nutrients. Many gimmicks marketed to the public are fakes. The overall market is huge because many people are worried about their weight and find it very difficult to control, with or without medical help. Evidence has been mounting that many more people are dieting than should be and that the resultant weight-cycling ("yo-yo dieting") is intrinsically harmful. At the same time, government officials have begun urging commercial weight-loss companies to investigate the actual impact of their programs and make meaningful data available to prospective clients.

General Information

Barrett S: Diet facts and fads.
In Barrett S (ed): The health robbers, 2nd edition, pp. 173–183.
Philadelphia, George F. Stickley Co., 1980.
Describes the pitfalls of fasting, supplemented fasting, low-carbohydrate (high-protein) diets, and overzealous high-carbohydrate diets. Provides a quick-reference guide to questionable products and promotions.

Mirkin G: Getting thin: All about fat – How you get it, how you lose it, how you keep it off for good.
Boston, Little, Brown and Company, 1983.
Debunks the gamut of diet and drug fads, exercise gimmicks, and cultural myths that hinder safe, lasting weight loss. Recommends a program of gradually increasing exercise combined with a diet aimed at producing gradual weight loss.

Fear of fat: the medical evidence.
Consumer Reports 50:455–457, August 1985.
Examines theories of obesity causes and means of reducing it. Also explores the debate over what constitutes an ideal weight. Includes a chart listing three interpretations of ideal weight based on age, gender, and height. Reviews hazards of obesity and fad and crash diets. Urges people to exercise more often.

Schwartz H: Never satisfied: A cultural history of diets, fantasies and fat.
New York, Macmillan, Inc., 1986.
Traces the history of American attitudes toward food, fatness, and dieting. Describes a shift from fictions related to food faddism to fictions related to scientific pronouncements about health. Notes that there has been no let-up in moneymaking activities by those who sense profits in weight control and diet promotions.

Commercial weight-loss programs.
National Council Against Health Fraud, Loma Linda, CA, 1987.
Position paper lists tips on evaluating commercial weight-loss programs. Disparages those that: (1) promise rapid loss, (2) have caloric intake below 800 calories per day, (3) create dependence on special products rather than prudent food choices, (4) fail to encourage permanent realistic lifestyle changes, (5) misrepresent salespeople as "counselors," (6) involve expensive contracts, (7) fail to note risks, (8) promote spurious pills or devices, (9) claim that "cellulite" exists in the body, or (10) claim that a "bulking agent" produces automatic weight loss.

AMA Council on Scientific Affairs: Treatment of obesity in adults.
JAMA 260:2547–2551, 1988.
States that prevention is the treatment of choice and that early identification of individuals at risk can be helpful in targeting those most likely to gain excessive weight. Discusses fasting, very-low-calorie diets, (balanced and unbalanced), and novelty diets. Recommends a comprehensive weight-reduction program that incorporates diet, exercise, and behavior modification.

Lamb L: The weighting game.
Secaucus, NJ, Lyle Stuart Inc., 1988.
Discusses the metabolic processes involved in determining body weight. Recommends a low-fat, high-carbohydrate program without excessive caloric restriction, plus exercise to increase the metabolically active muscle mass. Discusses the drawbacks of other diet programs and weight-loss aids.

Czajka-Norins DM, Parham ES: Fear of fat: Attitudes toward obesity.
Nutrition Today 25:26–32, January/February 1990.
Describes the role of the media in shaping people's attitudes toward body weight. Notes various ways that Americans are pressured to become thinner. Describes how the fashion, diet, and cosmetic industries are using insecurity about appearance to market products. Discusses how negative attitudes toward obesity may actually contribute to the problem by encouraging cyclic dieting, which stimulates fat deposition. Notes that television tends to portray eating as a responsibility-free and consequence-free activity.

Drewnowski A et al: Toward safe weight loss.
East Lansing, MI, Michigan Health Council, 1990.
Reports the conclusions of a task force to establish guidelines for weight-reduction programs. Provides guidelines for assessing risks related to the dieter's health, staffing of weight-loss programs, full disclosure to prospective clients, selection of weight-loss goals, nutrition recommendations, exercise, and psychological approaches. Recommends against the use of appetite-suppressant drugs and, in most cases, the use of formula products.

Bennion LJ, Bierman EL, Ferguson JM : Straight talk about weight control.
New York, 1991, Consumer Reports Books.
Provides detailed explanations of the definition, measurement, causes, and treatment of obesity. Covers pertinent research findings. Discusses the pros and cons of many types of weight-control methods. Emphasizes reducing calorie intake, increasing energy output, and maintaining positive eating habits.

Wooley SC, Garner DM: Obesity treatment: The high cost of false hope.
Journal of the American Dietetic Association 91:1248–1251, 1991.
States that it is widely agreed that obesity treatment generally is ineffective and, in many instances, may be destructive as well. Suggests that "the actual benefits of weight loss have been overstated and that the few individuals who experience treatment success may be consigned to a lifetime battle against biological mechanisms that operate to return them to their natural . . . weight." Describes how a typical person who fails might feel during and after the experience of dieting. States that possible negative consequences of dieting should be more seriously considered.

Papazian R: Never say diet?
FDA Consumer 25:8–12, October 1991.
Discusses recent research findings related to weight control. Notes that the location of body fat may be more important than the amount of extra weight—fat in the hips and thighs is less of a threat to health than abdominal fat. Cites research suggesting that lowering the fat content of one's diet may facilitate weight loss. Notes that three years after shedding 67 pounds on a liquid formula diet, Oprah Winfrey regained the weight and swore off dieting forever.

Methods for voluntary weight loss and control.
NIH Technology Assessment Conference Statement.
Bethesda, MD, National Institutes of Health, 1992.
Reports on a conference focused on: (1) the methods used to try to lose weight (2)

how successful these are, (3) the attributes of and barriers to success, (4) the beneficial and adverse effects of weight loss, (5) basic strategies for weight control, and (6) future directions for research. Notes that many people trying to lose weight don't need to do so, but most who need to do so are not succeeding. Notes that for most weight loss methods, there are few scientific studies evaluating their safety and effectiveness. Concludes that losing weight is not a simple problem of will power but a complex disorder of appetite regulation and energy metabolism.

Berg FM: Nondiet movement gains strength.
Obesity & Health 6:85–90, September/October 1992.
Reports that an "anti-diet" movement is growing out of concern by educators, health-care providers, and nutritionists that America's weight obsession is causing a major crisis. States that 40 percent of American women are dieting, but nearly two-thirds of them are not overweight. States that 61 percent of adolescent girls and 28 percent of boys have been on a weight-loss diet during the past year. Cites research showing that Miss America contestants and *Playboy* magazine centerfold models have become thinner during the past thirty years and are now at an anorexic level of 13 to 19 percent below their expected weight. Notes that expert opinion is shifting to the idea that overall wellness is more important than thinness. Describes new treatment programs focusing on: (1) feeling good about oneself, (2) eating well in a natural, relaxed way, and (3) being comfortably active.

Questionable Diets

Willis J: Diet books sell well but . . .
FDA Consumer 16:14–17, March 1982.
Describes the shortcomings of eleven fad diet plans.

Hegsted DM: Rating the diets.
Health 15:21-32, January 1983.
Describes advantages and disadvantages of Richard Simmons' Never-Say-Diet Diet, the Pritikin Diet, the Beverly Hills Diet, the University Diet, the Atkins Diet, the Cambridge Diet, the Stillman Diet, and the Scarsdale Diet. States that the Never-Say-Diet-Diet is sensible. Notes that the Pritikin Diet might be most successful but is too difficult for most people to follow. Criticizes the rest, calling the Beverly Hills Diet "a sure recipe for malnutrition if you stay on it long enough."

Bergland T: Rating the diets.
New York, Beekman House, 1983.
Analyzes and rates about 100 diets and diet programs.

*Fisher MC, LaChance PA: Nutrition evaluation
of published weight-reducing diets.
Journal of the American Dietetic Association 85:450–454, 1985.*
Discusses eleven published diet plans, using computer analyses made with the University of Massachusetts Nutrient Data Bank. Notes that the plans that emphasize ingesting foods from one food group or limit ingestion of a macronutrient result in the least adequate nutrient intakes.

*Van Itallie TB, Yang M: Cardiac dysfunction in obese dieters:
A potentially lethal complication of rapid, massive weight loss.
American Journal of Clinical Nutrition 39:695-702, 1984.*
Reports on the death of seventeen obese but otherwise healthy adults who died suddenly of ventricular arrhythmias during or shortly after completing rapid, massive weight reduction on a very-low-calorie liquid protein diet program. Notes that the danger appears greater for people who are slightly or moderately overweight than it does for those who are very overweight.

*Trubo R: Fad diets: Unqualified hunger for miracles.
Medical World News 27:44–46, 49–50, 52, 57–59, August 11, 1986.*
Surveys various aspects of the weight-loss marketplace, noting that the public consumes much of the information put in front of it, while physicians remain skeptical. Reports criticisms of the methods recommended by Fit for Life, the Rice Diet, the Rotation Diet, Dr. Berger's Immune Power Diet, and United Sciences of America. Notes that several experts had been unable to locate publishers for scientifically valid books on weight control.

*Harris LT: A spectrum of diet books.
Nutrition Forum 7:4–6, January/February 1990.*
Provides capsule reviews of ten diet books. Notes that the public is faced with many books that mix legitimate research findings with pseudoscience. Recommends The *Weighting Game, The New American Diet*, and The *I-Don't-Eat (But-Can't-Lose) Weight Loss Program*. Gives "borderline recommended" rating to *The T-Factor Diet, Elizabeth Takes Off,* and *The Stop-Light Diet for Children*. Does not recommend *The Two-Day Diet, Maximum Metabolism, How to Win at Weight Loss,* and *The Rice Diet Report*.

*Wadden TA, Van Itallie TB, Blackburn GL: Responsible and irresponsible
use of very-low-calorie diets in the treatment of obesity.
JAMA 263:83-85, 1990.*
States that very-low-calorie (VLC diets) usually contain 400 to 800 calories per day, most of them from high-quality proteins, plus vitamins and minerals, particularly

potassium. Notes that some programs use liquid formulas, while others utilize food sources (poultry, fish and lean meats). States that programs this drastic should be restricted to individuals who are at least 30 percent overweight and should be administered only under close medical supervision as part of a comprehensive program. Advises a weekly examination by a physician familiar with the metabolic effects of VLC diets, blood tests to detect potentially dangerous metabolic abnormalities, and behavior modification. States that patients in controlled investigations have typically consumed the diets for 12 to 16 weeks. Notes that weight gain is common after the eating of food is resumed, but it is more likely to occur with do-it-yourself programs than with medically supervised ones.

Pills, Potions, and Gimmicks

Drenick EJ: Bulk producers.
JAMA 234:271, 1975.
States that the idea that methylcellulose compounds are effective for appetite suppression is based on several misconceptions. Describes how the author demonstrated with x-ray examination that methylcellulose does not actually fill the stomach but quickly passes into the small intestine. Notes that the experimental subjects reported no reduction in appetite or hunger. Points out that there is no evidence that increasing the volume of a meal produces satiety in obese individuals.

Fenner L: Cellulite: hard to budge pudge.
FDA Consumer 14:4–9, May 1980.
Describes how the concept of "cellulite," has been marketed, noting that it is not a medical condition but a term coined in European salons and spas to describe deposits of dimpled fat found on the thighs and buttocks of many women. Notes that: (1) a double-blind study has shown that "cellulite" is ordinary fat; (2) dimpling occurs when fat pockets expand more than nearby fibers connecting the skin to deeper layers; (3) no equipment, exercise, or potion can remove fat exclusively from a single area of the body; and (4) a low-calorie diet-and-exercise program that produces general weight loss will reduce dimpling if the skin is sufficiently elastic to spring back when the amount of underlying fat is reduced.

The new diet pills.
Consumer Reports 47:14-16, January 1982.
Discusses criticisms of an FDA advisory panel report that judged benzocaine and phenylpropanolamine (PPA) to be safe and effective as diet aids. Notes that diet aid manufacturers were quick to capitalize on the panel's findings. Discusses studies of the prescription drug fenfluramine, which showed a rebound effect when the drug

was stopped. Concludes that PPA diet aids may suppress appetite for short periods, but there is no evidence that any diet pill promotes long-term weight control.

Bo-Linn GW et al: Starch blockers—their effect on calorie absorption from a high-starch meal.
New England Journal of Medicine 307:1413-1416, 1982.
Notes that "starch blockers" were claimed to contain an enzyme extracted from beans, which, when taken before meals, would block digestion of significant amounts of dietary starch. Notes that the enzyme works in the test tube, but the body produces more starch-digesting enzymes than starch-blocker pills could possibly block. Reports that no evidence of starch blockade was found in the feces of pill-takers. Warns that if undigested starch does reach the large intestine, it is fermented by bacteria normally present, leading to gas production and causing digestive disturbances.

Ballentine C: Spirulina, a miracle food it's not.
FDA Consumer 16:33–34, June 1982.
Notes that sales of spirulina soared in 1981 after *National Enquirer* ran a story promoting it as a diet pill containing phenylalanine, which "acts directly on the appetite center of the brain." Describes how one spirulina marketer was prosecuted and fined $225,000 for making false and misleading claims.

Willis, J: About diet wraps, pills and other magic wands for losing weight.
FDA Consumer 16:18–20, November 1982.
Discusses garments and body wraps claimed to "melt fat away" and several substances claimed to curb appetite or permit dieters to lose weight without changing their eating habits. The substances include phenylalanine, glucomannan, starch blockers, human chorionic gonadotropin (HCG), and spirulina.

Miller RW: EMS—Fraudulent flab remover.
FDA Consumer 17:29–32, May 1983.
States that electrical muscle stimulators are not "body shapers" and are neither safe nor effective for reducing pockets of fat under the skin. Notes that some EMS devices have legitimate medical uses, but their use at health spas and body salons is fraudulent. Describes how the FDA had carried out seizures against 19 firms that were selling or using EMS devices improperly, including one company marketing the "Europe Miracle Body Shaper" for home use.

Ballentine CL: Drugs and your waistline.
FDA Consumer 18:29–30, February 1984.

Surveys a range of diet drugs of varying degrees of effectiveness, noting claims made for them and describing their side effects. Discusses phenylpropanolamine (PPA), benzocaine, spirulina, glucomannan, and other bulk producing products, food supplements, and prescription drugs.

Ballentine CL: What's this glucomannan?
FDA Consumer 18:31, February 1984.
Describes glucomannan, a diet drug allegedly used by the Japanese. Notes side effects and general lack of effectiveness.

These eyes don't have it.
FDA Consumer 18:42–43, September 1984.
Describes how an optometrist marketed eyeglasses (the Vision Dieter) that had one lens tinted blue and the other tinted brown. States that they were promoted with claims that people wearing them for just two hours a day could control their appetite and lose weight. Notes that the FDA considered them illegal devices and took steps to have them seized and destroyed.

Lowell J: "Growth hormone releasers" don't cause weight loss.
Nutrition Forum 1:24, December 1984.
Describes claims made for amino acid products that are claimed to produce weight loss by releasing growth hormone. States that the products don't release growth hormone, but would be dangerous if they did so.

Pentel P: Toxicity of over-the-counter stimulants.
JAMA 252:1898–1903, 1984.
Notes that a recent survey had found that phenylpropanolamine (PPA) was the fifth most frequently used drug in the country. Notes that PPA was being used on the street as a substitute for less readily available amphetamines. Discusses the toxic effects, the most notable of which is increased blood pressure.

In One Ear...
FDA Consumer 19:42, February 1985.
Describes a device, the Acu-Thin Ear Stimulator, which was said to be based on acupuncture techniques. Notes that users were told to wear it in the ear, where it would stimulate pressure points that would suppress appetite. Describes how the FDA forced the manufacturer to stop marketing the device after a user was injured.

Uretsky SD: A pharmacist's guide to quack weight products.
American Pharmacy NS25:24–29, February 1985.

Discusses body wraps, ointments, Chinese teas, "growth-hormone releasers," guarana, phenylpropanolamine, cholecystokinin, spirulina, glucomannan, and dehydroepiandrosterone (DHEA) tablets.

Cunningham JJ: DHEA: Facts vs. hype.
Nutrition Forum 2:30–31, April 1985.
Describes how research on rats has been misinterpreted to suggest that dehydroepiandrosterone (DHEA), could produce weight control in humans. Notes that some "DHEA" pills sold in health food stores actually contain little or no DHEA. Cautions that pharmacologic dosages might be harmful. Reports that the FDA has ordered manufacturers and distributors to stop selling DHEA products as diet aids.

Roth WV et al: Weight reduction products and plans. Hearings before the Permanent Subcommittee on Investigations of the Committee on Governmental Affairs, U.S. Senate, May 14 and 15, 1985.
Washington, DC, U.S. Government Printing Office, 1985.
Describes Congressional inquiry into the diet and weight-loss industry, with emphasis on multilevel companies and mail-order products. Reports testimony by research scientists, FDA officials, a mail-order entrepreneur, and representatives of Herbalife International and Cambridge Plan International.

Willis J: The fad-free diet: How to take weight off (and keep it off) without getting ripped off.
FDA Consumer 19:26–29, July/August 1985.
Discusses the shortcomings of fad diets, amphetamines, human chorionic gonadotropin, (HCG), phenylpropanolamine (PPA), starch blockers, dehydroepiandrosterone (DHEA), cholecystokinin (CCK), arginine/ornithine combinations, spirulina, and glucomannan. Suggests that people who wish to lose weight pursue a sensible balanced diet under a physician's supervision.

Fitzgerald FT: Space-age snake oil: obesity and consumer fraud.
Postgraduate Medicine 78:231–233, 236, 240, September 1, 1985.
States that ads for weight-loss gimmicks typically offer: (1) a quick fix, (2) sexual allure, (3) no pain, strain, or hunger, (4) testimonials, (5) the imprimatur of experts, (6) figments of science, and/or (7) a guarantee. Describes the social pressure people are under to look attractive. Notes that desperate people often harm themselves trying to reduce.

Wycoff S: Diet fads waste money, not pounds.
Consumers Research 60:20–23, April 1986.

Summarizes information on starch blockers, bulk producing pills, grapefruit diet pills, other diet drugs, weight loss clinics, diet fads, body wraps, lotions, creams, and devices. Notes hazards arising from some diets, drugs, and devices. Discusses flaws in theories behind diet fads and other gimmicks.

Hecht A, Janssen W: Diet drug danger déjà vu.
FDA Consumer 21:22–27, February 1987.
Relates the history of 2,4-dinitrophenol, a highly toxic drug that was included in the "Chamber of Horrors" exhibit prepared by the FDA to help gain passage of the 1938 Food, Drug, and Cosmetic Act, after which use of this drug was banned. Notes that although dinitrophenol causes weight loss by accelerating metabolism, it also causes severe skin rashes, cataracts, agranulocytosis, jaundice, and other problems that can be fatal. Describes how in 1982, the FDA began receiving complaints of toxic reactions to dinitrophenol, which was being dispensed by Nicholas Bachynsky, MD, at his chain of weight-loss clinics in Texas. Describes actions taken by the Texas Attorney General to curb Dr. Bachynsky's use of the drug.

Thompson RC: Dangerous diet drugs from south of the border.
FDA Consumer 21:29–30, May 1987.
Focuses on Redotex, a Mexican diet product that contains thyroid hormone, a strong laxative, a circulatory stimulant, a tranquilizer, and a decongestant that can raise blood pressure. Notes that regulatory agencies have received reports of addiction, psychosis, blood pressure elevation, and even death among Redotex users. Describes actions by the FDA and the Mexican government to halt its distribution.

Beck M, Springen K, Beachy L, et al: The losing formula.
Newsweek 115:52–58, April 30, 1990.
Discusses Optifast, Slim-Fast, and various other programs that use liquid diet products. Quotes expert opinions that rapid weight loss tends to be less effective than gradual weight loss in the long run. Describes theories about the weight gain in "yo-yo" dieting.

Barrett S: The rise and fall of Cal-Ban 3000.
Nutrition Today 25:24-28, November/December 1990.
Describes the marketing of Cal-Ban 3000, a guar gum product that was promised to cause automatic weight loss without dieting or exercise. States that no long-term controlled test of guar gum as a weight-control agent had been reported in the scientific literature. Describes a series of state and federal regulatory actions that finally drove the product from the marketplace. Notes that when exposed to water, guar gum can swell to several times its original volume. Notes that several cases of

esophageal obstruction were reported among Cal-Ban users. Discusses "bulk-producers," "starch blockers," "growth-hormone releasers," and "sugar blockers," noting that none of these products work as advertised or produce weight loss.

Obesity Clinics

Hudnall M: How popular programs compare.
Environmental Nutrition 10:4–5, August 1987.
Compares the approaches of Optifast, Diet Center, Weight Watchers, TOPS, Nutri/System, Overeaters Anonymous, Registered Dietitians in private practice, Hospital weight-loss clinics, and residential facilities and spas. List questions that could help in making a choice.

Fatis M, Weiner A, Hawkins J, et al: Following up on a commercial weight loss program: Do the pounds stay off after your picture has been in the newspaper?
Journal of the American Dietetic Association 89:547–548, 1989.
Notes how commercial weight-loss programs are aggressively marketed, sometimes with before-and-after photographs. States that commercial programs typically fail to offer data that permits objective evaluation of long-term effectiveness. Describes a follow-up study in which thirty-one people whose pictures had appeared in local newspaper ads were interviewed about twenty months after they had reached their weight-loss goals. Reports that only eight had remained not more than 5 pounds above their initial weight-loss goal.

Miller A, Springen K, Buckley L, et al: Diets incorporated.
Newsweek 114:56–60, September 11, 1989.
Surveys the diet business. Lists and describes several popular diets. Discusses business methods of diet firms, cost of programs, and debates over the merits of Weight Watchers, Diet Center, the Kempner Rice Diet, Pritikin, Nutri/System, Optifast, United Weight Control, Jenny Craig Weight Loss Centers, Family Weight Loss Centers, Specialized Diet Consultants (Diet Cops), and Duke University Diet and Fitness Center. Notes harmful side effects from some diets. Notes how one reporter lost 47 pounds in 48 days at a University diet and fitness center.

Wyden R et al: Deception and fraud in the diet industry, Part I. Hearing before the Subcommittee on Regulation, Business Opportunities, and Energy, of the Committee on Small Business, House of Representatives, March 26, 1990.
Washington, DC, U.S. Government Printing Office, 1990.
Describes Congressional inquiry into the diet and weight-loss industry, with emphasis on commercial weight-loss clinics and physician-supervised weight-loss

programs. States opinion of subcommittee chairman Ron Wyden (D-OR) that "many products peddled in commercial clinics are untested, with little or no scientific proof of their safety and effectiveness. Most lay counselors and specialists in commercial diet clinics are undertrained lay people operating without any medical supervision. . . . Most commercial clinics promise fast, safe, easy weight loss. Most experts agree that fast weight loss is dangerous." Includes testimony by an assistant attorney general of Iowa who castigated the FDA for giving "purveyors of diet fraud full rein for nearly 30 years" to violate federal laws, with resultant consumer losses in the billions of dollars.

Wyden R et al: Deception and fraud in the diet industry, Part II. Hearing before the Subcommittee on Regulation, Business Opportunities, and Energy, of the Committee on Small Business, House of Representatives, May 7, 1990. Washington, DC, U.S. Government Printing Office, 1990.
Continues the inquiry described above with testimony by FDA officials, medical educators, representatives from seven weight-loss programs, and a consumer who states she was seriously harmed by one program.

Winner K: A weighty issue: Dangers and deceptions of the weight loss industry. New York, New York City Department of Consumer Affairs, 1991.
Describes an extensive undercover investigation of fourteen weight-loss centers in New York City. Notes that (1) few center representatives gave advance warning or openly discussed the safety risks of their program or of rapid weight loss in general, even when directly asked about possible problems; (2) some attempted to sell their services to people who had normal weight or were underweight; (3) some made quack biochemical claims about their products; and (4) some engaged in high-pressure sales tactics. Notes that following the study, the Department proposed regulations that would require weight-loss centers to (1) display a large sign stating that rapid weight loss can cause serious health problems, (2) advise consultation with a physician, (3) indicate that only permanent lifestyle changes can promote long-term weight loss, and (4) inform customers that information on dropout rates and staff qualifications were available on request.

Dieter beware! The complete consumer guide to weight-loss programs. Lynbrook, N.Y., Marketdata Enterprises, 1991.
Estimates that the weight loss and diet control industry sell over $30 billion worth of products, programs, and services. Describes the nature, marketing strategies, and history of many of these. Predicts that government regulation may increase as pressures mount for better data about program success rates, dropout rates, and disclosure to potential dieters of costs and possible adverse effects.

Saddler J: FTC targets thin claims of liquid diets.
The Wall Street Journal, pp. B1, B4, October 17, 1991.
Reports that the Federal Trade Commission charged the marketers of Optifast 70, Medifast 70, and Ultrafast with making deceptive claims that their programs are safe and effective over the long term. Notes that the three companies involved had signed consent agreements pledging that future claims about long-term loss will be based on studies of patients followed for at least two years. Notes that the FTC plans to look closely at other programs.

Silberner J: War of the diets.
U.S. News & World Report 112:55–60, February 3, 1992.
Reports how a panel of five experts rated the programs of Diet Center, Jenny Craig, Medifast, Nutri-System, Optifast, Physicians Weight Loss Centers, and Weight Watchers. Describes how the programs are marketed, noting that no research has been done comparing their results.

Part V:
Other "Alternative" Methods

Aromatherapy

Aromatherapy (sometimes written as aroma therapy) is described by its proponents as "the therapeutic use of the essential oils of plants." These oils are said to be very concentrated substances extracted from flowers, leaves, stalks, fruits, and roots, and also distilled from resins. They are said to represent the "life force" or "soul" of the plant. The oils are administered in small quantities through massage, or inhalation, or through creams and lotions. Occasionally, a product is taken internally.

One company that markets its products through health food stores also sells devices that "diffuse the essence, the spirit, the vital forces of the plant, creating a healthful environment." It also claims that inhaling the scents "balances the biological background," "revitalizes the cells," and produces a "strong energizing effect on the sympathetic nervous system." The American Aromatherapy Association offers "certification" based on attendance at two 3-day weekends plus submission of a thesis that includes case studies. The certification course includes such topics as internal methods of treatment, essential oils in healing, addressing common health problems, and how to market yourself. Another organization has offered "accredited certification" as an "Aromatherapist Practitioner," based on a correspondence course plus six seminars and two final exams.

There is no scientific evidence that the benefits achieved by aromatherapy are greater than those achieved by the power of suggestion. Even many adherents of aromatherapy restrict it to certain treatments, mainly to induce relaxation, and they fear that the more extreme claims made for it may discredit it.

Descriptive Literature

Freifeld K: Led by the nose.
Health 18:68, August 1986.
Describes the promotion of aromatherapy and lists several cosmetics and department store firms that market products. Quotes various industry spokespeople who claim that there is scientific research to support claims of benefit from aromatherapy products. However, none of the people making the claims could provide details or published reports.

Adler J, Brailsford K, King P: What kind of therapy smells?
Newsweek 109:62, March 2, 1987.

Briefly explains aromatherapy and its appeal. Mentions several department store chains and cosmetics firms that sell products for aromatherapy. Notes that "claims for aromatherapy are untested and tend to rely on examples drawn from the wisdom of the ancient Orient." Quotes a practitioner who states that the technique "addresses the nervous system and the energy fields of the body. It soothes the body, cleans the body, clears the body, and tones the body."

Stone J: Scents and sensibility.
Discover 10: 26-31, December 1989.
Describes research into the use of scents to influence human behavior and mood, improve productivity in the workplace, induce relaxation, and help people lose weight.

Larsen E: The nose knows.
Utne Reader, pp. 34-36, May/June 1991.
Describes commercial application of scents that are hoped to influence the behavior of shoppers and workers.

Krier BA: Health seekers use common scents.
Chicago Sun-Times, pp. 31-32, July 23, 1991.
Describes the use of aromatherapy as part of an enthusiast's daily regimen. Reports that the cosmetic company widely credited with popularizing aromatherapy in the United States did $50 million worth of business in 1990. Discusses the application of aromatherapy by various practitioners, especially physicians and chiropractors affiliated with Maharishi Ayur-Veda Health Centers and reports on proposals for regulation of aromatherapy by various agencies, especially the FDA.

Critical Literature

Aroma Therapy.
FDA Talk Paper, April 23, 1986.
Notes that aroma products are being introduced with claims or implications that their use will improve personal well-being in a variety of ways, such as "strengthening the body's self-defense mechanisms." Explains that the FDA has traditionally regarded perfumes as cosmetics—which the Food, Drug, and Cosmetic Act defines as articles to be introduced into or otherwise applied to the body to cleanse, beautify, promote attractiveness, or alter appearance. Claims that a perfume's aroma is good or beneficial is a cosmetic claim not requiring FDA approval before marketing. But a claim that a scent is effective in the prevention or

treatment of any health problem would be a drug claim that would require FDA approval.

Butler K: A consumer's guide to "alternative medicine."
Buffalo, Prometheus Books, 1992.
Notes that aromatherapy is alleged to prevent and cure scores of ailments including many serious diseases. States that there is no evidence to support these claims and that some may be based on placebo response. Notes that some therapists determine what oil to use by using a lock of hair or a handwriting sample from the patient in a dowsing (divining) ritual. Predicts that the cosmetics industry will attempt to market colognes, shampoos, aftershave lotions, and similar products with claims that they are stimulating, relaxing, or otherwise affect mood and thereby help health.

Baldness Remedies

Baldness cures have been marketed since ancient times. Until recently, however, no substance applied to the scalp has produced beneficial results. In 1988, the FDA approved topical minoxidil (Rogaine, manufactured by The Upjohn Company), which can help some people with thinning hair, but is expensive and must be applied indefinitely to sustain any gains that take place. Various types of hair transplantation can be useful in properly selected cases. In 1989, the FDA banned the sale of all nonprescription creams, lotions, or other externally applied products that are claimed to grow hair or prevent baldness.

Pinski JB, Pinski, KS: New aspects of hair transplantation.
Cutis 39:309–313, 1987.
Reviews a range of techniques in hair transplantation to produce a better hairline. Describes and discusses minigrafts, micrografts, and methods of applying such procedures.

Baldness, Is there hope?
Consumer Reports 53:543–547, September 1988.
Discusses two methods of treating baldness, minoxidil and hair transplants, focusing on the former. Describes the growth of interest in minoxidil after tests by Upjohn showed more hair growth in people who use minoxidil than in those using a placebo. Notes problems of hair loss following cessation of minoxidil treatment. Briefly discusses hair transplants, noting cost and possible complications.

Kligman AM, Freeman B: History of baldness, from magic to medicine.
Clinics in Dermatology 6:83–88, October–December 1988.
Surveys the history of attitudes toward baldness and efforts to treat it. Notes the association of hair with youthfulness, strength, good looks, and sometimes with status, profession, religion, manhood, and sexuality. Describes baldness treatments that have been popular at various times, noting theories behind the alleged cures. Mentions efforts by the FDA to combat fraudulent baldness cures.

Folkenberg J: Hair apparent? for some, a new solution to baldness.
FDA Consumer 22:8–11, December 1988/January 1989.
Notes the interest in minoxidil. Describes Upjohn's tests to determine Rogaine's efficacy. Reviews results of tests, noting differing interpretations of the results. Mentions side effects of minoxidil in a few users. Concludes that Rogaine may be useful to young men who have just started losing hair.

Katz HI: Topical minoxidil: review of efficacy and safety.
Cutis 43:94–98, 1989.
Reviews anecdotal reports by physicians and controlled trials sponsored by Upjohn. Notes that Upjohn studies show that a 2% minoxidil solution seems as effective as a 3% solution, but with less potential for systemic absorption. Discusses safety of minoxidil, noting that most side effects are minor, with only a few showing more serious problems. Concludes that minoxidil is safe and may be effective for some people, but not for most.

Bald-faced hair scam.
FDA Consumer 23:34–35, March 1989.
Describes FDA actions against two Canadian businessmen who apparently grossed more than $3 million during four years of selling a phony hair restorer by mail. Reports that the drugs were seized and the businessmen indicted for mail fraud, wire fraud, and violations of the Food, Drug, and Cosmetic Act..

Fleming RW, Mayer TG: New concepts in hair replacement.
Archives of Otolaryngology Head and Neck Surgery 115:278–279, 1989.
Reports on new techniques in hair replacement described at a recent International symposium on hair replacement surgery sponsored by the American Academy of Facial Plastic and Reconstructive Surgery. Discusses punch grafts, scalp reduction, Juri flaps, and expanders.

Shrank AB: Treating young men with hair loss.
British Medical Journal 298:847–848, 1989.
Briefly discusses wigs, hair transplants, and minoxidil lotion, noting shortcomings of each. Suggests that physicians discuss the options, but recognize that "except for the few who consider ample scalp hair essential for their work or self-esteem, young men are best advised to come to terms with their hair loss. Time spent—on reassuring patients that their natural hair loss is not the social disaster they believe and on explaining the problems and cost of treatments . . . may save the patient much trouble, anxiety, and money."

Burke KE: Hair loss, what causes it and what can be done about it.
Postgraduate Medicine 85:52–58, 67–73, 77, May 1, 1989.
Describes the growth of hair, noting racial and individual differences. Discusses different types of hair loss, noting causes and methods of treating them. Describes how the discovery that oral minoxidil (prescribed for high blood pressure) produced unwanted hair growth led to the testing of topical minoxidil. Suggests that minoxidil can be used to forestall balding at its early stages, while surgical procedures can be used for more extensive balding.

Hair Loss, New treatment for thinning or lost hair is an uncertain investment.
Mayo Clinic Health Letter 7:1–2, June 1989.
Describes how minoxidil is applied and possible theories about how it works. Notes that about one-third of users will grow new hair, mostly light coverage, though some will gain moderate to dense coverage. Mentions pitfalls: cost, slow hair growth, and the need to keep using the product indefinitely.

Olsen EA: Alopecia: evaluation and management.
Primary Care 16:765–787, 1989.
Notes that over half of all adults will experience hair loss at some point in their life. Reviews growth cycle in hair and explains different types and causes of hair loss, also noting gender differences. Discusses treatment for each type of hair loss.

Topical minoxidil does little for baldness.
Drug and Therapeutics Bulletin 27:74–76, September 18, 1989.
Reviews clinical data on minoxidil. Concludes that "topically applied minoxidil can increase hair growth but rarely enough to be of cosmetic value. Most responders lose the regrowth when treatment is stopped and even with continued use, the effect diminishes after one year. The cost of treatment and the small chance of growing and retaining regrown hair make it an indulgence that only the rich and patient can afford."

O'Loughlin S: Topical minoxidil for male pattern baldness.
Irish Medical Journal 84:3–4, March 1991.
Explains how hair growth occurs and how it changes over time. Describes how minoxidil is applied and discusses results. Notes that most users will have almost negligible hair growth, but some will have moderate hair growth, and a few will experience dense growth. Concludes that minoxidil has unimpressive results and high cost, but new-generation minoxidil-type drugs may yield better results.

Dardour JC: Treatment of male pattern baldness and
postoperative temporal baldness in men.
Clinics in Plastic Surgery 18:775–790, 1991.
Examines various plastic surgical methods of treating baldness.

Biofeedback Training

Biofeedback training is a technique in which a person uses information about a body function to attempt to gain control over that function. The practitioner connects the patient to an electronic device that measures blood pressure, pulse rate, muscle tension, skin temperature, perspiration, brain waves, or other variable bodily function. The patient receives information (feedback) on the changing levels of these activities from alterations in the instrument's signals, such as a flashing light, fluctuating needle, sound that rises or falls in pitch, or variable display on a television monitor. Relaxation techniques are used to effect changes in the signal and to identify which methods are most effective. The patient may ultimately learn to control the body function subconsciously without the machine.

The most common techniques of biofeedback include: (1) electromyographic biofeedback (EMG), in which an electrode picks up signals produced by microelectric pulses between nerve endings and muscle fibers; (2) temperature biofeedback, in which a thermal probe is placed on an affected body area to read skin temperature; and (3) electrodermal biofeedback or galvanic skin resistance (GSR), which uses a probe that responds to sweat. The variation used may depend on the ailment being treated. For example, EMG may be used in treating migraine headaches, while GSR may be utilized for conditions such as anxiety disorders or chronic pain.

Biofeedback was popularized before it had scientific support, and it still is abused by fringe practitioners. Nevertheless, the method has gained a measure of respectability. It has been utilized in helping patients control pain, anxiety, phobias, hypertension, sleep disorders, and some stomach and intestinal disorders. Some specialized techniques have been used to treat abnormal heart rhythms, epilepsy, Tourette's syndrome, fecal incontinence, and Parkinson's disease. Biofeedback practitioners may be physicians, psychologists, dentists, nurses, social workers, or other therapists. However, a buyer-beware situation still exists because untrained individuals with or without a professional degree can obtain a device and set up shop.

Critical Literature

Orne MT, Weiss T, Callaway E, et al: Biofeedback (Task Force Report #19). Washington, DC, American Psychiatric Association, 1980.
States that biofeedback therapy can be effective in the treatment of migraine

headaches, muscle-tension headaches, and some psychophysiological disorders. Expresses skepticism about links between biofeedback and metaphysical preoccupations such as "taking charge of one's body." Concludes: (1) biofeedback has not been found useful in severe psychiatric disorders but has been effective as an adjunct to psychiatric treatment to control anxiety and relieve specific psychosomatic complaints; (2) biofeedback is generally not effective unless patients practice the skill on a regular basis in their natural environment; (3) the few available studies indicate that hypnotic therapy, meditation, or relaxation training are equally effective; (4) there is no psychiatric condition for which biofeedback as such is the treatment of choice; (5) since medical and/or psychological training is needed for the overall management of patients who might be suitable for biofeedback, therapists should not be credentialed as independent professionals.

AMA Diagnostic and Therapeutic Technology Assessment (DATTA): Biofeedback. JAMA 250:2381, 1983.
Report of the American Medical Association's Office of Technology Assessment on the use of biofeedback as part of a program for headache treatment. Notes that there have been studies of the effectiveness of biofeedback in treating several clinical problems. Reviews positive and negative aspects of biofeedback, noting that it is safe and cost-effective, but is labor-intensive and requires special training. Notes that some poorly-trained practitioners claim it is a cure-all. Also notes the need for periodic retraining of the patient. Concludes that with appropriate safeguards and proper patient selection, biofeedback can be integrated into a successful therapeutic program for headaches.

Roberts AH: Biofeedback: research, training and clinical roles. American Psychologist 40:938–941, 1985.
Briefly reviews the history of biofeedback and the current relationships among research findings, clinical training, and clinical roles in behavioral medicine. Concludes that there is little relationship between research findings and the clinical practice of biofeedback. Urges graduate programs to teach students to think critically about such relationships.

Roberts AH: Literature update: Biofeedback and chronic pain. Journal of Pain and Symptom Management 2:169–171, Summer 1987.
Biofeedback has become a popular and widespread treatment modality for chronic pain. Although biofeedback does help some patients it is not known whether it is an essential or specific treatment for any chronic pain problem, or that it is superior to or less expensive than other treatments. Some reviewers note that biofeedback may even exacerbate pain problems in some chronic pain patients.
Miller L: What biofeedback does (and doesn't) do.

Psychology Today 23:22–24, November 1989.
Describes biofeedback training techniques and how they work. Describes a typical biofeedback training session. Offers tips on locating a biofeedback practitioner.

Masek B: Biofeedback.
Harvard Medical School Health Letter 15:1–4, August 1990.
Describes how the concept of biofeedback training emerged from experiments on rats performed during the 1960s. States that most people who go through biofeedback training use it to acquire deep relaxation skills, which could also be learned without electronic training. States that biofeedback training for this purpose typically takes six to ten sessions and is combined with other behavioral techniques such as behavior modification, relaxation training, or cognitive restructuring. States that people with Reynaud's syndrome (in which slight exposure to cold can cause painful constriction of blood vessels in the fingers) can be trained to protect themselves from attacks. States that biofeedback training may be effective against fecal incontinence, torticollis, and partial paralysis, but has limited value for preventing seizures, treating symptoms of hyperactivity, or regaining muscle control following spinal cord injury or stroke. Observes that battery-operated skin temperature monitors and devices that measure muscle or brain-wave activity have been marketed through the mail for home use. Cautions that these devices have not been systematically evaluated and are likely to "have a short working life before they wind up in a closet or attic, gathering dust."

Loening-Baucke V: Efficacy of biofeedback training in improving faecal incontinence and anorectal physiologic function.
Gut 31:1395–1402, 1990.
Describes a study of biofeedback training in seventeen women with fecal incontinence, eight of whom received biofeedback training. Concludes that biofeedback training is no better than conventional medical intervention.

Lee SW: Biofeedback as a treatment for
childhood hyperactivity: A critical review of the literature.
Psychological Reports 68: 163–192, February 1991.
Reviews thirty-six studies in which biofeedback was used to treat hyperactivity in children. Notes that most of the research had methodological flaws including small samples, few placebo control groups, diverse criteria for classifying a child as hyperactive, and lack of follow-up, and evaluation of whether the children adjusted in classroom and social situations. Most also use biofeedback in combination with other methods, making it difficult to establish the effectiveness of biofeedback training. Suggests that further research be done utilizing biofeedback training alone and with improved methodology and follow-up.

Proponent Literature

Lesko WA, Summerfield LM: The effectiveness of biofeedback and home relaxation training on reduction of borderline hypertension.
Health Education 19:19–23, October/November 1988.
Describes a clinical study of nondrug treatment of 112 adults with borderline hypertension. Compares the effectiveness of biofeedback, progressive relaxation, and exercise/nutrition, either alone or in various combinations. Notes that only 79 completed treatment, with the highest dropout rate among those with an exercise component. Concludes that relaxation training with or without biofeedback may help reduce high blood pressure.

Fishbain DA, Goldberg M, Khalil TM, et al: The utility of electromyographic biofeedback in the treatment of conversion paralysis.
American Journal of Psychiatry 145:1572–1575, 1988.
Reports how EMG biofeedback training was used to help four patients with conversion paralysis regain the use of their legs.

McGrady A, Higgins JT: Prediction of response to biofeedback-assisted relaxation in hypertensives: development of a hypertensive predictor profile (HYPP).
Psychosomatic Medicine 51:277–284, May/June, 1989.
Describes a study of thirty-nine hypertensive patients who were given biofeedback training. Concludes that high anxiety scores, forehead muscle tension, heart rate, hand temperature, plasma renin levels, and urinary and plasma cortisol may help determine whether biofeedback is likely to be effective.

Duckro PN, Cantwell-Simmons E: A review of studies evaluating biofeedback and relaxation training in the management of pediatric headache.
Headache 29:428–433, 1989.
Reviews seven studies published between 1984 and 1986 on relaxation training with or without biofeedback to help children control headaches. Concludes that behavioral treatment appears to be a potent alternative for the management of chronic headache in children.

Duchene P: Effects of biofeedback on childbirth pain.
Journal of Pain and Symptom Management 4:117–123, September 1989.
Describes a controlled study of forty women to determine whether EMG biofeedback can reduce pain during labor and delivery. Notes that the biofeedback group had shorter labor and required less medication. Notes some limitations on applicability of biofeedback training as part of childbirth.

Burgio KL, Engel BT: Biofeedback-assisted behavioral training for elderly men and women.
Journal of the American Geriatrics Society 38:338–340, 1990.
Reviews studies of biofeedback training to control urinary incontinence in patients with stress incontinence, urge incontinence, and incontinence following prostatectomy. Notes limitations, including the patient's tolerance for training.

Middaugh SJ: On clinical efficacy: Why biofeedback does—and does not—work.
Biofeedback and Self-Regulation 15:191–208, September 1990.
Discusses biofeedback, arguing that it only works if there is a match between what biofeedback contributes and what the patient needs. Compares several studies of the application of biofeedback training to solve various conditions. Argues that even studies showing negative results can be useful because they help to identify what types of patients can benefit by biofeedback training.

Cellular Therapy

Cellular therapy, also known as live cell therapy or fresh cell therapy, consists of injections of fresh embryonic animal cells, typically from sheep or cows. The product used is obtained from a specific organ or tissue said to correspond with the unhealthy organ or tissue of the recipient. Proponents claim that the recipient's body automatically transports the injected cells to the target organ, where they supposedly strengthen it.

Cellular therapy was developed in the early 1930s by Paul Niehans, MD, a Swiss physician. It soon became popular with a number of public figures as a means of rejuvenation. Wolfram Kuhnau, MD, a colleague of Dr. Niehans, introduced the treatment in Tijuana, Mexico in the late 1970s as a cancer treatment. It is also claimed to build the immune system and help victims of Down's syndrome, Alzheimer's disease, epilepsy, and various other diseases.

Cellular therapy has no proven benefit and has been reported to cause serious infections and allergic reactions. In 1985, the FDA banned importation into the U.S. of all cellular powders and extracts intended for injection. In 1987 the Federal Health Office of West Germany suspended the product licenses of a large number of whole-cell preparations.

Critical Literature

Lindeman B, Cubbison C: Cellular therapy: A shabby clinic offered rejuvenation but delivered death.
Today's Health 53:36–41, June 1975.
Vivid account of the death of two men who died from gas gangrene following injections of sheep cells at a Florida clinic. Notes that the doctor falsified the cause of death on the death certificate in an attempt to conceal what had happened.

Cell therapy rapped.
FDA Consumer 19:38, February 1985.
Reports on efforts by the FDA to ban the entry of all "cell therapy" powders and extracts intended for injection. Describes the method of producing such products and their hazards.

Cell therapy suspended.
Lancet, p. 503, August 29, 1987.

Discusses the West German Federal Health Office decision to suspend the product licenses of 235 whole-cell products, though numerous cell extracts remain unaffected. Notes the widespread use of such products, primarily by wealthy individuals and "misguided athletes," and the lack of evidence of any benefits. Reports on the hazards of using cellular treatments, as evidenced by the death of a popular woman athlete.

Saurat J-H, Didierjean L, Mérot Y, et al: Blistering skin disease in a man after injections of human placental extracts. British Medical Journal 297:775, 1988.
Describes the case of an elderly man who developed bullous pemphigoid after receiving two injections of human placental cells per month for a year and then a series of daily booster injections.

Tierney J: Buying time. In Health 4:35–44, January/February 1990.
Musings of a reporter who examined ways people try to delay or reverse the aging process. Includes interviews with several people who underwent cellular therapy costing $7,000 at a Swiss clinic.

Gelband H et al: Cellular treatment. In Gelband H et al: Unconventional cancer treatments, pp. 97–98. Washington, DC, U.S. Government Printing Office, 1990.
Describes the procedure for producing cellular products and injection of such products into patients. Reports claims made by proponents regarding the use of cellular treatment for various diseases. Notes that a 1957 survey of 179 German hospitals revealed 80 cases of serious immunologic reactions to cellular therapy, 30 of them fatal.

Last PM: Cell therapy: A cruel and dangerous deception. A drama in three acts. Journal of Paediatrics and Children's Health 26:197–199, August 1990.
Discusses the case of an Australian woman resident of a large nursing home who was treated for brain injury with a cellular injection administered by an Australian physician. Describes the preparation used, its composition, side effects, and alleged therapeutic properties. Notes the hazards associated with cellular therapy and the lack of evidence that it can help people. Discusses the need for greater vigilance on the part of nursing home and medical staffs on behalf of their patients and on the part of the government in banning the sale of such products in Australia.

Unproven methods of cancer management: Fresh cell therapy. Ca-A Cancer Journal for Clinicians 41:126–128, 1991.

"Alternative" Health Methods

Gives a brief history of the development and practice of cellular treatment by Dr. Paul Niehans and his followers. Notes the lack of scientific evidence of any benefits of such treatment. Mentions claims of its proponents. Discusses therapy's hazards, noting several deaths following such treatment.

Colonic Irrigation

Colonic irrigation is a procedure in which very large amounts of water are infused into the rectum through a tube, a few pints at a time, in an effort to wash away and remove the normal colonic contents. An ordinary enema involves a quart or so of water. A "high colonic" may involve twenty or more gallons. The contents of the high colonic enema may be pumped in with a machine or may be transmitted with an apparatus that relies on gravity. The water may be laced with coffee, herbs, enzymes, wheat or grass extract, or other additives. The procedure is said to "detoxify" the body, though no "toxins" have ever been specified or scientifically demonstrated. Practitioners who do the procedure and manufacturers of the equipment often advertise that "death begins in the colon" and that regular cleansing is necessary to maintain one's health.

Critical Literature

Eisele JW, Reay DT: Deaths related to coffee enemas.
JAMA 244:1608-1609, 1980.
Describes the cases of two women who had previously been treated by conventional therapy, but who turned to alternative clinics. At the clinic, they received coffee enemas and later suffered fatal results. Discusses the methods used in diagnosing the cause of death. Notes the popularity of naturopathic treatments, including coffee enemas.

Amebiasis associated with colonic irrigation – Colorado.
Morbidity and Mortality Weekly Report, March 13, 1981.
Describes the epidemiologic investigation of an outbreak of amebic dysentery associated with colonic irrigation at a chiropractic clinic. Ten patients had such fulminant disease that they developed bowel perforation and had to have a partial or total colectomy. Seven of these patients died.

Istre GR, Kreiss K, Hopkins RS, et al: An outbreak of amebiasis spread by colonic irrigation at a chiropractic clinic.
New England Journal of Medicine 307:339-342, 1982.
Provides further details on the outbreak reported above. Describes the apparatus used and the manner in which the infection was spread. Notes that the use of colonic machines are not routinely tested for cleanliness or evidence of fecal contamination. Urges stricter regulation of the procedure and its practitioners.

Zimmerman DR: High colonic quackery: A modern medicine show.
Rx Being Well 2:83–84, January/February 1984.
Describes the colonic enema procedure and its dangers. Debunks the theory of autointoxication.

Use of enemas is limited.
FDA Consumer 18:33, June 1984.
Discusses hazards of overuse of enemas and of colonic irrigation. Describes procedure used in colonic irrigation and the theory behind it. Mentions a chiropractic clinic in Colorado that offered colonic irrigation with a contaminated machine with fatal results. Reviews the case of Roy DeWelles, who sold a pressurized enema device. DeWelles had claimed that his device (the Detoxacolon) would cure 38 different diseases, ranging from asthma, anemia, and heart conditions to severe constipation, elongated colon, and cancer. For fifteen years he operated a clinic in Los Angeles where he treated cancer patients. The California Department of Health closed down the clinic after finding a one-in-seven incidence of death after the DeWelles treatment. He also operated a traveling clinic. He was finally put out of business by a conviction for mail fraud.

The case against colonic irrigation.
California Morbidity, September 27, 1985.
Reports that a California judge had issued an order to restrain a chiropractor from advertising or performing colonic irrigations. Notes the Colorado outbreak mentioned above plus other cases occurring under chiropractic care in California in 1981 and 1982. Concludes that contamination of the devices used is probably inevitable because the rectal tube is typically used for both fluid inflow and fecal expulsion. Also notes that colonic irrigation probably alters host defenses in otherwise healthy people by injuring the colon lining, removing protective mucus, and altering bacterial flora, all of which can facilitate disease if human pathogens are encountered. Recommends that the practice of colonic irrigation by chiropractors and others should cease because it can do no good, only harm.

Moxley JH: Issues in health fraud: Colonic irrigation.
Informational report of the AMA Council on Scientific Affairs, February 1987.
Explains the difference between therapeutic enemas administered by a physician and colonic irrigation administered by an "alternative" health care provider or self-administered. Summarizes the history of the theory of auto-intoxication, which viewed the contents of the bowel as pathological. The theory, which was disproven more than sixty years ago, held that impacted feces produce toxins that are absorbed through the intestinal lining and produce various diseases. Discusses colonic irrigation procedures and the health risks involved. States that despite the risks and

lack of proven benefit, many "alternative" practitioners promote colonic irrigation as a "natural" therapy that rids the body of poisons and assures health and longevity. Notes that patients who undergo this procedure seldom mention this to their physician. Suggests, for this reason, that patients with bloody diarrhea be asked if they are using it.

Renner JH: Doubly deadly: Fasting and colonics.
American Health 9:47, May 1990.
Reports a case of a woman who became comatose after taking colonics twice a day and fasting (consuming just water) to cleanse her bowels of "mysterious toxins," as recommended by her "nutritional advisor." Notes that both fasting and colonic irrigation can be deadly.

Dimethyl Sulfoxide (DMSO)

Dimethyl sulfoxide (DMSO) is an industrial solvent (similar to turpentine) that is a by-product of paper manufacturing. DMSO can penetrate the intact skin and carry other chemicals with it into the body. When administered to humans, it is absorbed rapidly and produces a garlic-like taste and odor on the breath and skin that can last as long as three days.

DMSO is claimed to relieve pain, reduce swelling, and speed healing of acute injuries and arthritis. It is popular among athletes as a treatment for sore muscles and other injuries. It is also offered by "alternative" cancer clinics for the treatment of arthritis, cancer, and other diseases. Its only approved uses in the United States are for treating interstitial cystitis (a rare type of bladder inflammation) and as a veterinary drug to reduce swelling due to trauma in horses and dogs. However, it is available in some health food stores, hardware stores, and other outlets where it is sold as a "solvent." A few states have passed laws permitting its manufacture and sale under certain circumstances.

In 1963 Stanley Jacob, MD, of the University of Oregon Medical School reported that DMSO could penetrate skin and produce local analgesia, decrease pain, and promote healing of injured tissue. That year the FDA approved an investigational new drug application and DMSO became widely used for the treatment of sprains, bruises, and minor burns. However, studies of the drug were not well-controlled, so it was impossible to judge whether reported improvement was due to the drug or some other factor. Experimental approval was withdrawn in 1965 after DMSO was found to cause eye damage in rabbits, but experimental status was restored after further studies found no such problem in humans.

In 1978, the FDA approved use of a 50% solution for instillation into the bladder to treat interstitial cystitis. Studies are continuing into the use of DMSO for the treatment of scleroderma and various other disorders, although its prominent odor makes it difficult to set up controlled studies. The Arthritis Foundation considers DMSO "still experimental" and warns that industrial-grade DMSO should never be used because contaminants could produce serious reactions. The AMA, the National Cancer Institute, and the American Academy of Pediatrics, have also published statements that DMSO is an unproven modality.

Critical Literature

Dimethyl sulfoxide (DMSO).
The Medical Letter 22:94–95, 1980.
Concludes: "Dimethyl sulfoxide in high concentrations may prove to be effective in diminishing pain, muscle spasm and swelling associated with various acute inflammatory conditions and soft-tissue injuries, and as a vehicle for enhancing the penetration of other topical drugs. Its usefulness for treatment of amyloidosis, scleroderma, and other disorders requires further study. There is no convincing evidence that DMSO is effective for treatment of any type of arthritis. Its safety has not been established for any indication and DMSO preparations that have not been purified for human use could be dangerous."

Hecht A: DMSO: No proof of miracles.
FDA Consumer 14:28–29, September 1980.
Chronicles the use of DMSO and its regulatory status. Notes that a recent "60 Minutes" broadcast and congressional hearings had catapulted DMSO into the limelight. Notes that Mexican clinics purported to be dispensing DMSO are actually dispensing steroids, phenylbutazone, tranquilizers, and dipyrone, some of which are dangerous.

Dimethyl sulfoxide: Controversy and current status – 1981.
Proceedings of the AMA House of Delegates, pp. 207–210, December 6–9, 1981.
Notes the growing controversy over the use of DMSO, with the media hailing it as a wonder drug and others calling it a hoax. Reviews the industrial use of DMSO and the results of research studies conducted up to 1980. Discusses legal and regulatory actions by the FDA and others. Reports that three DMSO products were currently available: a 50% solution for treatment of interstitial cystitis, a 90% solution for veterinary use, and an impure 99% solution for use by industry as a degreaser solvent. This latter product is also sold by various stores and by mail order for treatment of various diseases. Concludes that further studies are needed to judge DMSO's safety and effectiveness.

Garmon L: Judging DMSO: There's the rub.
Science News. 122:398–399, 408, 1982.
Explores the controversy over the use of DMSO for treating arthritis, bursitis, and muscle aches. Describes many research studies that are under way. Notes that ten states have legalized the manufacture, prescription, and use of DMSO in concentrations and applications other than the one approved by the FDA.

*American Academy of Pediatrics, Committee on Drugs
and Committee on Sports Medicine: Dimethyl sulfoxide (DMSO).
Pediatrics. 71:76–77, 1983.*
Reviews research status of DMSO. Discusses DMSO's side effects of skin irritation and "musty, garlicy " breath odor. Concludes that veterinary and industrial-strength DMSO products are not safe for human use and that their effectiveness for treating sprains and strains has not been established.

*Unproven methods of cancer management, dimethyl sulfoxide (DMSO).
Ca—A Cancer Journal for Clinicians 33:122–125, 1983.*
Notes that DMSO was being used as a cancer treatment at the Degenerative Disease Medical Center, run by Mrs. Mildred Miller, and at clinics affiliated with the Metabolic Research Foundation, run by Harold Manner, PhD. Mentions unsuccessful efforts by the former to force insurance companies to pay for DMSO cancer treatments. Notes that the FDA has approved a 50% sterile aqueous solution of DMSO for the symptomatic relief of interstitial cystitis, but this concentration was not considered strong enough to be potentially helpful in dealing with the pain of chronic illnesses. Concludes that there is no evidence that DMSO alone or combined with laetrile and procaine hydrochloride results in objective benefit in the treatment of cancer in humans.

*Ballentine C: When a book is a label.
FDA Consumer 17:34–35, October 1983.*
Describes how the FDA had seized copies of a book promoting DMSO along with a large supply of DMSO from a company that had been marketing DMSO with claims that it was good for treating backache and arthritis. Notes that although the FDA succeeded in stopping this particular promotion, the case caused the agency to reevaluate its policy toward seizing books as labeling.

*Trice JM, Pinals RS: Dimethyl sulfoxide: A review
of its use in the rheumatic disorders.
Seminars in Arthritis and Rheumatism. 15:45–60, 1985.*
Cites 117 references. Describes the chemical composition of DMSO and its effects on the body. Discusses the use of DMSO for relief of pain and inflammation, osteoarthritis, rheumatoid arthritis, progressive systemic sclerosis, amyloidosis, and several other disorders. Discusses effects on the immune system. Notes the difficulty of doing double-blind studies because DMSO's odor makes it easily distinguishable. Concludes that DMSO's therapeutic role and legitimacy in medical practice remain in limbo.

Gelband H et al: Dimethyl sulfoxide (DMSO).
In Gelband H et al: Unconventional cancer treatments, pp. 99–100, 1990.
Washington, DC, U.S. Government Printing Office.
Describes the industrial and laboratory uses of DMSO as a solvent. Describes claims made for DMSO by unconventional practitioners. States that animal research has not suggested any practical use for treating cancer in humans.

Arthritis Foundation: Unproven remedies resource manual.
Atlanta, Arthritis Foundation, 1991
Cites eighteen scientific studies of DMSO in animals and humans. Notes that it reduced inflammation in some types of animals but worsened it in others. States that most reports claiming benefit for arthritis have been testimonial. States that the evidence for effectiveness against scleroderma has been conflicting. Concludes that DMSO should be considered experimental for treating arthritis and musculoskeletal injuries. Warns that industrial-grade DMSO should never be used because contaminants can produce serious reactions.

Questionable Approaches to Mental and Emotional Help

Many unproven techniques are marketed to the public with claims that they can solve emotional problems, enhance interpersonal relations, and/or increase mental and physical functioning. This section discusses a variety of items that have been subjected to critical evaluation. Additional items are covered in the section on New Age and Occult Practices.

General Literature

Silver LB: The "magic cure": A review of the current controversial approaches for treating learning disabilities.
Journal of Learning Disabilities 20:498–504, 512, 1987.
Reviews proven and unproven approaches to the treatment of learning disabilities. States that special education and various types of psychotherapy are valid approaches. Notes that medications may make a hyperactive child more available for learning but do not directly treat learning disability. Defines "neurophysiological retraining" as a group of approaches based on the idea that stimulating specific sensory inputs or exercising specific muscles can retrain, recircuit, or in some way improve the functioning of part of the central nervous system. States that three such approaches, optometric visual training, patterning (Doman/Delacato method), and therapy for "cerebellar-vestibular dysfunction" are not supported by scientific evidence. Also criticizes applied kinesiology, skull-bone manipulation, megavitamin therapy, the Feingold diet, and sugar-restrictive diets.

Scott WC: Alternative psychological methods in patient care.
Informational Report of the AMA Council on Scientific Affairs
Chicago, American Medical Association, February 1990.
Reviews 104 reports bearing on psychological techniques and the immune system ("psychoneuroimmunology"), the "relaxation response," meditation, relaxation techniques, autogenic training, biofeedback training, guided imagery, hypnosis, and various combinations of these approaches. Concludes that evidence exists to suggest that these techniques may affect many body systems and exert some benefits, but current research in this area is inadequate, inconclusive, and replete with methodological inadequacies, poorly defined terms, and inconsistent results.

Astrologic Counseling

Carlson S: Astrology.
Experientia 44:290–297, 1988.
Reviews the history and modern practice of astrology and concludes that it is big business. Expresses concern that advice from astrologers may seriously impact the welfare of those who rely on it. States that a typical individual counseling session costs $50 to $200, and often even more. States that many astrologers hold themselves to be better than conventional counselors. Describes the theories of astrology and the evidence demonstrating them to be wrong. States that an astrologer who is a skilled counselor and a caring person may benefit clients, but most astrologers have no training in counseling and "a few are outright charlatans who use astrology to bilk the gullible." States that a person with a real problem who seeks astrological counseling is courting disaster and that unregulated astrology is a threat to public health. States that astrologers should be held to the same standards as accredited professionals and stopped from advertising abilities that they cannot demonstrate.

Firewalking

Seminars are being taught in which walking across hot coals is used as the keystone of a self-improvement program. Promoters of this practice claim that special techniques enable students to walk on hot coals, and that these techniques can be applied to solve many problems of ordinary life. The leading American proponent is Anthony Robbins, author of *Unlimited Power.*

Leikind BJ, McCarthy WJ: An investigation of firewalking.
Skeptical Inquirer 10:23–34, Fall 1985.
Reports on the authors' investigation of firewalking in Los Angeles as taught by Anthony Robbins at the Robbins Research Institute. States that firewalking is claimed to cure impotence and chronic depression and to help people overcome fears, stop smoking and overeating, study more effectively, increase self-confidence, and enable people to instantly know the most effective ways to communicate with and persuade others. Describes the physics of firewalking, explaining that heat transfer from porous coals is usually not rapid and that a thin layer of water vapor that forms between the foot and the coals further impedes heat transfer. Concludes that a Robbins seminar may temporarily increase the self-esteem of its participants who succeed in walking safely across the coals, but may lower the self-esteem of others who balk or get burned. Warns that since the seminar is based on a false premise

(successful firewalking is attributed to mental strength), the rest of the program should be considered untrustworthy.

Dennett MR: Firewalking: Illusion or reality?
Skeptical Inquirer 10:36–40, Fall 1985.
States that firewalking has been claimed not only to increase self-confidence but also to cure failing eyesight and to send malignant tumors into remission. Describes the author's personal experience and his observations of others involved in the practice. Notes that many people have been burned, a few of them seriously.

Pankratz L: Fire walking and the persistence of charlatans.
Perspectives in Biology and Medicine 32:291–298, Winter 1988.
Describes early investigations of firewalking. Notes how easy it is for skilled magicians (and charlatans) to fool untrained observers.

Meditation

Meditation is generally defined as a class of techniques intended to influence an individual's consciousness through the regulation of attention. It may involve lying quietly or sitting in a particular position; attending to one's breathing (yoga); adopting a passive attitude; attempting to be at ease; or repeating a word aloud or to oneself (transcendental meditation).

Woodrum E: The development of the transcendental meditation movement.
The Zetetic 1:38–48, Spring/Summer 1977.
Traces the history of transcendental meditation (TM) and its importation into the United States during the early 1960s. States that the movement expanded by emphasizing practical, physiological, material, and social benefits of TM for conventional persons, with almost no other-worldly references. States that "average meditators" have practical motivations for practicing TM, which they regard simply as a useful mental exercise, but members of the small inner movement have philosophical motivations and regard TM primarily as a path to "cosmic consciousness." [Note: *The Zetetic* was renamed *Skeptical Inquirer* after its first year of publication.]

Bjork RA et al: In the mind's eye: Enhancing human performance.
Washington, DC, National Academy Press, 1991.
Reports on an investigation into techniques that are alleged to influence learning, memory, tension levels, tolerance to pain, and other aspects of performance. Concludes with respect to meditation that people who meditate regularly may have a more restful lifestyle and that a variety of relaxation techniques may help reduce

stress. States, however, that there is no reason to believe that meditation is more effective than simply resting to reduce stress or that meditation alone provides lasting benefits such as reducing high blood pressure or other unhealthful responses to stress.

Neural Organizational Technique

Cooke P: The Crescent City cure.
Hippocrates 2:60–70, November/December 1988.
Describes the controversy surrounding the treatment of about fifty children who had various types of learning disabilities, including Down's syndrome. States that the program was based on Neural Organization Technique (NOT), a method developed by chiropractor Carl Ferreri and said to be used by hundreds of chiropractors worldwide. Describes proponents' claims that "blocked neural pathways" can be corrected by adjusting bones of the skull—by rubbing or squeezing the patient's head, pulling on the ears, pressing on the roof of the mouth, or pushing on the eyes. Reports that many of the children found the treatment painful.

Past-Life Therapy

Past-life therapy is based on the idea that psychological disorders arise from the influence of traumas and personality traits from one's past lives intruding on the subconscious. Proponents say they use hypnosis, meditation, or guided imagery to "regress" the patient to earlier incarnations ("past lives") which, when brought to consciousness, resolve the problems they have been causing. There is no scientific evidence that these notions are valid.

Spanos NP: Past-life hypnotic regression: A critical view.
Skeptical Inquirer 12:174–180, Winter 1988.
Notes that some people who have been hypnotized and asked to regress past their birth times report that they experience past lives. States that "age-regression suggestions are invitations to become involved in the make-believe game of being a child once again. People who accept this invitation do not, in any literal sense, revert back to childhood. Instead they . . . become temporarily absorbed in the fantasy situation of being a child." Cites experiments in which people who are informed that they have "hidden selves" carry the experimenter's wish to display them. Describes experiments in which people reported "past-lives" whose characteristics varied according to instructions given by the experimenters. Notes that subjects who seem most imaginative and hypnotizable report the most vivid past-life fantasies, and that subjects who believed in reincarnation were most likely to believe that the fantasies were related to an actual past life.

Reichian Therapy (Orgone Therapy)

Wilhelm Reich, MD, a former associate of psychiatrist Sigmund Freud, claimed to have discovered "orgone energy," the most powerful force in the universe, and wrote extensively of its manifestations. Soon after coming to the United States in 1934, Reich designed and built "orgone energy accumulators." Most of them were boxes of wood, metal and insulation board about the size of a telephone booth. He claimed that a person sitting inside the box would absorb orgone, which would cure virtually every illness, including cancer. In 1954 the FDA obtained an injunction ordering Reich to stop marketing his devices. When he violated the injunction, he was prosecuted for contempt of court and sent to prison, where he died in 1956. During the late 1960s, disciples founded the *Journal of Orgonomy* and the American College of Orgonomy, both of which are still active.

Gardner M: Reich the rainmaker: The orgone obsession.
Skeptical Inquirer 13:26–30, Fall 1988.
Traces the actions of Wilhelm Reich as he became progressively grandiose and delusional. Describes some of the activities of his modern-day followers.

Self-Help Books

Thousands of self-help books, audiotapes, and videotapes have been marketed to the public with claims that they can help people function better mentally, improve relationships with others, relieve anxiety or depression, or achieve other desirable emotionally-related goals. These claims should be viewed with caution. Although some of these materials may be helpful, most have not been tested for validity.

Rosen GM: Self-help treatment books and the
commercialization of psychotherapy.
American Psychologist 42:46–51, January 1987.
States that self-help books are more likely to help when people are under treatment than when used alone. Notes that many self-help materials are promoted with extravagant and ethically questionable claims. Notes that few do-it-yourself books have provisions to protect readers against failing to comply with instructions. Should treatment failure occur, the readers may inappropriately blame themselves, become skeptical that they can be helped, and fail to seek professional help. The author has been chairman of the American Psychological Association's Task Force on Self-Help Therapies.

Gambrill E: Self-help books: Pseudoscience in the guise of science.
Skeptical Inquirer 16:389–399, Summer 1992.

Notes that many self-help books exaggerate people's ability to alter themselves or their environment and that failure to achieve unrealistic goals offered by these books can make people more depressed.

Subliminal Tapes

Thousands of videotapes and audiotapes containing repeated messages are being marketed with claims that they can help people lose weight, stop smoking, enhance athletic performance, quit drinking, think creatively, raise I.Q., make friends, reduce pain, improve vision, restore hearing, cure acne, conquer fears, read faster, speak effectively, handle criticism, relieve depression, enlarge breasts, and do many other things. At least one company sells subliminal tapes for children, including a toilet-training tape for toddlers. Many tapes contain music said to promote relaxation. Most of the tapes are said to contain messages that are inaudible or barely audible, but some are fully audible. Videotapes may feature images, said to be relaxing, combined with repeated messages shown so briefly that they cannot be seen.

Merikle PM: Subliminal auditory messages: An evaluation.
Psychology and Marketing 5:355–372, 1989.
Describes how the author tested "subliminal" audiotapes from several companies and concluded that they contained no embedded messages that could conceivably influence behavior.

Greenwald AG, Spangenberg ER, Pratkanis AR: Double-blind tests of subliminal self-help audiotapes.
Psychological Science 2:119–122, 1991.
Another research team tested volunteers for a study of tapes said to improve memory and self-esteem—but switched the tapes for half of the participants. Regardless of the tape used, about half claimed to achieve the results they were told to expect—but objective tests of memory and self-esteem showed no change.

Bjork RA et al: In the mind's eye: Enhancing human performance.
Washington, DC, 1991, National Academy Press.
Although many people claim that subliminal self-help tapes contribute to self-improvement, there is no scientific evidence to support such claims

Moore TE: Subliminal perception: Facts and fallacies.
Skeptical Inquirer 16:273–281, 1992.
States that there is no scientific evidence that inaudible messages are unconsciously or subconsciously perceived or can influence behavior.

Therapeutic Touch

Therapeutic touch was developed during the 1970s by Dolores Krieger, PhD, RN, who for many years was professor of nursing at New York University. Its proponents claim that it is possible to use one's hands to detect when someone is ill, pinpoint areas of pain, reduce anxiety, and stimulate the sick person's recuperative powers. They also claim that their maneuvers produce changes in the body's "energy field" that can be demonstrated with Kirlian photography (see page 107). Most practitioners of therapeutic touch are nurses, many of whom consider themselves "holistic."

As taught by Dr. Krieger, therapeutic touch involves four steps: (1) "centering," a meditative process said to align the healer with the patent's energy level; (2) "assessment," said to be performed by using one's hands to detect forces emanating from the patient; (3) "unruffling the field," said to involve sweeping "stagnant energy" downward to prepare for energy transfer; and (4) transfer of energy from practitioner to patient. "Non-contact therapeutic touch" is done the same way, except that the "healer's" hands are held a few inches away from the body.

There is no scientific evidence that the "energy transfer" postulated by proponents actually exists. No study of therapeutic touch has been reported in a reputable scientific journal, but it is safe to assume that any reactions to the procedure are psychological responses to the "laying on of hands." Reiki, a similar practice alleged to heal by transferring "universal life energy" from practitioner to patient, is said to have been used in Oriental countries for thousands of years.

Critical Literature

Rojas L: Touchy subject.
Rocky Mountain Skeptic 20(6): 1–7, 1992.
Reports how the author, a registered nurse, became concerned about the encroachment of pseudomedicine into the nursing profession and asked why the Colorado Board of Nursing had endorsed courses in resonance balancing, crystal healing, reflexology, applied kinesiology, life energy balancing, healing colors, and therapeutic touch for continuing education credit. Describes the current situation, focusing upon therapeutic touch. Notes that following a meeting with members of the Rocky Mountain Skeptics, the Board appointed a subcommittee to study the matter.

Weider B: Therapeutic touch.
Shape, p. 32, May, 1992.
States that therapeutic touch is taught at nursing schools nationwide and has an estimated 30,000 practitioners. Notes that since the practice is unlicensed, "anyone can hang out a shingle and call herself a 'therapist.'" Notes that spokespeople at the American Medical Association and the American Psychiatric Association were unfamiliar with therapeutic touch. Cites a proponent's claim that practitioners scan the patient's energy flow and move it to areas where it can ease pain or heal.

Detecting science fraud and abuse.
NCAHF Bulletin Board, p. 2, May/June 1992.
Describes the problem of "true-believers" who are so certain that their views are correct that they suspend objectivity and engage in "wishful science." Notes that "true believers" typically: (1) hold a double-standard in which they demand absolute proof of regular health care, but will accept flimsy evidence for the validity of their beloved procedures; (2) demand that their methods be disproved by others, rather than operating according to the scientific dictum that no procedure should be considered safe or effective until it has been proven to be so; (3) argue against the use of untreated controls in clinical trials, declaring that to do so is unethical because it withholds a beneficial treatment from the control group; (4) organize pressure groups to advance their procedures. Illustrates these points with a study of wound-healing study purporting to show the value of non-contact therapeutic touch, noting that although the study appears well-designed, it should be viewed with great skepticism because of its astounding hypothesis. Notes that since the quality of an experiment cannot be absolutely certain from reading a written report, no such finding should be accepted unless it is replicated by qualified experts.

Proponent Literature

Krieger D: The therapeutic touch.
Englewood Cliffs, NJ, Prentice-Hall Inc., 1979.
Describes the author's association with healers who used "laying on of hands," and how she gradually combined their approach with ideas from yoga, Ayurvedic medicine, Chinese medicine, and Tibetan medicine. States that she has taught her techniques to thousands of nurses and explained the method on radio and television throughout the country, in workshops, and in many public articles. Reports that she had become interested after participating in a study in which people who were touched by a healer reported that they felt better. Notes that during the next few weeks she "was astounded by the number of medical reports or first person reports that told either of an amelioration of symptoms or actual disappearance of

symptoms. . . . Pancreatitis, brain tumor, emphysema, multiple endocrine disorders, rheumatism, arthritis, and congestive heart disease were but a few." Describes self-tests purported to demonstrate the existence of "energy flow in the empty space beyond the skin boundaries of your hands." Presents more than forty brief reports from people (identified only by their initials) who describe their thoughts and experiences using therapeutic touch.

Krieger D: Living the therapeutic touch: Healing as a lifestyle.
New York, Dodd Mead & Company, 1987.
Elaborates on the author's theories and techniques of therapeutic touch. Claims that the process manipulates "life-giving or healing energies," which are called "prana" in Sanskrit and "Ch'i" or "Qi" in Chinese. States that the energy is transformed by "complex non-physical structures," which, in Sanskrit, are called "chakras."

Part VI:
Appendices

Appendix 1: Organizations Skeptical of "Alternative" Methods

Hundreds of organizations can give good advice about health matters related to their scope of activity. The ones listed here either have a special interest in consumer protection or have issued position papers or other literature critical of various "alternative" methods. Additional information about many of these organizations can be found in the *Encyclopedia of Medical Organizations and Agencies* [Gale Research, Inc., Detroit], which is available at many libraries.

Consumer Protection Organizations

American Council on Science and Health (ACSH)
1995 Broadway, New York, NY 10023
(212) 362-7044
Evaluates issues involving food, drugs, chemicals, the environment, lifestyle, and health. Has more than 200 prominent scientific and policy advisors. Publishes *Priorities* magazine and produces frequent peer-reviewed reports. Hosts seminars and press conferences, serves as a clearinghouse for the news media, and answers individual inquiries from the public.

Children's Healthcare Is A Legal Duty (CHILD), Inc.
Box 2604, Sioux City, IA 51106
(712) 948-3295
Opposes child abuse and neglect associated with religious practice, particularly the avoidance of medical care by families involved in faith healing.

Committee for the Scientific Investigation of Claims of the Paranormal (CSICOP)
P.O. Box 703, Amherst, NY 14226
(716) 636-1425
Encourages critical investigation of paranormal and fringe-science claims. Is composed of prominent scientists, educators, and journalists, and is assisted by more than fifty scientific and technical consultants. Publishes *Skeptical Inquirer* and *Skeptical Briefs* and maintains subcommittees on astrology, education, paranormal health claims, and parapsychology. Groups similar to CSICOP exist in many areas of the United States and in several foreign countries.

Consumer Health Information Research Institute (CHIRI)
3521 Broadway, Kansas City, MO 64111
(816) 444-8615
Promotes consumer and patient education activities, including studies of misinformation, fraud and quackery. Maintains a publications list and can answer individual questions.

Consumers Union (CU)
101 Truman Ave., Yonkers, NY 10703
(914) 378-2000
Conducts research and produces *Consumer Reports, Consumer Reports on Health, Consumers Union News Digest,* and many books, pamphlets, films, newspaper columns, radio and television programs, and teaching aids. CU's Washington office monitors government activities and represents consumers through lawsuits and testimony before regulatory agencies.

Council of Better Business Bureaus
4200 Wilson Boulevard, Arlington, VA 22203
(703) 276-0100
Keeps track of complaints against businesses and may issue a report when many people complain about a company. Issues occasional pamphlets related to health frauds and quackery. Has teamed with the FDA to issue educational materials urging advertising managers to screen out misleading ads for health products.

National Association for Chiropractic Medicine (NACM)
P.O. Box 794, Middleton, WI 53562
(608) 767-3539
Provides referrals to scientifically oriented chiropractors for treatment or insurance claim reviews. Its members limit their practice to musculoskeletal problems and have denounced unscientific methods used by many of their colleagues. The group's application form includes a pledge to "openly renounce the historical chiropractic philosophical concept that subluxation is the cause of disease."

National Consumers League
815 15th St., N.W., Washington, DC 20005
(202) 639-8140
Addresses many issues, most of them economic, and presents its views to Congress and various government agencies. Publishes *Consumers' Almanac,* a monthly newsletter, and shoppers' guides, some of which cover health-related issues.

National Council Against Health Fraud (NCAHF)
P.O. Box 1276, Loma Linda, CA 92354
(714) 824-4690
NCAHF Resource Center
2800 Main St., Kansas City, MO 64108
(816) 753-8850
NCAHF Task Force on Victim Redress
P.O. Box 1747, Allentown, PA 18105
(215) 437-1795
Has more than 1,000 members and has chapters in 13 states. Activities include a bimonthly newsletter, a media clearinghouse, consumer complaint referral services, legislative action, research on questionable methods of health care, and seminars for professionals and the general public. Also maintains task forces to conduct extensive investigations and issue position papers. Its Task Force on Victim Redress helps victims of quackery who want to file suit. Other task forces cover acupuncture, chiropractic, nutrition diploma mills, diet and behavior, broadcast media abuse, dubious dental practices, vitamin abuse, "ergogenic aids," herbs, medical neglect of children, cancer quackery, and the quality of information in health periodicals.

Public Citizen Health Research Group (HRG)
2000 P St., N.W.
Washington, DC 20036
(202) 833-3000
Publishes *Public Citizen Health Resources Group Health Letter*, monitors government health agencies, analyzes proposed legislation, testifies at hearings, and files lawsuits when it believes that government agencies are too lax in protecting consumers from dangerous foods, drugs, or medical practices. Also investigates and issues reports on the effectiveness of state licensing boards and on various other economic and quality-of-care issues.

Professional, Voluntary, and Business Organizations

American Academy of Allergy and Immunology
611 East Wells St., Milwaukee, WI 53202
(414) 272-6071   (800) 822-2762

American Association of Retired Persons (AARP)
601 E St., N.W.
Washington, DC 20049
(202) 728-4780

American Cancer Society
1599 Clifton Road, N.E., Atlanta, GA 30329
(404) 320-3333   (800) 255-2352

American College of Physicians
Independence Mall West, 6th St. at Race, Philadelphia, PA 19106
(215) 351-2400

American Diabetes Association
P.O. Box 25757, Alexandria, VA 22313
(703) 549-1500   (800) 232-3472

American Dietetic Association
216 West Jackson St.
Chicago, IL 60606
(312) 899-0040   (800) 366-1655

American Heart Association
7320 Greenville Ave., Dallas, TX 75231
(214) 373-6300   (800) 242-1793

American Medical Association Library Answer Center
515 North State St., Chicago, IL 60610
(312) 464-4818

American Society of Clinical Oncology
435 N. Michigan Ave., Chicago, IL 60611
(312) 644-0828

Arthritis Foundation [also has chapters in many cities]
1314 Spring St., N.W., Atlanta, GA 30309
(404) 872-7100   (800) 283-7800

National Cancer Institute
9000 Rockville Pike, Bethesda, MD 20892
(800) 638-6694

National Council on Patient Information and Education
666 Eleventh St., N.W., Suite 810, Washington, DC 20001
(202) 347-6711

National Multiple Sclerosis Society
205 East 42nd St., New York, NY 10017
(212) 986-3240 (800) 624-8236

Government Agencies

Federal Trade Commission (FTC)
6th and Pennsylvania, Washington, DC 20580
(202) 326-2222

National Association of Attorneys General (NAAG)
444 N. Capitol St., Washington, DC 20001
(202) 628-0435

National Health Information Center (NHIC)
P.O. Box 1133, Washington, DC 20013-1133
(800) 336-4797
Helps callers locate sources of information about health matters. [Caution: People who inquire about "alternative" practices may be referred to proponent organizations.]

New York City Department of Consumer Affairs
42 Broadway
New York, NY 10004
(212) 487-4444

Office of the Inspector General (OIG)
General Services Administration, Attention: Hotline Officer
18th and F Streets, N.W., Washington, DC 20405
(800) 424-5210

U.S. Food and Drug Administration (FDA)
5600 Fishers Lane, Rockville, MD 20587
(301) 443-3170

U.S. Postal Service (USPS)
475 L'Enfant Plaza, Washington, DC 20260
(202) 268-5400

Appendix 2: Publications Skeptical of "Alternative" Methods

Many publications offer reliable health news and other information. The ones listed below have shown consistent interest in investigating questionable and controversial health matters.

Magazines

Consumer Reports
P.O. Box 53029, Boulder, CO 80322.
Covers a moderate number of topics related to health and nutrition.

FDA Consumer
Superintendent of Documents, P.O. Box 371954, Pittsburgh, PA 15250.
Covers nutrition, food safety, drugs, and government regulatory actions.

Health
P.O. Box 54218, Boulder, CO 80322.
Features well-researched articles about health issues. Formerly called *Hippocrates* and *In Health*.

Living Well
P.O. Box 7550, Red Oak, IA 51591.
Published by *Good Housekeeping* in cooperation with the American Medical Association. Outstanding coverage of a wide variety of health topics.

Obesity and Health
Healthy Living Institute, RR#2, Box 905, Hettinger, ND 58639.
Covers research developments, government actions, dubious products and services, and other topics related to weight-control..

Priorities
American Council on Science and Health, 1995 Broadway, New York, NY 10023.
Focuses on controversies involving life-style, environmental chemicals, and quackery.

Skeptic
2761 N. Marengo Ave., Altadena, CA 91001.
Features critical analyses of paranormal and pseudoscientific claims.

Skeptical Inquirer
Box 703, Buffalo, NY 14226.
Features critical analyses of paranormal and pseudoscientific claims.

Newsletters

CNI Nutrition Week
Community Nutrition Institute, 2001 S St., N.W., Washington, DC 20009.
Covers economic and political issues related to nutrition.

Consumer Protection Report
National Association of Attorneys General
444 N. Capitol St.
Washington, DC 20001
Covers state enforcement of state and federal consumer protection laws, including some cases involving health frauds.

Consumer Reports on Health
Box 36356, Boulder, CO 80322.
Presents detailed reports on health strategies, with occasional reports on quackery.

Diet Busine$$ Report
Marketdata Enterprises, 181 S. Franklin Ave., Suite 608, Valley Stream, NY 11581.
Tracks marketing and business aspects of the diet industry, with considerable material about questionable products and practices.

Environmental Nutrition
2112 Broadway, New York, NY 10023.
Provides critical reviews of books espousing dubious diet and nutrition practices. Attacks some forms of nutrition quackery, but is not consistently critical of unproven uses of dietary supplements.

Harvard Health Letter
P.O. Box 420300, Palm Coast, FL 32142.
Features superb analyses of controversial issues, particularly those involving recently published research.

Healthline
Mosby Year Book, 11830 Westline Industrial Drive, St. Louis, MO 63146.
General health information with occasional articles on quackery.

Lawrence Review of Natural Products
Facts and Comparisons, 111 West Port Plaza, Suite 423, St. Louis, MO 63146.
Authoritative monthly monographs on herbs and other naturally occurring products.

Mayo Clinic Health Letter
P.O. Box 53889, Boulder, CO 80322.
Solid, practical information with occasional reports on quackery.

The Medical Letter on Drugs and Therapeutics
1000 Main St., New Rochelle, NY 10801.
Provides authoritative evaluations, mostly of drugs, but occasionally covers supplement products, herbs, and therapeutic diets.

NCAHF Newsletter
P.O. Box 1276, Loma Linda, CA 92354.
Covers a wide variety of events related to quackery and health frauds.

Nutrition Forum
P.O. Box 1747, Allentown, PA 18105.
Features in-depth reports and undercover investigations related to quackery and health frauds.

Skeptical Briefs
P.O. Box 703, Buffalo, NY 14226
Newsletter of the Committee for the Scientific Investigation of Claims of the Paranormal. Contains at least one article on quackery in each issue.

Public Citizen Health Research Group Health Letter
2000 P St., N.W., Washington, DC 20036
Focuses on health practices and products that it considers ineffective, misleading, dangerous, and/or unethical.

Tufts University Diet and Nutrition Letter
P.O. Box 57857, Boulder, CO 80322.
Solid, practical information, with occasional reports related to quackery.

University of California at Berkeley Wellness Letter
P.O. Box 420148, Palm Coast, FL 32142.
Solid, practical information with frequent reports related to quackery.

Appendix 3: Organizations That Promote "Alternative" Methods

Academy of Orthomolecular Medicine
Alliance for Alternatives in Healthcare
American Academy of Environmental Medicine
International Academy of Holistic Health and Medicine
American Academy of Otolaryngic Allergy
American Association for Acupuncture and Oriental Medicine
American Association of Ayurvedic Medicine
American Association of Naturopathic Physicians
American Association of Nutritional Consultants
American Association of Oriental Healing Arts
American Association of Orthomolecular Medicine
American Botanical Council
American Chiropractic Association
American College of Advancement in Medicine
American College of Orgonomy
American Herbal Products Association
American Herbalists Guild
American Holistic Medical Association
American Holistic Medical Foundation
American Holistic Nurses Association
American Institute of Homeopathy
American Naprapathic Association
American Natural Hygiene Society
American Nutritional Consultants Association
American Nutritional Medical Association
American Quack Association
American Schizophrenia Association
Association of Health Practitioners
Cancer Control Society
Center for Advancement in Cancer Education
Center for Frontier Sciences (Temple University)
Center for Medical Consumers
Center for Science in the Public Interest [organic foods]
Citizens for Health
Committee for Freedom of Choice in Medicine

Confederation of Health Organizations
Council for Responsible Nutrition
Dietary Supplement Coalition
Feingold Association of the United States
Foundation for Alternative Cancer Therapy, Ltd.
Foundation for the Advancement of Innovative Medicine
Herb Research Foundation
Holistic Dental Association
Human Ecology Action League (HEAL)
Huxley Institute for Biosocial Research
International Academy of Nutrition and Preventive Medicine
International Alliance of Nutri-Medical Associations
International Association of Cancer Victors and Friends
International Association of Dentists and Physicians.
International Chiropractors Association
International Foundation for Homeopathy
Life Extension Foundation (of Hollywood, Florida)
International Health Foundation
Linus Pauling Institute
National Academy of Research Biochemists
National Center for Homeopathy
National Council for Improved Health
National Health Care Alliance
National Health Federation
National Institutes of Health Office on Unconventional Medical Practices
National Nutritional Foods Association
National Progressive Health Political Action Committee
National Wellness Coalition
Nutrition for Optimal Health Association
Nutritional Health Alliance
Orthomolecular Medical Society
People Against Cancer
People's Consortium for Medical Freedom
People for Reason in Science and Medicine
People's Medical Society
Physicians Committee for Responsible Medicine
Price-Pottenger Nutrition Foundation
Project Cure
Touch for Health Foundation
World Chiropractic Alliance
World Research Foundation

Appendix 4: Publications That Promote "Alternative" Methods

Books

Kruger H: Other healers other cures
Indianapolis, Bobbs-Merrill Company, 1974

Shealy N, Freese AS: Occult medicine can save your life
Columbus, OH, Brindabella Books, 1975

Kaslof LJ (ed.): Wholistic dimensions in healing
Garden City, NY, Doubleday & Company, 1978

Otto HA, Knight JW: Dimensions in wholistic healing
Chicago, Nelson-Hall, 1979

Pizer H: Guide to the new medicine
New York, William Morrow, 1982

Inglis B, West R: The alternative health guide
New York, Alfred A. Knopf, 1983

Lowe C, Nechas JW, et al: Whole body healing
Emmaus, PA, Rodale Press, 1983

Bauman E et al (eds.): The holistic health lifebook
Lexington, MA, The Stephen Greene Press, 1984

Bliss E (ed.): The new holistic health handbook
Lexington, MA, The Stephen Greene Press, 1985

Grossman R: The other medicines
Garden City, NY, Doubleday & Company, 1985

Porkert M, Ullman C: Chinese Medicine
New York, William Morrow, 1988

Atkins RC: Dr. Atkins' health revolution
Boston, Houghton Mifflin, 1988

Drury N, Drury S: Illustrated dictionary of natural health
New York, Sterling Publishing Co., 1989

Fulder S: The handbook of complementary medicine
Falmouth, England, Hodder and Stoughton, 1989

Ley BM (ed.): Health talks
Fargo, ND, Christopher Lawrence Communications, 1989

Olsen KG: The encyclopedia of alternative health care
New York, Simon and Schuster, 1989

Heimlich J: What your doctor won't tell you
New York, HarperCollins, 1990

Greenberg K: Challenging orthodoxy
New Canaan, CT, Keats Publishing, Inc., 1991

Magazines

The American Chiropractor
Better Nutrition for Today's Living
Body, Mind & Spirit
The Choice
Choices
Delicious!
East West Natural Health
Explore!
FACT
Flex
Frontier Perspectives
Health Consciousness
Health Counselor
Health Freedom News
Health Science

Health World
Herbalgram
Holistic Medicine
The Human Ecologist
Innovation
Let's Live
Longevity
Muscle & Fitness
New Age Journal
New Body
Nutrition & Fitness
Nutritional Perspectives
Penthouse
Senior Health
Total Health
Townsend Letter for Doctors
Vegetarian Times
Your Health

Newsletters

Alternatives
Antha
Atkins Health Letter
Cancer Chronicles
Forefront
Fountain
Health & Healing
HealthFacts
Health Resource Newsletter
Men's Health Newsletter
Natural Fitness Newsletter
Natural Living Newsletter
New Millenium
Nutrition News (published by Siri Khalsa)
People's Medical Society Newsletter
Pure Facts
Second Opinion

Newspapers

The Chiropractic Journal
Dynamic Chiropractic
Health News & Review
Health Store News
Nutrition Health Review

Trade Publications

Health Foods Business
Natural Food and Farming
Natural Foods Merchandiser
Organic Times
Whole Foods

Journals

ACA Journal of Chiropractic
Chiropractic Research Journal
Chiropractic Technique
Digest of Chiropractic Economics
International Journal of Biosocial and Medical Research
Journal of Applied Nutrition
Journal of Manipulative Physiology and Therapeutics
Journal of Naturopathic Medicine
Journal of Optimal Nutrition
Journal of the Advancement of Medicine
Today's Chiropractic

Appendix 5: Glossary of "Alternative" Methods and Terms

Each of the items below has one or more of the following characteristics: (1) its rationale or underlying theory is not consistent with accepted scientific beliefs; (2) it has not been demonstrated safe and/or effective by well-designed studies; or (3) its promotion involves deception and/or misinformation.

Absent healing: A form of faith healing done without the presence of the healer. Usually said to involve the power of prayer or projection of positive and healing thoughts to the ailing person. Also called remote healing.

Acupressure (shiatsu): A technique that uses finger pressure instead of needles at "acupuncture points."

Acupuncture: A system of treatment purported to balance the body's "life force" by inserting needles into or beneath the skin (or by using other forms of stimulation) at various points where imaginary horizontal and vertical lines ("meridians") meet on the surface of the body. These points are said to represent various internal organs. Although acupuncture can sometimes relieve pain, there is no evidence that it can influence the course of any organic disease.

Alexander technique: A system of training claimed to improve posture and movement during the activities of daily life. Instead of concentrating on contracting muscles that hold the anatomy in place, the Alexander technique aims to release muscles that are interfering with good body mechanics, and to "restore tone to muscles that are slack." The technique does not work directly upon emotional health but is claimed to improve it through kinesthetic awareness.

Amino acid analysis of urine: A procedure claimed by its proponents to be useful in uncovering a wide range of nutrition and metabolic disorders. As with hair analysis, the test report may be accompanied by a lengthy computer printout containing speculations about the patient's state of health.

Anthroposophical medicine: A set of practices based on the occult philosophy of Rudolph Steiner (1861–1925) and said to relate humankind to the natural environment, with emphasis on color, rhythm, and spirituality. Its practitioners frequently prescribe homeopathic remedies, herbs, study of musical instruments, social service projects, prayer, and meditation. The remedies are claimed to restore balance either by strengthening the therapeutic "etheric body" or by moderating the animalistic "astral body."

Applied kinesiology: A pseudoscience based on the belief that every organ dysfunction is accompanied by a specific muscle weakness that can be diagnosed by various tests. (Note: Kinesiology, which is the study of the mechanics and anatomy of motion, is a legitimate science.)

Aromatherapy: An approach based on the theory that massaging various plant oils into the skin or inhaling their odors can help heal hundreds of diseases and conditions.

Astrology (medical): Use of a horoscope to determine the diseases and infirmities to which a person is predisposed. Stellar patterns at the time of birth are believed to indicate potential illness, which may be triggered by subsequent transit of the planets over sensitive areas of the natal chart. "Medical astrologers" may claim (based on "astrological influences") that a part of the body is prone to weakness at certain times or that particular times (based on the phases of the moon) may be ideal for surgery or fertility planning. Some also give dietary advice.

Auriculotherapy: A variant of acupuncture based on the belief that the body is "represented" by various points on the ear. According to proponents, the arrangement corresponds to an inverted fetus, with the head near the earlobe. Proponents claim that acupuncturing specific sites on the ear can alleviate ailments that originated in "corresponding" parts of the body and that diagnosis can be performed by examining the ear for signs of tenderness or variations in electrical conductivity.

Autogenic therapy: Relaxation and meditation techniques claimed to facilitate self-balance or self-healing. It is based on exercises in which the trainee repeats a specific phrase while thinking about a part of the body. It has been claimed to be effective against alcoholism, obesity, asthma, diabetes, arthritis, and anxiety, as well as for improving concentration and general performance.

Autointoxication: A theory that stasis causes the contents of the intestines to putrefy, forming toxins that are absorbed and cause chronic poisoning of the body. This theory was popular around the turn of the century but was abandoned by the scientific community during the 1930s. No such "toxins" have ever been identified, and careful observations have shown that the bowel habits of individuals in good health can vary greatly.

Ayurvedic medicine: A set of practices promoted by transcendental meditation (TM) organizations. Ayurveda (meaning "life knowledge") is said to be based on a traditional Indian approach that includes meditation, purification procedures, rejuvenation therapies, herbal and mineral preparations, exercises and dietary advice based on "Ayurvedic body type."

Bach flower remedies: Extracts of various flowers whose scents are claimed to restore health by correcting negative emotional states that underlie all disease. The method was developed by Edward Bach, a physician who practiced homeopathy.

Bates method: A system of relaxation exercises claimed to cure poor vision. The method is based on the mistaken belief that the dimensions of the eyeball and the shape of the lens have nothing to do with poor eyesight. The exercises include: (1) palming (staring at a black object, then closing the eyes and recalling the blackness), (2) shifting the gaze continually from object to object, and (3) staring directly into the sun (a hazardous procedure).

Biofeedback: A relaxation technique that can help people learn to control certain body functions. The patient is connected to a device that continuously signals the heartbeat, skin temperature, degree of muscle contraction, or other mechanism. The patient is instructed to relax so that the signals decrease to a desirable level. Biofeedback can help people achieve deep relaxation, but the same mental state can be accomplished without electronic monitoring. In 1980, the American Psychiatric Association concluded that there is no psychiatric condition for which biofeedback as such is the treatment of choice. In scientific hands, biofeedback has achieved a measure of respectability for the treatment of psychophysiologic symptoms. However, claims that biofeedback fosters "personal growth," "self-understanding," "stabilization of the autonomic system," or the like are simplistic and unproven.

Biorhythms: A pseudoscience based on the theory that human behavior is influenced by regular body rhythms that begin at the moment of birth.

"Candidiasis hypersensitivity": A fad diagnosis based on the idea that multiple common symptoms are caused by sensitivity to the common fungus, *Candida albicans.*

Cell salts: A set of twelve salts claimed to be effective against a wide variety of diseases. The theory behind their use is that the basic cause of disease is mineral deficiency, correction of which will enable the body to heal itself.

Cellular therapy: Injections of animal cells into the human body, claimed by various proponents to cure disease, rejuvenate or "revitalize" the body, and prolong life. The cells are commonly obtained from freshly slaughtered sheep fetuses, but other animals can be used. The method is also called "cell therapy" and "live-cell therapy."

"Cellulite" removers: Various gadgets, creams, and potions claimed to remove the dimpled fat found on the thighs and buttocks of many women. "Cellulite" is not a medical term. Biopsies have shown that it is simply ordinary fatty tissue that bulges outward while the skin remains partially bound by fibers to the underlying tissues. No externally applied nonsurgical treatment can remove fat selectively from one part of the body.

Chelation therapy: A series of intravenous administrations of a synthetic amino acid (EDTA) plus various other substances.

Chinese Medicine: See Oriental Medicine

Chiropractic: A broad spectrum of practices related to the false premise that spinal misalignments ("subluxations") are the cause, or the underlying cause, of most ailments.

Christian Science: A religious denomination that rejects scientific medical care in favor of spiritual healing. It contends that illness is an illusion caused by faulty beliefs, and that prayer heals by replacing bad thoughts with good ones.

Clinical ecology: A pseudoscience based on the premise that multiple symptoms are triggered by hypersensitivity to common foods and chemicals.

Colonic irrigation: A "high colonic" enema performed by passing a rubber tube into the rectum for a distance of up to 20 or 30 inches. Warm water is pumped in and out through the tube, a few pints at a time, typically using 20 or more gallons. Some practitioners add herbs, coffee, or other substances to the water. The procedure is said to "detoxify" the body, though no "toxins" have ever been specified or scientifically demonstrated.

Complementary medicine: A term used by unscientific practitioners who claim to "integrate" both alternative and orthodox methods into their practice.

Cranial osteopathy: A pseudoscience based on the notion that manipulation of the bones of the skull can cure various ailments. This notion is false because the bones of the skull are firmly attached to each other. Also called craniopathy

Cryonics: The practice of freezing the head and brain or the entire human body, as soon as possible after death, with the hope of eventually restoring life. Proponents claim that it is possible to preserve the basic biological components of the brain and that future technology may be able to repair brain damage. There is no evidence that cryonic technology works in laboratory animals. Even if the rest of a person's body could be revived after hundreds of years, the brain could not. Brain cells deteriorate within minutes after death, and any still viable when the body is frozen would be burst by the freezing process.

Crystal healing: A variety of practices based on the idea that crystals, especially quartz crystals, possess an energy field that can heal disease.

Cytotoxic testing: A test performed by adding samples of the patient's blood plasma and white blood cells to samples of dried foods on a special microscope slide. The white cells are examined over a period of time to see whether they have changed their shape or disintegrated. Controlled experiments have shown that cytotoxic testing is not reliable for determining food allergies.

Dianetics: An approach described by its proponents as a pastoral counseling method for locating and eliminating unwanted emotional and psychosomatic problems. The goal of therapy is to erase traumatic memories through a procedure in which an auditor may use an "E-meter" (a device that measures changes in skin resistance to electricity) to help the patient recall traumatic events.

Electrodiagnosis: The use of a machine to diagnose "electromagnetic energy imbalances." Using a probe connected to the machine, the practitioner touches the patient's hands and feet and interprets numbers that appear on a computer screen or other indicator. Devices of this sort are used to diagnose supposed allergies, vitamin deficiencies, and "degeneration" or "inflammation" of the body's organs.

Energy medicine: An umbrella term for various practices said to be based on the practitioner's ability to view or sense an individual's "energy field" or "etheric body." Some practitioners claim to rely on psychic ability, while others use electrodiagnostic devices.

"Environmental medicine": An designation used by clinical ecologists to make themselves sound more respectable.

Ergogenic aids: Various concoctions of vitamins, minerals, and/or amino acids that are marketed with false claims that they can increase stamina and endurance and help build stronger muscles. Some are falsely touted to be "natural steroids" or "growth-hormone releasers."

Faith healing: A variety of approaches based on the idea that prayer, divine intervention, or the actions of an individual healer can cure or relieve illness.

Feingold diet: A diet based on the idea that salicylates and artificial food colors and flavors cause children to be hyperactive. Although many parents who have followed the diet have reported improvement in their children's behavior, controlled experiments have failed to support the Feingold hypothesis.

Feldenkrais: A system of exercise therapy said to improve posture, breathing, coordination, and self-image. It is claimed to reestablish connections between the brain and the muscles and nerves that have been altered by physical trauma, chronic tension, or bad habits.

"Glandulars": Raw glandular or organ tissues that have been dehydrated and made into tablets or capsules. They are claimed to "support" corresponding organs within the body. However, they exert no special physiological function because they contain no hormones and are digested before being absorbed into the body.

"Growth-hormone releasers": Amino acid supplements touted as weight loss or sports nutrition aids. Claims for them are based mainly on faulty extrapolation from experiments with animals. There is no evidence that these products, taken by mouth, actually release growth hormone in humans, produce weight loss, or enhance athletic ability.

Hair analysis: A test misused by unscientific practitioners to diagnose "mineral imbalances" or the presence of "toxic minerals." The test is usually obtained by sending a small amount of hair from the nape of the neck to a commercial laboratory for analysis. The laboratory report may suggest what supplements should be taken.

"Health food:" A term implying that a food has special properties beyond the mere nutrients it contains.

Herbal crystallization analysis: A bogus test performed by adding a solution of copper chloride to a dried specimen of the patient's saliva on a slide. The resultant crystal patterns are then matched to those of dried herbs to determine supposed body problem areas and the herbs for treating them.

Hellerwork: A method of massage that combines deep tissue massage with movement reeducation and a guided verbal dialogue.

Herbology: Self-study of herbs, herbalism, and herbal therapy. It is generally based on outdated concepts, such as the "doctrine of signatures," astrological notions, and folklore.

"Holistic" approach: A slogan used to suggest that a practitioner treats the "whole person," with due attention to emotional factors as well as the person's lifestyle. Most practitioners who call themselves "holistic" use unscientific methods for diagnosis and treatment.

Homeopathy: A pseudoscience based on the idea that symptoms can be cured by taking infinitesimal amounts of substances that, in larger amounts, can produce similar symptoms in healthy people. Homeopathic theory states that the more dilute the remedy, the more powerful it is.

Iridology: A pseudoscience based on the idea that each area of the body is represented by a corresponding area in the iris (pupil) of the eye. Practitioners claim to diagnose nutritional imbalances that can be treated with vitamins, minerals, herbs, and similar products.

Keyes technique: A nonsurgical alternative for treating advanced periodontal disease (pyorrhea). The technique includes microscopic examination of the plaque and cleaning the teeth and gums with a mixture of salt, baking soda and peroxide. Well-designed studies have found that surgical treatment is more effective for advanced periodontal disease and that the baking soda mixture is less convenient and no more effective than ordinary toothpaste.

Kirlian photography: A method alleged by some faith healers to register their healing force ("aura") in photographs taken with a special apparatus. It is also used as a diagnostic method in which characteristics of the "aura" are claimed to indicate various states of health. Critics have demonstrated that the nature of the pictures produced can be controlled by the degree of finger pressure applied to the apparatus and that the photographic images are also affected by perspiration.

Lingual test for vitamin C. A procedure in which a drop of test solution is placed on the tongue and observed for color change. There is no scientific evidence that the test indicates the vitamin C status of the body.

Live-cell analysis: A test performed by examining the patient's blood under a dark-field microscope to which a television monitor has been attached. Both practitioner and patient can then see blood cells and debris, which appear as dark bodies outlined in white. Proponents claim that the procedure is useful in diagnosing vitamin and mineral deficiencies, tendencies toward allergic reactions, liver weakness, and many other health problems that are treatable with food supplements.

Macrobiotic diet: A semi-vegetarian diet claimed by its proponents to improve health and prolong life. Proponents suggest that the diet is effective in preventing and treating cancer, AIDS, and other serious diseases. There is no evidence to support these claims. Some versions of the macrobiotic diet contain adequate amounts of nutrients, but others do not.

Magnetic healing: An approach claimed to heal illness with magnetic forces. The devices used have included copper bracelets, crosses, magnetic rings, hand-held magnets, and magnets attached to clothing, held against the skin with adhesive, or placed under one's bedding. Modern proponents claim that magnets can be used for diagnosis of "magnetic deficiency states" as well as for treatment of disease.

Mail-order diet pills: Various products claimed to suppress appetite or alter metabolism. They include vitamin concoctions, "fat-burners," products claimed (falsely) to suppress appetite by filling up the stomach, and substances claimed (falsely) to block the absorption of sugar, starch, or fat. Ads for these products typically offer effortless weight loss of a pound a day or more.

Mental imagery: A procedure in which detailed mental images are used in an attempt to control a situation. For example, cancer patients may imagine that their white blood cells are little knights in white armor attacking their tumors, which they picture as black dragons. New Age devotees may imagine that they have spirit guides and work to put as much detail as possible into the fantasized image.

Mercury-amalgam toxicity: A "fad" diagnosis made by unscientific dentists who tell patients that their "silver" (mercury-amalgam) fillings are making them ill and should be replaced.

Metabolic therapy: A loosely defined treatment program based on the idea that cancer, arthritis, and other chronic illnesses result from a disturbance of the body's ability to protect itself. The program is claimed to detoxify the body and strengthen the immune system. Its components, which vary from practitioner to practitioner, may include megadoses of vitamins, oral enzymes, pangamic acid, coffee enemas, a low-protein diet, and laetrile (for cancer).

Naprapathy: A variant of chiropractic based on the philosophy that contractions of the body's soft tissue cause illness by interfering with neurovascular function. Its proponents claim that gentle stretching of ligaments, muscles and other connective tissue of the spine and joints of the body can restore health by relieving such interference. Naprapathic practice also includes nutritional, postural, and exercise counseling. Its practitioners are not licensed.

"Natural" food: A loosely-defined term suggesting that a product has been minimally processed and contains no "artificial" additives.

Natural hygiene: A form of naturopathy that emphasizes fasting and food-combining, a dietary practice based on the incorrect notion that certain food combinations can cause or correct ill health.

Naturopathy: A system of treatment based on the belief that the cause of disease is violation of nature's laws. Naturopaths believe that diseases are the body's effort to purify itself, and that cures result from enhancing the body's ability to heal itself. Naturopathic treatments can include "natural food" diets, vitamins, herbs, tissue minerals, cell salts, manipulation, massage, exercise, diathermy, colonic enemas, acupuncture, and homeopathy. Like some chiropractors, many naturopaths believe that virtually all diseases are within the scope of their practice. Naturopaths are licensed to practice in several states. Recently, despite the unscientific nature of their beliefs, the U.S. Secretary of Education granted approval for an accrediting agency for naturopathic schools.

Negative ion generator: A device that produces negatively charged particles (ions), which combine with dust particles and cause them to cling to room surfaces rather than floating freely through the air. Large, expensive devices that clean the air of pollen, dust, and other allergens, are used to create "clean rooms" for manufacturing sensitive electronic devices. Proponents of negative ion therapy (aeroiontherapy) claim that small-sized generators can prevent illness by neutralizing positive ions with negative ones, but these devices cannot actually produce enough ions to change the air in a room effectively. In addition, scientific studies have failed to support the claims of negative ion proponents. The FDA has warned that negative ion generators have no proven health benefits and that no health-related claim can be made without premarket approval.

Neural organization technique: A method claimed to treat learning disorders and other problems of the brain and nervous system by manipulating the sphenoid bone of the skull.

Nutripathy: A pseudoscience in which treatment with supplements and other measures is related to a formula devised by Cary Reams. Proponents claim that the formula, derived from the results of nonstandard urine and saliva tests, reveals energy input and energy use within the body. Reams, a self-professed biophysicist, was prosecuted for practicing medicine without a license during the 1970s.

"Organic" food: A loosely defined term suggesting that the food has been grown without the use of pesticides or manufactured fertilizers. Although the foods themselves cannot be distinguished from "ordinary" foods, they usually cost more.

Oriental medicine: Chinese, Taoist, or other Far Eastern traditional medicine that integrates vitalism, nature worship, herbalism, martial arts, and other lore. Its practices includes acupuncture, dietary procedures, and pulse diagnosis.

Orthomolecular therapy: A treatment approach that supposedly provides the correct amounts of nutritionally "right" molecules normally found in the body. Its practitioners prescribe large doses of vitamins, minerals, and various other substances. It is sometimes referred to as megavitamin therapy.

Passive exercise: A purported method of weight control claimed to take the strain out of exercise by doing it for you. Offered at slenderizing salons, this approach typically involves a table that rocks or shakes or a motor-driven rowing machine or bicycle. Passive exercise may produce temporary relaxation, but it cannot cause weight loss. That requires active exercise in which calories are burned as a result of physical exertion.

Past-life therapy: A form of psychotherapy based upon a belief in reincarnation. Proponents claim that illness and unhappiness are the result of negative experiences in a past life that scar the psyche. Patients usually are hypnotized and asked to travel back in time to a previous existence. Fantasies experienced in the highly suggestible trance-state are treated as reality and "relived" until they lose their emotional impact. Among other things, critics point out that although patients can describe their supposed past lives in great detail, they are not able to speak outdated languages or read outdated writings from those time periods.

Polarity therapy: A system of manipulation, stretching exercises, clear thinking, and diet claimed to restore health by removing blocks and restoring the flow of "life energy" between the positive (head) and negative poles (feet) of the body.

Provocation-neutralization: A test in which the patient reports symptoms that occur within ten minutes after various substances are administered under the tongue or injected into the skin. If symptoms occur, the test is considered positive and lower concentrations are given until a dose is found that "neutralizes" the symptoms.

Psychic healing: A term used by its proponents to characterize any form of healing that is not medical and cannot be explained in terms of current medical knowledge. Includes such methods as faith healing, laying on of hands, remote healing, and shamanic practices.

Psychic surgery: A procedure in which sleight-of-hand is used to create an illusion that patients can be cured with surgery that leaves no skin wound. Skilled observers have noted that animal parts or cotton wads soaked in betel juice (a red dye) were palmed and then exhibited as "diseased organs" supposedly removed from the patient's body.

Psychoneuroimmunology: A set of theories and practices based on the hope that brain functioning affects the immune system in ways that can be modified by "positive thinking." Some proponents claim that positive thinking can materially effect the natural course of serious diseases, such as cancer. No convincing evidence has been published to support this idea. In addition, some studies have found no evidence of altered immunity or higher cancer incidence in people who are severely depressed.

Qigong (pronounced "chi-gung"): An ancient form of Chinese medical practice purported to influence the "life force" (Qi) flowing through channels ("meridians") in the body. Internal Qigong involves deep breathing, concentration, and relaxation techniques used by individuals for themselves. External Qigong is performed by "Qigong masters" who claim to cure a wide variety of diseases with energy released from their fingertips.

Radionics: Practices based on the unsubstantiated theory that diseases can be diagnosed and treated with devices that tune into vital energy patterns emitted by pathogens or diseased body organs. Radionics theory was originated by Albert Abrams, MD, whom the AMA considered the "dean of gadget quacks." Abrams developed various devices that supposedly detected diseases by their vibratory rates (radio frequencies), and cured them by emitting disease-destroying vibrations.

Radiesthesia: Practices based on claims that "sensitive" individuals can diagnose illness by using a pendulum, dowsing rod, or other indicator to detect electromagnetic "vibrations" emanating from a sample of blood, hair, fingernail clippings, saliva, urine, or a personal object, such as a picture, article of clothing, or jewelry.

Raw milk: Milk in its natural (unpasteurized) state. Contaminated raw milk can be a source of harmful bacteria, such as those that cause dysentery and tuberculosis. "Certified" milk is unpasteurized milk with a bacteria count below a specified standard, but it can still contain significant numbers of disease-producing organisms. In 1987, the FDA banned the interstate sale of raw milk and raw milk products packaged for human consumption.

Rebirthing: A bodywork technique that uses hyperventilation to induce an altered state of consciousness that supposedly enables the subject to overcome traumatic memories and achieve spiritual renewal. It is usually done with the subject resting on a mat or in a hot tub.

Reflexology: A system of diagnosis and treatment based on the theory that pressing on certain areas of the hands or feet can help relieve pain and remove the cause of disease in other parts of the body.

Reichian therapy: A method based on the notions of Wilhelm Reich, MD, a psychoanalyst who believed that the ego, id, and superego "inhabit" a body. He claimed that sitting in a specially designed box would enable people to accumulate "orgone energy," which would cure virtually every illness.

Reiki: A healing system alleged to "utilize universal life force energy to vitalize and balance the entire physical/mental, emotional. spiritual dynamic." Proponents also state that reiki is "a powerful tool for stress-reduction and relaxation, as well as a complete preventative self-health care method."

Rolfing (structural integration): A form of massage claimed to lengthen, straighten, and balance the body in relation to the pull of gravity. Therapeutic effects are said to result from bringing the head, shoulders, chest, and legs into vertical alignment.

Spot-reducing aids: A variety of products claimed to remove fat from parts of the body to which they are applied. These include vibrators, body wraps, and skin creams. Nothing applied to the outside of the body can reduce the fat content of the underlying body part. The only ways to accomplish this are through overall weight reduction or—in carefully selected cases—with plastic surgery such as liposuction. Exercise devices claimed to trim the abdomen, thighs, or arms are also dubious. Although exercise can tighten muscles in these areas, it cannot remove the fat between the muscles and the skin. This is illustrated by the fact that tennis players, who spend large amounts of time exercising only one arm, have equal amounts of fat in both arms.

Silva mind control: A system of meditation and autosuggestion claimed to help people enter a state of deep relaxation in order to bring about various improvements in one's life.

Subliminal tapes: The notion that the mind can be unconsciously influenced by messages that are below the threshold of sensation.

Subluxation": A nebulous term used by many chiropractors to represent the basic or underlying cause of disease. Some chiropractors consider subluxations to be spinal bones (vertebrae) that are misaligned or out-of-place. Others use the term to mean "fixations" (reduction of movement). Some chiropractors claim that their "subluxations" can be seen on x-ray films, while others claim that additional findings are needed to diagnose them. Subluxation is also a legitimate medical term for partial dislocation.

Therapeutic touch: A system in which the hands are used to "direct human energies to help or heal someone who is ill." Proponents claim that healers can detect and correct "energy imbalances" by stroking the body or placing their hands above the afflicted part. Healing supposedly can result from a transfer of "excess energy" from healer to patient.

Tissue salts: A set of twelve products containing various homeopathic dilutions of inorganic minerals found in the body. Advocates of their use claim that the basic cause of disease is mineral deficiency, correction of which will enable the body to heal itself.

Transcendental meditation (TM): An experience, based on repetition of a meaningless word, in which participants supposedly enter a state of "pure or transcendental consciousness" that produces relaxation, clearer and more powerful thinking, lowered blood pressure, confidence, and tranquility.

Visual training: "Vision therapists" claim to strengthen eyesight through a series of exercises and the use of eyeglasses. Their training sessions may take place several times a week and cost thousands of dollars for a series. They emphasize exercises that involve hand-eye coordination, watching a series of blinking lights, focusing on a string of objects, and even sleeping in a certain position. Often they prescribe bifocal and prism glasses for nearsightedness. They claim that these methods can improve school and athletic performance, increase I.Q., help overcome learning disabilities, and help prevent juvenile delinquency. However, there is no scientific evidence to support these claims.

Yoga: A variety of approaches based on ancient Indian beliefs about human existence. Proponents claim that various exercises can improve physical and emotional health by bringing harmony and balance to the individual. The recommended exercises include yogic breathing, meditation, other relaxation techniques, bending, stretching, holding various postures, dietary measures, and "emotion culturing" (evoking positive emotions and diffusing negative ones).

Zone therapy; *see* **Reflexology**

Index

Abrams, Dr. Albert, 335
Absent healing, 325
Accreditation, 27
  of acupuncture schools, 39
  of chiropractic schools, 47
  of naturopathy schools, 100
Accupath 1000, 215
Acu-Thin Ear Stimulator, 271
Acupressure, 39, 325
Acupuncture, 7, 28, 39–44, 57, 325
  complications, 41
Advertising
  "ergogenic aids," 195
  food, FTC investigation, 196
  mail-order health products, 30
  nonprescription drugs, 23
  quack claims, 18
  in tabloids, 22
  vitamins, 176–177
Aeroionotherapy, 333–334
AIDS, unproven remedies, 150–156
AIDS Coalition to Unleash Power (ACT-UP), 150, 156
Airola, Paavo, 114, 203, 205
Alcott, William, 14
Alexander technique, 325
Alivizatos, Dr. Hariton, 128–130
Allergies, food, 237–238
Aloe vera, 77
Alta-Dena Certified Dairy, 194
"Alternative" methods
  definitions relating to, 4–7, 31
  lure of, 9–10, 16, 23
  NIH panel, 33
  organizations promoting, 32–33, 319–320
  organizations skeptical of, 311–315
  patients' attitudes toward, 20–21, 115–116, 118, 137
  physicians' attitudes toward, 93

promotion by media, 3
proposed classification, 26
publications promoting, 324
publications skeptical of, 316–318
why people choose, 9, 18, 90–91, 119–120, 121, 164
Alternative Therapies, Unproven Methods, & Health Fraud, 3
AMA; *see* American Medical Association
Amalgameter, 189
American Association of Naturopathic Physicians, 100
American Association of Nutritional Consultants, 189
American Biologics Hospital, 117
American Cancer Society
  definition of questionable method, 6
  nutrition guidelines, 125
American Council on Science and Health, 311
American Dietetic Association, 199, 204
American Holistic Health Sciences Association, 189
American Holistic Medical Association, 81
American Medical Association (AMA)
  and "alternative" psychological methods, 300
  Bureau of Investigation, 11
  concern about health fraud, 11–12, 33–34
  Council on Foods and Nutrition, 247
  Council on Scientific Affairs, 12, 183, 211, 224, 265, 294, 300
  Department of Investigation, 11–12
  Diagnostic and Therapeutic Technology Assessment (DATTA), 12, 133
  Division of Library and Information Management, 12
  and DMSO, 297
  and hair analysis, 211, 213, 214

American Medical Association (cont'd.)
  Historical Health Fraud and Alternative
    Medicine Collection, 12, 15
  and homeopathy, 88
  Medical Code of Ethics, 11
  and multiple chemical sensitivity
    syndrome, 224
  National Congresses on Medical
    Quackery, 33–34
  and obesity treatment, 265
  Propaganda Department, 11
  suits against, by chiropractors, 48, 49, 52
American Medical News, 12
American Natural Hygiene Society, 97
American Nutritional Medical Association, 189
American Quack Association, 32
Amino acid analysis of urine, 325
Amino acids, safety of, 201–202
Anthroposophic medicine, 325–326
Antiquackery activities, 33–36
Applied kinesiology, 29, 57, 208–209, 300, 326
Aromatherapy, 279–281, 326
Arthritis, unproven approaches, 163–169, 299
  prevalence, 163–164, 165, 167
Asai, Kazuhiko, 198
Aslan, Dr. Anna, 191
Asthma, dangerous remedies, 24
Astrological counseling, 301
Astrology, 26, 106, 326
  psychic, 110
Atikian, Sonia and Khachadour, 79
Atkins, Dr. Robert, 33
Aura, 107, 331
Auriculotherapy, 39, 40, 326
Autogenic therapy, 326
Autointoxication, 326–327
Avogadro's number, 85, 89
Ayurvedic medicine, 45–46, 327
Azarcón, 71

Bach flower remedies, 327
Bachynsky, Dr. Nicholas, 273

"Balancing body chemistry," 28
Baldness remedies, 282–284
Barnes, Dr. Carl, 132
Barrett, Dr. Stephen, 17, 33, 36, 46, 213, 216
Bastyr College, 100
Bates method, 327
Bee pollen, 198, 199
Benzocaine, 269
Berger, Dr. Joel, 232
Berger, Dr. Stuart, 204, 237
Bernadean University, 187
Beverly Hills Diet, The, 97
Biofeedback training, 285–289, 327
Bio-Medical Center, 131
Biorhythms, 106, 327
Bland, Dr. Jeffrey, 186
Body wraps, 270
Brinkley, John R., 14
Bristol Cancer Help Center, 122
British Medical Association, 6
Bulk-producers, 269, 271, 274
Burton, Dr. Lawrence, 114, 131, 134
Burzynski, Dr. Stanislaw, 126, 127
"Buyer's clubs," 150, 156

Cal-Ban 3000, 273–274
Cambridge Plan International, 272
Cameron, Dr. Ewan, 145
Cancer
  clinical trials, 113
  and diet, 118, 124–126
  incidence, 113–114
  questionable treatment, 113–156
    antineoplastons, 126–126
    characteristics, 114–124, 136
    claims for, 115
    Gerson therapy, 114, 127–128
    Greek Cancer Cure, 128–130
    Hoxsey cancer treatment, 130–131
    "hyperoxygenation therapies," 147
    immunoaugmentative therapy (IAT), 22, 114–115, 131–134
    insurance reimbursement, 114–115
    laetrile, 135–139

"Alternative" Health Methods / 341

Livingston-Wheeler therapy, 139–140
macrobiotic diet, 250–252
metabolic therapy, 140–142
OTA report, 122–123, 134
prevalence, 124
proponent literature, 148–149
proponent organizations, 147–148
psychological approaches, 121, 142–144
Revici method, 144–145
"shaving" chemotherapy, 117
vitamin C megadoses, 145–146
Cancer Control Society, 136, 205
Candida albicans, 225
"Candidiasis hypersensitivity," 225–228. 232–233, 327
CANHELP, 148
Canthaxanthin, 200
Carnitine, 261
Carotid body resection, 238–239
Cavanaugh, Beth, 184–185
Cayce, Edgar, 109
Cell salts, 328
Cell Tech, Inc., 256
Cellular therapy, 290–292, 328
"Cellulite," 265, 269, 328
Chakras, 308
Chandler, Jennie, 14
Channeling, 104, 107
Chelation therapy, 157–162, 328
oral, 159
Ch'i, 7, 39, 308
Children's Healthcare Is A Legal Duty (CHILD), 311
Chinese medicine, 39, 57, 100
Chiropractic, 7, 47–57, 328
criticism of, 50–53
history of, 48–49
and homeopathy, 93
and nutrition, 53
spinal manipulation, studies of, 54–56
Cho Low Tea, 30
Chopra, Dr. Deepak, 45, 46
Christian Science, 58–62, 328
Christian Science Sentinel, 58

Chronic fatigue syndrome, 228–229
Clinical ecology, 218, 220–221, 328
Club SeneX, 192
Coalition for Alternatives in Nutrition and Healthcare, 32
Cold reading, 109
Colgan, Michael, 202
Colonic irrigation, 10, 293–295, 328
Comfrey, 78
Committee for Freedom of Choice in Cancer Therapy, 148
Committee for Freedom of Choice in Medicine, 148
Committee for the Scientific Investigation of Claims of the Paranormal (CSICOP), 104, 107, 311
Commonweal Cancer Help Program, 143
Complementary method, definition, 5, 329
Consumer Health Information Research Institute, 312
Consumer Reports, 17
Consumers Union, 194, 312
Council for Responsible Nutrition, 177, 178, 205
Council of Better Business Bureaus, 312
Cramp, Dr. Arthur J., 11
Cranial osteopathy, 28, 329
Cranton, Dr. Elmer M., 157
Credentials, bogus, 102, 203, 204
Crook, Dr. William G., 226
Cryonics, 329
Crystal healing, 108, 110, 329
Cult, definition, 5
Curanderos, 71
Cytotoxic testing, 236–237

Davis, Adelle, 199, 202, 205
De Wells, Roy, 294
Dehydroepiandrosterone (DHEA), 272
Dentistry, dubious, 27–29
Dentistry, "holistic," 28, 29
Dermatron, 215
DeVita, Dr. Vincent, 117
Diagnostic tests, dubious, 93, 189, 208–217
amino acid analysis of urine, 325

Diagnostic tests, dubious (cont'd.)
applied kinesiology; see Applied kinesiology
cytotoxic testing, 236–237
electroacupuncture, 210–215
electrodiagnosis, 329
for food allergies, 224–238
hair analysis, 209–215
herbal crystallization analysis, 216
iridology, 94–96, 199, 257
lingual vitamin C test, 216–217
live-cell analysis, 217
National Vitamin Gap Test
Nutritional Fitness Profile, 174–175
provocation and neutralization, 219, 223, 335
Yeast Test, 174
Dianetics, 329
Diet(s)
and behavior, 204
and cancer, 118, 124–126
and criminal behavior, 244–245
fad, 264–269
Feingold, 242–244, 300, 330
Gerson, 127, 128
and hyperactivity, 242–244
macrobiotic, 247–252
primitive, myths about, 176
vegetarian, 169, 258–263
Dietary Supplement Coalition, 205
Dimethyl sulfoxide (DMSO), 296–299
Dinitrophenol, 273
DiOrio, Father, 67
DMSO, 296–299
Doctrine of Signatures, 78
Doman/Delacato method, 300
Donsbach, Kurt, 102
Donsbach University, 190, 205
Doshas, 45
Dr. Berger's Immune Power Diet, 237
Drown, Ruth, 15

E-meter, 329
East West Journal, 247

East West Natural Health, 247
Eddy, Mary Baker, 58
EDTA, 157
Electric muscle stimulators, 270
Electroacupuncture, 28, 215–216
Emery, Eugene, Jr., 67
Energy medicine, 329–330
Enforcement actions
effectiveness, 18, 175, 254
by FDA, 125, 174, 192, 198, 228, 270, 271, 273, 283, 290, 298, 304
by FTC, 186, 212–213, 276
by state and local agencies, 30, 152, 192–193, 237, 255, 273
Enrich International, 256
"Environmental medicine," 330
Environmental Protection Agency, 180
Enzymatic Therapy, Inc., 174
Eosinophilia-myalgia syndrome, 201
"Ergogenic aids," 194–195, 330

Fad diagnoses, 218–233
"candidiasis hypersensitivity"; see "Candidiasis hypersensitivity"
chronic fatigue syndrome, 228–229
"environmental illness," 218–225, 233
"hypoglycemia," 229–230
"hypothyroidism," 218, 233
"mercury-amalgam toxicity," 230–232, 233, 332
Faddism
definition, 5
food, 175–176
Faith healing, 63–68, 330
danger to children, 60, 61, 62, 63, 65
Federal Trade Commission
impact on quackery, 18, 32
enforcement actions, 186, 212–213, 276
Feingold, Dr. Benjamin, 242
Feingold Association of the United States, 242
Feingold diet, 242–244, 300, 330
Feldenkrais, 330
Ferreri, Carl, 303

Feverfew, 77
Fiber, dietary, 125–126
Firewalking, 26, 301–302
Fit for Life, 97, 98
Fluoridation, opposition to, 27–28, 29
Folk medicine, 69–73
Food and Drug Administration
   Dietary Supplement Task Force, 205
   enforcement actions; *see* enforcement actions, by FDA
   and homeopathy, 27, 85–86, 88
   impact on quackery, 18, 32
   pesticide report, 180
   top ten health frauds, 23
Food(s)
   advertising, FTC investigation, 196
   "health," 195–196
   "natural," 333
   "organically grown," 178–180
   pesticide levels, 180
   safety, 179, 180
Food combining, 98
Food faddism, 14
Foster, Peter, 30
Foundation for the Advancement of Innovative Medicine (FAIM), 32–33
Fox, Dr. Ross, 129
Fraud, definition, 5
Fredericks, Carlton, 202, 205
Freeman, Hobart, 65
Freireich Experimental Plan, 15

Gamma-hydroxybutyrate, 201
Garlic, 198
Germanium sesquioxide, 147, 198, 200
Gerovital, 191–193
Gerson, Dr. Max, 127, 128
Gerson therapy, 114
Giller, Dr. Robert, 204
"Glandulars," 330
Glomectomy, 238–239
Glucomannan, 271
Grant, W.V., 66, 67
Great Earth International, 186, 187, 203

Green, Dr. Saul, 149
"Growth-hormone releasers," 271, 274, 330
Guess, Dr. George A., 92
Guide to the American Medical Association Historical Health Fraud and Alternative Medicine Collection, 12, 15

Hahnemann, Dr. Samuel, 85, 92
Hair analysis, 54, 330
Hall, G. Stanley, 14
Harrell, Dr. Ruth, 182
Hatch, Sen. Orrin, 206
Health Alternatives Legal Foundation, 32
Health food industry, overview, 173
Health food stores, advice from, 155, 184–187
"Health foods," 195–196, 197–198, 331
Health fraud and quackery, 13–36; *see also* Quackery
"Health freedom," 16, 33, 115, 123, 135, 136
Health from God's Pharmacy, 77
Health Products & Promotions Information Network, 34
Health Science, 97
Hellerwork, 331
Herbal crystallization analysis, 206, 331
Herbalife International, 255, 272
Herbert, Dr. Victor, 36, 81
Herbology, 28, 331
Herbs, 74–80
Hohensee, Adolphus, 15
Holbrook, Martin L., 14
Holistic, definition, 6, 331
"Holistic medicine," 81–84, 109, 331
Holmes, Oliver Wendell, 86–87
Homeopathy, 85–93, 331
   and electrodiagnosis, 215–216
Honest Herbal, The, 74, 80
Houdini, Harry, 65
Hoxsey, Harry, 15, 130–131
Hughes, Mark, 255

Hunter, Charles and Frances, 66
Hutchinson, Woods, 14
Hydrogen peroxide treatment, 147
Hyperactivity
    and food additives, 242–244
    and sugar, 245–246
Hypoglycemia, fad diagnosis,
Hypothyroidism, fad diagnosis, 218, 233

Immunoaugmentative therapy (IAT), 22, 114–115, 131–134
"Innate Intelligence," 7, 47
International Association of Cancer Victors and Friends, 147
International Journal of Biosocial Research, 204
Interro, 215–206
Iridology, 94–96, 199, 257, 331

Jacob, Dr. Stanley, 296
JAMA; Journal of the American Medical Association, 12
Jarvis, Dr. William T., 36
Jensen, Bernard, 94, 96

Keller, James Gordon, 116
Kelley, William D., 114
Kellogg, John Harvey, 14
Ketoconazole, 226
Keyes technique, 331
Kirlian photography, 26, 107, 306, 331–332
Km, 257
Knight, J.Z., 104
Krebs, Ernst T., Jr., 135
Krebs, Dr. Ernst T., Sr., 135
Krieger, Dr. Dolores, 306, 307–308
Kuhlman, Kathryn, 64
Kuhnau, Dr. Wolfram, 290
Kushi, Michio, 247, 251
Kushi Institute, 247, 250, 251

Laetrile, 135–139
Lane, Dr. Henry, 94
Lawrence Review of Natural Products, The, 74
Learning disabilities, unproven treatment, 300
Lecithin, 198
LeShan, Dr. Lawrence, 143
Let's Have Healthy Children, 199
Lieberman, Shari, 204
"Life energy," 7
Life Extension: A Practical Scientific Approach, 190, 191
Life-extension claims, 190–193
Life Extension Foundation, 191
Light Force, 256
Liquid diet products, 273
Live cell analysis, 217, 332
Livingston-Wheeler, Dr. Virginia, 139–140
Longevity, bogus claims for, 190
Lourdes, 64
L-tryptophan, 201
Lust, Benedict, 100

Macfadden, Bernarr, 14
MacLaine, Shirley, 104, 105
Macrobiotics, 247–252, 332
Magnetic healing, 332
Maharishi Mahesh Yogi, 45
Manipulation spinal, 7, 51, 52, 54–56
Manner, Dr. Harold, 140–141, 298
Martin, Gary, 203
Materia medica, 85
Matol Botanical International, 257
McCoy, Bob, 15
McGrady, Pat, 148
Media, promotion of "alternative" methods, 3
Medicine shows, 14
Meditation, 45, 302
Megavitamin therapy, 173, 180–184, 244
Melton, J. Melton, 104
Mendelsohn, Dr. Robert, 205
Mental imagery, 143, 332
"Mercury-amalgam toxicity," 230–232, 233, 332
"Meridians," 39, 335

"Alternative" Health Methods / 345

Metabolic Intolerance Test, 236
"Metabolic therapy," 140–142, 333
MetPath Laboratories, 134
Mexican clinics, 24, 116–117, 120, 127, 135, 140–142
Milk
  certified, 193, 336
  raw, 193–194, 336
Miller, Mildred, 298
Mindell, Earl, 203
Minoxidil, 282–284
Moxibustion, 39
Multilevel marketing, 253–257
"Multiple chemical sensitivity (MCS)," 218, 219, 224, 233
Multiple sclerosis, 27
Museum of Questionable Devices, 15

Naprapathy, 333
National Association for Chiropractic Medicine, 312
National Center for Nutrition and Dietetics, 345
National Consumers League, 312
National Council Against Health Fraud (NCAHF), 35, 313
  and acupuncture, 43
  and chiropractic, 50–51
  and commercial weight-loss programs, 265
  Task Force on Victim Redress, 35
National Health Council, 34
National Health Federation, 32, 147
National Institutes of Health, 33
National Nutritional Foods Association, 100, 207
National Research Council, 224–225, 233
National Vitamin Gap Test, 174
"Natural food," 196, 333
"Natural health" movement, 14, 175
Natural Hygiene, 97–99, 333
Nature's Sunshine, 257
Naturopathy, 7, 100–103, 333
Negative ion generator, 333–334

Nelson, Mildred, 130
Neural organization technique, 303, 334
Nevada Clinic, 215
"New Age" practices, 81, 104–110
New York City Department of Consumer Affairs, 31, 155–156, 178–179, 195, 275
Nichols, Mary Gove, 14
Niehans, Dr. Paul, 290
Nixon, President Richard M., 39
Nolen, Dr. William, 67, 132
Nontraditional method, definition, 6
Nu Skin International, 257
Null, Gary, 205
Nutri-Books Corp., 206
Nutripathy, 203, 334
Nutrition fads and fallacies, 173–176
"Nutrition insurance," 176–178
Nutrition Labeling and Education Act, 205
Nutrition
  dubious credentials, 187–190
  sources of reliable advice, 189
Nutritional Health Alliance, 205–206
Nutritional products, illegal sales of, 53–54, 174, 185–186
Nutritional Science Association, 188
Nutritionist licensing, need for, 188–189
Nutritionists Institute of America, 187

Obesity
  attitudes toward, 265, 267
  clinics, 274–276
Occult and New Age practices, 104–110
Ohsawa, George, 247
Olsen, Kristin, 205
Omnitrition, 256
"Organically grown foods," 178–180, 196, 334
"Orgone energy," 7, 336
Orgone therapy, 304
Oriental medicine, 334
"Orthomolecular therapy," 173, 180–184, 334
Ozone therapy, 147

PABA, 192
Palmer, Bartlett Joshua, 49
Palmer, Daniel David, 47, 49, 56
Paranormal beliefs, extent of, 105–106
Passive exercise, 334
Past-life therapy, 26, 303, 334
Pau d'arco, 76
Pauling, Dr. Linus, 145, 202
Pearson, Durk, 191, 205
Pepper, Rep. Claude, 10, 18, 31
Pesticides, 180
PharmTech Research, 125
Phenylpropanolamine, 269–270, 271
Physician Data Query (PDQ) system, 113
Placebo effect, 8, 13, 91, 223
Polarity therapy, 335
Pollen, bee, 198, 199
Popoff, Peter, 65
Prana, 7, 308
Prayer, effect on healing, 68
Procaine, 192
Protein supplements, 196
Provocation and neutralization test, 219, 223, 335
Proxmire Amendment, 206
"Psychic surgery," 69, 142, 335
Psychoneuroimmunology, 335
Public Citizen Health Research Group, 313
Pulse diagnosis, 45
Pure Facts, 242
Pyridoxine; *see* Vitamin B$_6$

Qi, 7, 39, 335
Qigong, 26, 335
Quack (s)
  characteristics of, 8, 19, 25–26, 188, 190
  definition, 5
Quackery
  antiquackery activities, 33–36
  avoiding, 25, 26
  bogus devices, 20
  cancer; *see* Cancer, questionable treatment
  characteristics of victims, 8, 34, 35
  conferences about, 33–34, 35, 152, 156
  cost of, 13, 18
  definition, 5
  dental; *see* Dentistry, dubious
  device museum, 15
  difficulty in spotting, 8
  and the elderly, 23, 24, 32
  examples of dubious products, 10–11
  FDA top ten health frauds, 23
  government regulation, 9, 30–32; *see also* Enforcement activities
  government reports, 10, 18, 31, 122–123, 135
  harmful effects, 8–9, 19, 22
  history of, 13–15
  impact of federal agencies, 18
  in Iowa, 20
  and the media, 3, 104
  mail-order, 29–30, 332
  misconceptions about, 7–9, 20
  in Nevada, 19
  and nonprescription drugs, 23
  and patient education, 34, 35, 118, 123
  persistence of, 17
  in Rhode Island, 24
  strategies used by promoters, 6, 15–16, 36, 136
  surveys of extent, 16, 23–24
  teenage involvement, 21
  victims, 22, 25, 79, 83–84, 102, 130, 132, 141, 145, 163, 189, 199, 256, 257, 293
  vulnerability to, 8, 9, 17
  weight-loss; *see under* Weight control
Questionable method, definition, 6
Quimby, Phineas Parker, 58

Radiesthesia, 336
Radionics, 335
Randi, James, 65, 67
Raw milk, 193–194, 336
Rea, Dr. William, 223
Reams, Cary, 203, 334
Rebirthing, 336
Recommended Dietary Allowances (RDAs), 177

Redotex, 273
Reference Daily Intake (RDI), 207
Reflexology, 29
Reich, Dr. William, 304, 336
Reichian therapy, 304, 336
Reiki, 336
Renner, Dr. John, 151
Reverend Ike, 64
Revici, Dr. Emmanuel, 144–145
Robbins, Anthony, 96, 301
Roberts, Oral, 64
Rockland Corporation, 256
Rodale, J.I., 202
Rolfing, 336
Rose, Dr. Louis, 67
Roy, Leo, 114

Sagan, Dr. Carl, 4
Salani, Raymond J., Jr., 190
Sargenti root canal therapy, 29
Sassafras tea, 79
Sattilaro, Dr. Anthony, 251
Schauss, Alexander, 204
Scheel, John, 100
Scientific method, 3–4, 18
Self-help books, 304–305
Shaklee Corporation, 254
Shaw, Sandy, 191, 205
Shelton, Herbert, 97, 98
"Sick Building Syndrome," 242
Siegel, Dr. Bernie, 142–143, 144
Silva mind control, 337
Simonton, Dr. O. Carl, 142, 143
"60 Minutes," 230–232
Smith, Dr. Lendon, 203
Spirulina, 270
Spot-reducing aids, 336–337
"Starch blockers," 270, 274
Steiner, Rudolph, 326
Straus, Charlotte Gerson, 127
"Stress vitamins," 177
Structural integration, 336
Subliminal tapes, 305, 337
"Subluxations," chiropractic, 47, 50, 51, 54, 337

Sugar, and hyperactivity, 245–246
Sunrider International, 256, 257
Swan, Dr. Rita, 62

Tabloid newspapers, misinformation in, 22
Testimonials, 8, 253, 254, 272
 and Christian Science, 58, 68–69
Therapeutic touch, 306–308, 337
Tissue salts, 337
TMJ quackery, 29
Transcendental meditation (TM), 45, 302, 337
Treben, Maria, 77
True believers, 8
Truss, Dr. C. Orian, 226
Twitchell, David and Ginger, 60
Tyler, Dr. Varro, 74

U.S. Centers for Disease Control, 201
U.S. Postal Service, impact on quackery, 18, 32
Ullman, Dana, 92–93
"Unicorn horn," history of, 13
United Sciences of America, 255–256
Unproven method, definition, 5
Unscientific methods, definitions, 4–7

Vega device, 215
Vegetarian diet, 258–263
Vegetarian diet, and arthritis, 169
Vis Medicatrix Naturae, 7
Visual training, 300, 337–338
"Vital energy," 39
"Vital force," 100
Vitalism, 7
Vitamin(s)
 A, toxicity, 199, 200
 B_6, 183–184,
  toxicity, 199–200
 B_{12}, deficiency, 249
 "B_{17}"; see Laetrile
 C
  and AIDS, 151
  and cancer, 145–146
  lingual test, 216–217, 332

Vitamins (cont'd.)
  and "health foods," 173–207
  myths encouraging use, 173
  "stress," 177
"Vitamiticians," 187
Voll, Dr. Reinold, 215
von Peczely, Ignatz, 94, 95

Weight control
  clinics, 274–276
  general information, 264–267
  pills, potions and gimmicks, 269–276
  questionable diets, 267–269

Why Your Child Is Hyperactive, 242
Wigmore, Ann, 152
Winfrey, Oprah, 266
Winter, Dr. Benjamin, 239

Yiamouyiannis, Dr. John, 29
"Yo-yo" dieting, 264
Yoga, 302, 338
Yoswick, Chester, 188
Young, Dr. James Harvey, 15

Zen macrobiotic diet, 202, 247
Zone therapy; *see* Reflexology